IMMUNOTHERAPY OF
LYMPHOID MALIGNANCIES

IMMUNOTHERAPY OF LYMPHOID MALIGNANCIES

Edited by

Peter Hillmen
Thomas E. Witzig

CLINICAL PUBLISHING

OXFORD

Distributed worldwide by
Taylor & Francis Ltd
Boca Raton · London · New York · Washington, DC

Clinical Publishing
an imprint of Atlas Medical Publishing Ltd

Oxford Centre for Innovation
Mill Street, Oxford OX2 OJX, UK

Tel: +44 1865 811116
Fax: +44 1865 251550
Web: www.clinicalpublishing.co.uk

Distributed by:

Taylor & Francis Ltd
6000 Broken Sound Parkway NW, Suite 300
Boca Raton, FL 33487, USA
E-mail: orders@crcpress.com

Taylor & Francis Ltd
23–25 Blades Court
Deodar Road
London SW15 2NU, UK
E-mail: uk.tandf@thomsonpublishingservices.co.uk

A catalogue record for this book is available from the British Library

ISBN 1 904392 52 0

The publisher makes no representation, express or implied, that the dosages in this
book are correct. Readers must therefore always check the product information and
clinical procedures with the most up-to-date published product information and data
sheets provided by the manufacturers and the most recent codes of conduct and safety
regulations. The authors and the publisher do not accept any liability for any errors in
the text or for the misuse or misapplication of material in this work

Project manager: Gavin Smith
Typeset by Mizpah Publishing Services Private Limited, Chennai, India
Printed in Spain by T G Hostench SA, Barcelona, Spain

Contents

Contributors

KRISTIE A. BLUM MD, Assistant Professor of Internal Medicine, Division of Hematology and Oncology, The Ohio State University, Columbus, Ohio, USA

BRETT THOMAS BRINKER MD, Hematology/Oncology Fellow, Division of Hematology/Oncology, Northwestern University Feinberg School of Medicine, Chicago, Ilinois, USA

JOHN C. BYRD MD, Associate Professor of Medicine and Medicinal Chemistry, D. Warren Brown Professor in Leukemia Research, Director of Hematologic Malignancies, Division of Hematology and Oncology, The Ohio State University, Columbus, Ohio, USA

BRUCE D. CHESON MD, Professor of Medicine, Division of Hematology/Oncology, Georgetown University, Lombardi Comprehensive Cancer Center, Washington, DC, USA

BERTRAND COIFFIER MD, Professor of Haematology, Depertment of Haematology, Hospices Civils de Lyon and University, Lyon, France

MORTON COLEMAN, MD, The Center for Lymphoma and Myeloma, Division of Hematology and Oncology, Department of Medicine, Weill Medical College of Cornell University and New York Presbyterian Hospital, New York, New York, USA

MYRON STEFAN CZUCZMAN MD, Head, Lymphoma/Myeloma Service, Associate Professor of Medicine, Division of Medical Oncology, Roswell Park Cancer Institute, Buffalo, New York, USA

JULIE P. DEANS PhD, Associate Professor, AHFMR Senior Scholar Chair, Immunology Research Group, Department of Biochemistry and Molecular Biology, University of Calgary, Calgary, Alberta, Canada

JULIAN DECTER MD, The Center for Lymphoma and Myeloma, Division of Hematology and Oncology, Department of Medicine, Weill Medical College of Cornell University and New York Presbyterian Hospital, New York, New York, USA

NANCY DRISCOLL RPA-C, Division of Haematology and Oncology, Long Island Jewish Medical Center, New York, New York, USA

VIVIANE DUBRUILLE PhD, Doctor of Haematology, Hotel Dieu, University Hospital, Nantes, France

MARTIN J. S. DYER MA, DPhil, FRCP, FRCPath, Professor of Haemato-Oncology, MRC Toxicology Unit / Leicester University, Leicester, UK

CHRISTOS EMMANOUILIDES MD, Associate Professor, Division of Hematology and Oncology, UCLA, currently: Interbalkan European Medical Center-Oncology, Pylaia, Thessaloniki, Greece

RICHARD R. FURMAN MD, The Center for Lymphoma and Myeloma, Division of Hematology and Oncology, Department of Medicine, Weill Medical College of Cornell University and New York Presbyterian Hospital, New York, New York, USA

DAVID M. GOLDENBERG MD, Immunomedics, Inc., Morris Plains, New Jersey, USA

LEO I. GORDON MD, Abby & John Friend Professor of Cancer Research, Chief, Division of Hematology/Oncology, Northwestern University Feinberg School of Medicine, Division of Hematology/Oncology, Chicago Ilinois, USA

TERRY J. HAMBLIN DM, FRCP, FRCPath, FMedSci, Professor of Immunohaematology, University of Southampton, Department of Haematology, Royal Bournemouth Hospital, Bournemouth, UK

JEAN-LUC HAROUSSEAU MD, Professor of Haematology, Hotel Dieu, University Hospital, Nantes, France

FRANCISCO J. HERNANDEZ-ILIZALITURRI MD, Assistant Professor of Medicine, Department of Medical Oncology. Member of the Tumor Immunology Program, Department of Immunology, Roswell Park Cancer Institute, Buffalo, New York, USA

PETER HILLMEN MRCP, MRCPath, PhD, Department of Haematology, Pinderfields Hospital, Wakefield, UK

IVAN D. HORAK MD, Immunomedics, Inc., Morris Plains, New Jersey, USA

ANDREW JACK BSc, MB, ChB, PhD, Consultant Haematopathologist, Haematological Malignancy Diagnostic Service (HMDS), Leeds General Infirmary, Leeds, UK

ANDRZEJ J. JAKUBOWIAK MD, PhD, Assistant Professor of Internal Medicine, University of Michigan Medical Center, Ann Arbor, Michigan, USA

DALE M. JANSON RPA-C, MBA, Division of Haematology and Oncology, Long Island Jewish Medical Center, New York, New York, USA

MARK S. KAMINSKI MD, Professor of Internal Medicine, University of Michigan Medical Center, Ann Arbor, Michigan, USA

MICHAEL KEATING MD, Professor of Medicine, Department of Leukemia, University of Texas M.D. Anderson Cancer Center, Houston, Texas, USA

PETER MCLAUGHLIN MD, Professor of Medicine, Department of Lymphoma/Myeloma, University of Texas MD Anderson Cancer Center, Houston, Texas, USA

JOHN P. LEONARD MD, The Center for Lymphoma and Myeloma, Division of Hematology and Oncology, Department of Medicine, Weill Medical College of Cornell University and New York Presbyterian Hospital, New York, New York, USA

THOMAS S. LIN MD, PhD, Assistant Professor of Internal Medicine, Division of Hematology and Oncology, The Ohio State University, Columbus, Ohio, USA

BLANCHE H. MAVROMATIS MD, Assistant Professor of Medicine, Lombardi Comprehensive Cancer Center, Washington, DC, USA

HÅKAN MELLSTEDT MD, PhD, Professor of Oncologic Biotherapy, Department of Oncology (Radiumhemmet), Karolinska University Hospital Solna, Stockholm, Sweden

SUSAN M. O'BRIEN MD, Professor, Department of Leukemia, University of Texas M.D. Anderson Cancer Center, Houston, Texas, USA

DILIP V. PATEL MD, Division of Haematology and Oncology, Long Island Jewish Medical Center, Albert Einstein College of Medicine, Bronx, New York, New York, USA

Karl S. Peggs BM, BCh, MA, MRCP, MRCPath, Senior Lecturer in Bone Marrow Transplantation, Department of Haematology, University College Hospital, Royal Free and University College London Medical School, London, UK

Kanti R. Rai MD, Chief, Division of Haematology and Oncology, Long Island Jewish Medical Center, Albert Einstein College of Medicine, Bronx, New York, New York, USA

Farhad Ravandi MD, Assistant Professor of Medicine, Department of Leukemia, University of Texas M.D. Anderson Cancer Center, Houston, Texas, USA

Nancy Lou Tuinstra RN, Mayo Clinic College of Medicine, Nuclear Medicine, Rochester, Minnesota, USA

William A. Wegener MD, Immunomedics, Inc., Morris Plains, New Jersey, USA

Thomas E. Witzig MD, Professor of Medicine, Division of Internal Medicine and Hematology, Mayo Clinic, Rochester, Minnesota, USA

Karen W. L. Yee MD, Fellow, Department of Leukemia, University of Texas M.D. Anderson Cancer Center, Houston, Texas, USA

1

The history of immunotherapy for lymphoid malignancies

H. Mellstedt

INTRODUCTION

It has been a dream for a long time for immunotherapists to treat and cure patients with malignancies by using immunotherapeutic drugs.

The first attempt to vaccinate patients with cancer dates back to the end of the 18th century (1777) when the surgeon to the Duke of Kent, Dr. Nooth, immunised himself with tumour cells with the aim of preventing cancer, a brave and visionary experiment.

At the beginning of the 20th century, Paul Ehrlich coined the term 'The Magic Bullet', i.e. antibodies that could trace invaders and destroy them. During the first half of that century, there were several reports on a limited number of patients with lymphomas and chronic lymphocytic leukaemia (CLL) treated with serotherapy. De Carvalho [1] treated patients with leukaemia and lymphoma with hyperimmune gamma globulin raised in horses and donkeys against leukaemic cells. Some major and long-lasting responses were seen. CLL patients were also treated with isologous sera against normal lymphocytes. Healthy individuals were immunised with allogeneic lymphocytes and plasmapheresed. Sera with high titres of cytotoxic antibodies were transfused to end-stage CLL patients. In some, there were short falls in the peripheral blood white cell count [2]. In Sezary's syndromes, anti-thymocyte globulin and anti-lymphocyte globulin were shown to be effective in some patients [3, 4].

Modern immunotherapy of haematological malignancies, especially lymphoid disorders, began in the early 1970s. An overview of early clinical studies is presented in this chapter with the focus on interferons, monoclonal antibodies (MAbs) and vaccines.

INTERFERONS

Interferons are cytokines which have been shown to have many effects on the immune system. They were found to stimulate the activity of natural killer (NK) and T cells, as well as up-regulate surface structures on tumour cells and immune cells, such as tumour antigens and major histocompatibility complex (MHC) molecules. We have since learnt a lot more about effects of interferons on other systems, but their effects on the immune system were the main reasons why interferons were considered candidates for immunotherapy.

Håkan Mellstedt, MD, PhD, Professor of Oncologic Biotherapy, Department of Oncology (Radiumhemmet), Karolinska University Hospital Solna, Stockholm, Sweden.

During the 1960s, techniques for the production of natural interferons were established and large amounts of natural interferons could be produced by infection of buffy coat white cells with Sendai virus [5] as well as spontaneously produced by the lymphoma cell line Namalwa [6]. The Finnish virologist Cantell and his colleagues [5] pioneered the production of natural α-interferon.

The first report on treatment of patients with multiple myeloma using natural α-interferon was published in 1979 by Mellstedt and colleagues [7] and showed tumour responses (>50% reduction of the M-component) in preferentially IgA and Bence Jones' myeloma, a finding which was later confirmed for natural α-interferon but not for recombinant α-interferon [8]. In a subsequent randomised study, Mellstedt and colleagues [9] showed that natural α-interferon therapy induced the same response rate as melphalan/prednisone therapy in IgA and Bence Jones' myeloma but a lower response in IgG myeloma. By increasing the dose from 3×10^6 to 10×10^6 U/day for 7 consecutive days every third week, both the response and the toxicity profile increased [10]. When melphalan/prednisolone was combined with α-interferon, the response rate increased from 48 to 66% [11]. Similar results were obtained with other chemotherapy regimens [12].

The first report of the use of α-interferon as maintenance therapy for multiple myeloma in remission after chemotherapy was published in 1990 by Mandelli and co-workers [13] and showed that the response duration time (26 vs. 14 months; p = 0.002) and overall survival (52 vs. 39 months; p = 0.05) increased in the treatment group when compared with a group receiving no treatment.

The use of α-interferon had earlier been explored in non-Hodgkin lymphomas (NHLs) of the B-cell type. A consistent finding was that low-grade lymphomas responded, but not high-grade lymphomas. The first report was published in 1978 by Merigan and colleagues [14]. Later, extended phase II trials showed a beneficial effect in low-grade lymphomas but mainly only partial remissions. Higher doses, i.e. up to 50×10^6 U/m^2 three times per week, improved the response rate but with considerable toxicity [15–17]. In lymphomas of T-cell origin [mucosis fungoides, Sezary's syndrome, cutaneous T-cell lymphoma (CTCL)] the effect of α-interferon was more impressive, with one third being complete responders in those receiving the highest dose [18–20].

α-interferon was also subsequently tested in combination with standard chemotherapy for various lymphomas of T- and B-cell origin. Response rate increased but so did toxicity. The best responding subgroup was follicular NHL [21].

The best clinical effect in lymphoid malignancies was noted in hairy cell leukaemia. The first report was published in 1984 by Quesada and colleagues [22]. The majority of the patients responded, although only with a partial remission. Complete responders varied from 5 to 40%. Hairy cell leukaemia was the first approved indication for α-interferon worldwide.

Approval of α-interferon for NHL and myeloma differed between countries. α-interferon is only in use for some selected groups of NHL (see separate chapter in this volume) and is still under investigation by a few groups as maintenance therapy for multiple myeloma patients after high-dose chemotherapy and stem cell rescue.

MONOCLONAL ANTIBODIES

In 1975, Köhler and Milstein [23] described the hybridoma technique for the production of monoclonal antibodies (MAbs). This allowed for the first time the production of MAbs of pre-defined specificity.

Initial reports using MAbs in mouse lymphoma models were highly encouraging. Bernstein and colleagues [24, 25] used MAbs to a differentiation antigen to treat transplanted murine leukaemia and showed that MAbs could eradicate both local and systemic disease. One problem in this model was the emergence of antigen-negative lymphoma cells which caused recurrent disease.

Initial experiments in man in the early 1980s were performed in conditions of bulk, almost overwhelming disease, and the preliminary results were not at all encouraging. First experiments were performed in patients with NHL of the B-cell type and acute lymphoblastic leukaemia with antibodies against various differentiation antigens both on normal and malignant lymphocytes [26, 27]. A wide range of similar experiments performed around this time showed that the clinical effects of unconjugated murine MAbs were limited to short reductions in the peripheral blood white cell count with little or no effect on solid masses or bone marrow infiltration [28].

In marked contrast to these results, it was possible in some B-NHL patients to induce remission with small doses of MAbs directed against the idiotypic determinant of the tumour-associated immunoglobulin [29]. Whilst the remissions induced by this approach were long lasting, the remission rate was low and the amount of effort required to generate patient-specific MAbs precluded more general use. The initial enthusiasm to use MAbs as therapeutic tools for the treatment of malignancy therefore waned.

Many groups abandoned clinical attempts with unconjugated MAbs and began to focus on conjugated MAbs. Whether labelled with radioisotope, prodrug or drug toxin, this approach depends on the toxicity of the conjugated moiety relegating the role of antibody to that of a passive vector. Some of these approaches have yet to be assessed in lymphoid malignancies. A few successes have been seen later which will be summarised in this book.

Many barriers to effective therapy with unconjugated MAbs were soon recognised and impressive results with MAbs started to emerge.

Naked MAbs have dramatically changed the therapeutic milieu in the management of lymphoma. Rituximab is a chimeric MAb directed against the CD20 antigen expressed by most B cells at different stages of development. Its clinical activity led to FDA approval for the management of follicular lymphoma and this was reported in a multicenter phase II pivotal trial in 1998 [30]. The overall response rate was 48% with 6% complete remissions (CR). A median time to progression of 12 months was noted. Similarly, activity in aggressive lymphomas was reported by Coiffier and co-workers [31]. The overall response rate was 31% with 14% CR and a median time to progression of 246 days. In small lymphocytic lymphomas/CLL, a higher dose and more frequent dosing than the standard dose was required to achieve a response [32].

The first study of chemotherapy-rituximab combination in low-grade lymphoma was presented by Czuczman and colleagues [33, 34]. The overall response rate was 100% with 58% CR and a median time to progression of 63 months.

The first randomised phase III study combining rituximab with chemotherapy in diffuse large cell lymphomas was reported by GELA (Groupe d'Etude des Lymphomes de l'Adulte). Complete response rates were 64 and 77% in the CHOP (cyclophosphamide, doxorubicin, oncovin, prednisolone) and CHOP-rituximab arms, respectively. More importantly, 2-year overall survival was 61% in the CHOP arm and 73% in the CHOP-rituximab arm. These differences were statistically significant [35].

In 1979, Herman Waldmann from the University of Cambridge, UK, immunised rats with human lymphocytes and carried out a fusion that was to yield a diverse range of antibodies. All lytic antibodies recognised the same antigen, CD52. Anti-CD52 IgM antibodies (Campath-1M) were originally chosen for clinical development as they efficiently activated complement and induced depletion of T cells. This antibody was used for T-cell depletion in bone marrow transplants. Later, IgG versions (IgG_{2A}/IgG_{2B}) were produced which could deplete leukaemic B cells from the circulation of B-prolymphocytic leukaemia (B-PLL) patients, probably through antibody-dependent cellular cytotoxicity (ADCC). Results with the anti-CD52 IgG_{2B}-version (Campath-1G) in patients with a variety of lymphoproliferative diseases showed that this MAb could readily deplete malignant cells from the peripheral blood, bone marrow and spleen. However, lymph nodes were relatively unaffected [36]. Later, genetically reshaped Campath-1H (humanised) induced remission in 2 patients with advanced NHL of the B-cell type [37].

Based on the initial promising results with Campath-1H, the pharmaceutical company Burroughs-Wellcome initiated extended phase II trials in NHL in Europe and the USA in 1991. Due to the overall impression by the company that the effect was not as they had expected, the study in Europe was closed in 1995. We had at that time in our centre noted that patients with refractory CLL of the B-cell type responded very well to Campath-1H. When we analysed all 40 B-CLL patients included in this first trial, 42% of the patients refractory to alkylating agents responded to Campath-1H [38]. This was later confirmed by Keating and co-workers [39] in the pivotal study of CLL patients resistant to fludarabine for registration of Campath-1H by FDA. In 1996 it had already been shown by our group that if Campath-1H was given as first-line therapy to CLL patients in a small pilot study (n = 9), 80% of the patients responded [40]. In the phase II European multicentre study, patients with advanced low-grade NHL previously treated with chemotherapy were also included. A total of 50 patients were enrolled: 14% of the patients with B-cell lymphoma achieved a partial remission. It was also noticed in this study that mycosis fungoides appeared to respond very well. Four out of eight patients responded with 2 CR [41]. Subsequently, the superior effect of Campath-1H in patients with mycosis fungoides/ Sezary's syndrome was confirmed in a phase II study including 22 patients with an overall response rate of 55% and 32% CR [42].

VACCINES

Tumour vaccines are active immunotherapies whereby the host is induced to produce an immune response against autologous tumour cells. The different types of vaccines are quite variable and include those directed at known tumour-specific antigens (e.g., idiotype) as well as whole tumour cells. The immune response might be enhanced by using co-stimulatory agents such as key-hole limpet haemocyanin (KLH), adjuvant cytokines such as granulocyte macrophage colony-stimulating factor (GM-CSF), interleukin (IL)-2 or IL-12 or *ex vivo* expanded dendritic cells (DC).

B-cell malignancies are clonal disorders with all tumour cells expressing the same tumour-specific immunoglobulin, the unique variable region of which is termed an idiotype that can serve as a target for immunotherapy. The concept of active idiotype vaccination was pioneered in a murine multiple myeloma model [43]. Weekly immunisations with tumour-derived paraprotein in Freund's adjuvant-induced protective immunity against MOPC-315 and MOPC-460 plasmacytoma cells in syngeneic Balb/c mice [44]. Anti-idiotype antibody and thymus-derived idiotype-specific T helper cells were required to develop protective tumour immunity [45]. Similarly, studies in the murine BCL-1 lymphoma model demonstrated efficient protection of mice against BCL-1 tumour challenge after immunisation with idiotype protein [46]. Similar principles apply to the murine 38C13 lymphoma model. Vaccination with KLH-coupled idiotypes induced protective immunity against a subsequent tumour challenge in syngeneic mice [47]. In this model, cure of pre-established tumours required a combination of chemotherapy and idiotype vaccination [48].

Most laboratory and clinical research experience in the management of B-cell malignancies has been on idiotype vaccines. Idiotypic vaccination in NHL achieved the first unprecedented success. Kwak and co-workers [49] demonstrated for the first time that an idiotypic vaccine formulation administered following conventional chemotherapy was capable of inducing idiotype-specific immune responses in 7 out of 9 follicular lymphoma patients, from whom each respective idiotype had been previously obtained. The main characteristics of this vaccine formulation were represented by both the use of KLH as the immunological carrier for the idiotype and that of Syntex adjuvant formulation (SAF)-1 as an immunological adjuvant [49].

In an extended follow-up, 32 patients with follicular lymphoma in first remission were immunised with the idiotype, and 45% mounted an anti-idiotype response. Freedom from disease and overall survival was superior in patients who developed an immune response

[50]. Several investigators have reported early clinical experiences with this approach. Induction of an immune response seems more frequent and the most prominent clinical effects have been noted in patients with minimal tumour burden. Loading of the idiotype onto autologous DC increases the immune response several fold [51]. Prospective randomised trials are in progress to evaluate the clinical efficacy of idiotype vaccination in low-grade lymphoma in CR.

The first to show the expression of idiotypic structures on the myeloma clone in humans was Mellstedt and colleagues [52] in 1974. The first idiotype immunisation study in multiple myeloma was published by Mellstedt and colleagues in 1996 [53]. A transient immune response could be noticed in 2 of 5 patients immunised with the idiotype alone absorbed onto alum. In a subsequent study using the autologous idiotype as a vaccine together with the adjuvant cytokine GM-CSF, all 5 immunised patients mounted a CD4 as well as CD8 idiotype-specific T-cell response and a major tumour response (>50% reduction of the M-component) could be noticed in one of the patients [54].

The first study using DCs pulsed with idiotype was published in 1998 by Wen and collaborators [55] and showed that this approach was also feasible in myeloma and may result in an enhanced immune response.

Idiotype immunisation of sibling donors of myeloma patients has also been undertaken. Before transplant, the donors were immunised with the patient's idiotype. After transplant, it could be shown that the idiotype-specific T cells were transferred to the recipient [56].

So far, vaccine development in B-cell malignancies has only been focused on the use of individual idiotypes, which might not be an optimal immunogenic antigen in man. In the future, many other antigenic structures will be explored, such as whole tumour cells, MUC-1, etc.

SUMMARY

Modern immunotherapy for lymphoid malignancies began around 1970. Two major achievements have facilitated the progress of immunotherapy. The most important was our increased knowledge of the function of the immune system and the interaction between tumour cells and immune functions. The other was in techniques for producing immunotherapeutics. The first products were natural products e.g. interferons, but recombinant protein technologies were soon introduced. Technologies for producing large amounts of MAbs for clinical use, especially chimeric and humanised antibodies, have also been instrumental and the future of immunotherapy looks bright. Looking back at the last 30–35 years, progress during the 1970s was slow and many of the strategies which were born during this decade have since been discarded. However, the developments made then have helped us to learn a lot and the progress made during the 1990s and the first years of the 21st century has been tremendous. It is no exaggeration to state that the use of antibodies, vaccines, cytokines and other biological products will increase dramatically during the decades to come and thus improve the therapeutic outcome for patients with lymphoid malignancies.

REFERENCES

1. De Carvalho S. Preliminary experimentation with specific immunotherapy of neoplastic disease in man. I. Immediate effects of hyperimmune equine gamma globulins. *Cancer* 1963; 16:306–330.
2. Lazlo J, Buckley C, Amos D. Infusion of autologous immune plasma in chronic lymphocytic leukemia. *Blood* 1968; 31:104–110.
3. Barret A, Bridgen D, Roberts T, Staughton R, Byrom N, Hobbs J. Anti-lymphocyte globulin in the treatment of advanced Sezary's syndrome. *Lancet* 1976; 1:940–941.

4. Edelson R, Raafat J, Berger C, Grossmann M, Troja C, Hardy M. Anti-tumor cytoglobulin in the management of cutaneous T-cell lymphoma. *Cancer Treat Rep* 1979; 63:675–680.
5. Strander H, Cantell K, Carlstrom G, Jakobsson PA. Clinical and laboratory investigations on man: systemic administration of potent interferon to man. *J Natl Cancer Inst* 1973; 51:733–742.
6. Finter N, Fantes K, Johnston M, Christofinis G, Ball G. The Namalva line of lymphoclastoid cell as a source of large amounts of human interferon. Symposium on interferons and the control of cell-virus interactions, Rehovot, Israel, 1977, May 2–6.
7. Mellstedt H, Ahre A, Bjorkholm M, Holm G, Johansson B, Strander H. Interferon therapy in myelomatosis. *Lancet* 1979; 1:245–247.
8. Ludwig H, Cortelezzi A, Scheithauer W, Van Camp BG, Kuzmits R, Fillet G *et al.* Recombinant interferon alfa-2C versus polychemotherapy (VMCP) for treatment of multiple myeloma: a prospective randomized trial. *Eur J Cancer Clin Oncol* 1986; 22:1111–1116.
9. Ahre A, Bjorkholm M, Mellstedt H, Brenning G, Engstedt L, Gahrton G *et al.* Human leukocyte interferon and intermittent high-dose melphalan-prednisone administration in the treatment of multiple myeloma: a randomized clinical trial from the Myeloma Group of Central Sweden. *Cancer Treat Rep* 1984; 68:1331–1338.
10. Ahre A, Bjorkholm M, Osterborg A, Brenning G, Gahrton G, Gyllenhammar H *et al.* High doses of natural alpha-interferon (alpha-IFN) in the treatment of multiple myeloma – a pilot study from the Myeloma Group of Central Sweden (MGCS). *Eur J Haematol* 1988; 41:123–130.
11. Osterborg A, Bjorkholm M, Bjoreman M, Brenning G, Carlson K, Celsing F *et al.* Natural interferon-alpha in combination with melphalan/prednisone versus melphalan/prednisone in the treatment of multiple myeloma stages II and III: a randomized study from the Myeloma Group of Central Sweden. *Blood* 1993; 81:1428–1434.
12. Ludwig H, Cohen A, Huber H, Hachbaur D, Jungi W, Senn H *et al.* Interferon alfa-2b with VMCP compared to VMCP alone for induction and interferon alfa-2b compared to controls for remission maintenance in multiple myeloma: interim results. *Eur J Cancer* 1991; 27:40–46.
13. Mandelli F, Avvisati G, Amadori S, Boccadoro M, Gernone A, Lauta VM *et al.* Maintenance treatment with recombinant interferon alfa-2b in patients with multiple myeloma responding to conventional induction chemotherapy. *N Engl J Med* 1990; 322:1430–1434.
14. Merigan TC, Sikora K, Breeden JH, Levy R, Rosenberg SA. Preliminary observations on the effect of human leukocyte interferon in non-Hodgkin's lymphoma. *N Engl J Med* 1978; 299:1449–1453.
15. Horning SJ, Merigan TC, Krown SE, Gutterman JU, Louie A, Gallagher J *et al.* Human interferon alpha in malignant lymphoma and Hodgkin's disease. Results of the American Cancer Society trial. *Cancer* 1985; 56:1305–1310.
16. Sherwin SA, Knost JA, Fein S, Abrams PG, Foon KA, Ochs JJ *et al.* A multiple-dose phase I trial of recombinant leukocyte A interferon in cancer patients. *JAMA* 1982; 248:2461–2466.
17. O'Connell MJ, Colgan JP, Oken MM, Ritts RE, Jr, Kay NE, Itri LM. Clinical trial of recombinant leukocyte A interferon as initial therapy for favorable histology non-Hodgkin's lymphomas and chronic lymphocytic leukemia. An Eastern Cooperative Oncology Group pilot study. *J Clin Oncol* 1986; 4:128–136.
18. Foon KA, Bunn PA, Jr. Alpha-interferon treatment of cutaneous T cell lymphoma and chronic lymphocytic leukemia. *Semin Oncol* 1986; 13(suppl 5):35–39.
19. Kohn EC, Steis RG, Sausville EA, Veach SR, Stocker JL, Phelps R *et al.* Phase II trial of intermittent high-dose recombinant interferon alfa-2a in mycosis fungoides and the Sezary syndrome. *J Clin Oncol* 1990; 8:155–160.
20. Olsen EA, Rosen ST, Vollmer RT, Variakojis D, Roenigk HH, Jr, Diab N *et al.* Interferon alfa-2a in the treatment of cutaneous T cell lymphoma. *J Am Acad Dermatol* 1989; 20:395–407.
21. Chisesi T, Capnist G, Vespignani M, Dini E. The role of interferon alfa-2b and chlorambucil in the treatment of non-Hodgkin's lymphoma. *Cancer Treat Rev* 1988; 15(suppl A):27–33.
22. Quesada JR, Reuben J, Manning JT, Hersh EM, Gutterman JU. Alpha interferon for induction of remission in hairy-cell leukemia. *N Engl J Med* 1984; 310:15–18.
23. Köhler G, Milstein C. Continuous cultures of fused cells secreting antibody of predefined specificity. *Nature* 1975; 256:495–497.
24. Bernstein ID, Tam MR, Nowinski RC. Mouse leukemia: therapy with monoclonal antibodies against a thymus differentiation antigen. *Science* 1980; 207:68–71.
25. Badger CC, Bernstein ID. Therapy of murine leukemia with monoclonal antibody against a normal differentiation antigen. *J Exp Med* 1983; 157:828–842.

26. Nadler LM, Stashenko P, Hardy R, Kaplan WD, Button LN, Kufe DW *et al*. Serotherapy of a patient with a monoclonal antibody directed against a human lymphoma-associated antigen. *Cancer Res* 1980; 40:3147–3154.

27. Ritz J, Pesando JM, Sallan SE, Clavell LA, Notis-McConarty J, Rosenthal P *et al*. Serotherapy of acute lymphoblastic leukemia with monoclonal antibody. *Blood* 1981; 58:141–152.

28. Ritz J, Schlossman SF. Utilization of monoclonal antibodies in the treatment of leukemia and lymphoma. *Blood* 1982; 59:1–11.

29. Miller RA, Maloney DG, Warnke R, Levy R. Treatment of B-cell lymphoma with monoclonal anti-idiotype antibody. *N Engl J Med* 1982; 306:517–522.

30. McLaughlin P, Grillo-Lopez AJ, Link BK, Levy R, Czuczman MS, Williams ME *et al*. Rituximab chimeric anti-CD20 monoclonal antibody therapy for relapsed indolent lymphoma: half of patients respond to a four-dose treatment program. *J Clin Oncol* 1998; 16:2825–2833.

31. Coiffier B, Haioun C, Ketterer N, Engert A, Tilly H, Ma D *et al*. Rituximab (anti-CD20 monoclonal antibody) for the treatment of patients with relapsing or refractory aggressive lymphoma: a multicenter phase II study. *Blood* 1998; 92:1927–1932.

32. Byrd JC, Murphy T, Howard RS, Lucas MS, Goodrich A, Park K *et al*. Rituximab using a thrice weekly dosing schedule in B-cell chronic lymphocytic leukemia and small lymphocytic lymphoma demonstrates clinical activity and acceptable toxicity. *J Clin Oncol* 2001; 19:2153–2164.

33. Czuczman MS, Grillo-Lopez AJ, White CA, Saleh M, Gordon L, LoBuglio AF *et al*. Treatment of patients with low-grade B-cell lymphoma with the combination of chimeric anti-CD20 monoclonal antibody and CHOP chemotherapy. *J Clin Oncol* 1999; 17:268–276.

34. Czuczman M, Grillo-Lopez AJ, White CA *et al*. Progression free survival after six years follow up of the first clinical trial of rituximab/CHOP chemoimmunotherapy. *Blood* 2001; 98:601a.

35. Coiffier B, Lepage E, Briere J, Herbrecht R, Tilly H, Bouabdallah R *et al*. CHOP chemotherapy plus rituximab compared with CHOP alone in elderly patients with diffuse large-B-cell lymphoma. *N Engl J Med* 2002; 346:235–242.

36. Dyer MJ, Hale G, Hayhoe FG, Waldmann H. Effects of CAMPATH-1 antibodies in vivo in patients with lymphoid malignancies: influence of antibody isotype. *Blood* 1989; 73:1431–1439.

37. Hale G, Dyer MJ, Clark MR, Phillips JM, Marcus R, Riechmann L *et al*. Remission induction in non-Hodgkin lymphoma with reshaped human monoclonal antibody CAMPATH-1H. *Lancet* 1988; 2:1394–1399.

38. Osterborg A, Dyer MJ, Bunjes D, Pangalis GA, Bastion Y, Catovsky D *et al*. Phase II multicenter study of human CD52 antibody in previously treated chronic lymphocytic leukemia. European Study Group of CAMPATH-1H Treatment in Chronic Lymphocytic Leukemia. *J Clin Oncol* 1997; 15:1567–1574.

39. Keating MJ, Flinn I, Jain V, Binet JL, Hillmen P, Byrd J *et al*. Therapeutic role of alemtuzumab (Campath-1H) in patients who have failed fludarabine: results of a large international study. *Blood* 2002; 99:3554–3561.

40. Osterborg A, Fassas AS, Anagnostopoulos A, Dyer MJ, Catovsky D, Mellstedt H. Humanized CD52 monoclonal antibody Campath-1H as first-line treatment in chronic lymphocytic leukaemia. *Br J Haematol* 1996; 93:151–153.

41. Lundin J, Osterborg A, Brittinger G, Crowther D, Dombret H, Engert A *et al*. CAMPATH-1H monoclonal antibody in therapy for previously treated low-grade non-Hodgkin's lymphomas: a phase II multicenter study. European Study Group of CAMPATH-1H Treatment in Low-Grade Non-Hodgkin's Lymphoma. *J Clin Oncol* 1998; 16:3257–3263.

42. Lundin J, Hagberg H, Repp R, Cavallin-Stahl E, Freden S, Juliusson G *et al*. Phase 2 study of alemtuzumab (anti-CD52 monoclonal antibody) in patients with advanced mycosis fungoides/Sezary syndrome. *Blood* 2003; 101:4267–4672.

43. Lynch RG, Graff RJ, Sirisinha S, Simms ES, Eisen HN. Myeloma proteins as tumor-specific transplantation antigens. *Proc Natl Acad Sci USA* 1972; 69:1540–1544.

44. Sakato N, Eisen HN. Antibodies to idiotypes of isologous immunoglobulins. *J Exp Med* 1975; 141:1411–1426.

45. Sakato N, Semma M, Eisen HN, Azuma T. A small hypervariable segment in the variable domain of an immunoglobulin light chain stimulates formation of anti-idiotypic suppressor T cells. *Proc Natl Acad Sci USA* 1982; 79:5396–5400.

46. George AJ, Tutt AL, Stevenson FK. Anti-idiotypic mechanisms involved in suppression of a mouse B cell lymphoma, BCL1. *J Immunol* 1987; 138:628–634.

47. Kaminski MS, Kitamura K, Maloney DG, Levy R. Idiotype vaccination against murine B cell lymphoma. Inhibition of tumor immunity by free idiotype protein. *J Immunol* 1987; 138:1289–1296.

48. Campbell MJ, Esserman L, Levy R. Immunotherapy of established murine B cell lymphoma. Combination of idiotype immunization and cyclophosphamide. *J Immunol* 1988; 141:3227–3233.

49. Kwak LW, Campbell MJ, Czerwinski DK, Hart S, Miller RA, Levy R. Induction of immune responses in patients with B-cell lymphoma against the surface-immunoglobulin idiotype expressed by their tumors. *N Engl J Med* 1992; 327:1209–1215.

50. Hsu FJ, Caspar CB, Czerwinski D, Kwak LW, Liles TM, Syrengelas A *et al*. Tumor-specific idiotype vaccines in the treatment of patients with B-cell lymphoma – long-term results of a clinical trial. *Blood* 1997; 89:3129–3135.

51. Hsu FJ, Benike C, Fagnoni F, Liles TM, Czerwinski D, Taidi B *et al*. Vaccination of patients with B-cell lymphoma using autologous antigen-pulsed dendritic cells. *Nat Med* 1996; 2:52–58.

52. Mellstedt H, Hammarstrom S, Holm G. Monoclonal lymphocyte population in human plasma cell myeloma. *Clin Exp Immunol* 1974; 17:371–384.

53. Bergenbrant S, Yi Q, Osterborg A, Bjorkholm M, Osby E, Mellstedt H *et al*. Modulation of anti-idiotypic immune response by immunization with the autologous M-component protein in multiple myeloma patients. *Br J Haematol* 1996; 92:840–846.

54. Osterborg A, Yi Q, Henriksson L, Fagerberg J, Bergenbrant S, Jeddi-Tehrani M *et al*. Idiotype immunization combined with granulocyte-macrophage colony-stimulating factor in myeloma patients induced type I, major histocompatibility complex-restricted, CD8- and CD4-specific T-cell responses. *Blood* 1998; 91:2459–2466.

55. Wen YJ, Ling M, Bailey-Wood R, Lim SH. Idiotypic protein-pulsed adherent peripheral blood mononuclear cell-derived dendritic cells prime immune system in multiple myeloma. *Clin Cancer Res* 1998; 4:957–962.

56. Kwak LW, Taub DD, Duffey PL, Bensinger WI, Bryant EM, Reynolds CW *et al*. Transfer of myeloma idiotype-specific immunity from an actively immunised marrow donor. *Lancet* 1995; 345:1016–1020.

2

Immunological markers of lymphoid malignancy

A. Jack

AN INTEGRATED APPROACH TO THE DIAGNOSIS OF LYMPHOID MALIGNANCY

In the past hundred years there have been numerous classifications of lymphoproliferative disorders. Some of these, such as the National Cancer Institute Working Formulation, the Kiel classification and the French-American-British (FAB) classification of leukaemia have had a major influence on the development of haematological oncology. Many other classifications have been largely forgotten. The publication of the Revised European American Lymphoma (REAL) classification [1] followed by the World Health Organisation (WHO) Classification of Haematological Malignancies in 2001 marked a turning point in the development of haematopathology. For the first time, the largely artificial distinction between lymphomas and lymphoid leukaemias was recognised so that they were considered as different presentations of the same entity. For example, this recognition has effectively ended the confusion caused by the arbitrary separation of B-cell chronic lymphocytic leukaemia (B-CLL) and small lymphocytic lymphoma. The second major impact of the WHO classification was to change the approach to the laboratory diagnosis of leukaemia and lymphoma with much greater emphasis on immunophenotyping, in particular, and other biological parameters. The WHO classification defines each of the diagnostic entities in terms of morphology, immunophenotype, cytogenetics and clinical features. This means that laboratory and clinical protocols can be developed that allow the diagnosis to be approached independently through these routes. Ensuring that the results of these investigations are concordant is now the major guarantee that a particular diagnosis is accurate. This represents an important practical advance towards improving the reliability of the laboratory diagnosis of leukaemia and lymphoma; an area where there has been considerable cause for concern in the past. Effective immunophenotyping is critical to the success of this approach to diagnosis. In the past decade, the number of antibodies that can be used as diagnostic reagents has grown and this has been accompanied by improvements in both immunocytochemistry and flow cytometric techniques. At the same time, there has been a growth in understanding of the detailed immunophenotypes associated with the diagnostic entities of the WHO classification. In many cases it is now possible to make a firm diagnosis based on immunophenotypic criteria alone and this provides a very effective check on the accuracy of a morphologically based diagnosis.

One of the weaknesses of the WHO classification is that although many of the entities can be diagnosed accurately and reproducibly, they are also highly heterogeneous with

Andrew Jack, BSc, MB, ChB, PhD, Consultant Haematopathologist, Haematological Malignancy Diagnostic Service (HMDS), Leeds General Infirmary, Leeds, UK.

respect to clinical behaviour and response to treatment. This means that in many cases, the routine immunophenotypic analysis of lymphoproliferative disorders needs to be extended to include prognostic markers that can be used to stratify patients according to their likely response to treatment. As more therapeutic monoclonal antibodies enter clinical practice, it will become important to assess accurately the extent of expression of cellular targets both at presentation and relapse. It is also becoming clear that in many cases, the immunophenotype is predictive of the presence of specific cytogenetic abnormalities. This can be useful in designing protocols to make the best use of relatively expensive cytogenetic and molecular investigations and to provide a further level of cross-validation of their results.

IMMUNOPHENOTYPING METHODS IN HAEMATOPATHOLOGY

Determination of an accurate immunophenotype in each tumour depends on the integrated use of immunocytochemistry and flow cytometry. These are complementary techniques and each has its strengths and weaknesses. Both techniques have undergone considerable development in recent years and the optimal overall approach to immunophenotyping continues to evolve.

The most important advance in immunocytochemistry has been the expansion of antibodies that can be used on paraffin-embedded sections. This has meant that immunocytochemistry performed on cryostat sections, which was formerly essential for a number of important markers, is now very rarely used in routine diagnosis. The increasing number of antibodies available has been complemented by improving techniques. The most important of these is the use of unmasking processes that expose antibody-binding sites that are obscured by extensive protein cross-linking during formaldehyde fixation. This can be carried out by heating dewaxed sections in a citrate buffer using either a microwave oven or pressure cooker or by the use of proteolytic enzymes. Heat-based methods are now used wherever possible because they can be more easily controlled and give more reproducible results than enzymatic approaches. A variety of methods designed to increase the sensitivity of the technique have also been developed in recent years.

These developments have expanded greatly the applicability of immunocytochemistry for the diagnosis of leukaemia and lymphoma. However, there are still a number of important limitations. The quality of results that can be obtained using immunocytochemistry on fixed tissue depends critically on the way that the biopsy was obtained and initially processed. Optimum results depend on controlled fixation. In the case of a large specimen, such as a whole lymph node, this means that the biopsy should be sliced before fixation and thin slices placed in fixative for a maximum of 24 h. Similar constraints also apply to tissue processing. To do this effectively usually requires unfixed tissue to be dissected in the laboratory. This, together with the requirements of polymerase chain reaction (PCR) and fluorescent in situ hybridisation (FISH) studies, means that the need to obtain fresh tissue samples has actually increased in recent years, in spite of the decline in the use of cryostat sections for immunocytochemistry. The second major limitation of immunocytochemistry is that most routine methods are effectively limited to one colour. Most markers used in the diagnosis of leukaemia and lymphoma are not entirely lineage specific and this means that links between one marker and another have to be based on morphology; this can be difficult and unreliable and is again highly dependent on the quality of the tissue processing. Current attempts to resolve this problem have centred on the use of multi-colour immunoflourescence labelling [2] but much simpler enzyme-based methods are also possible if combination of antibodies to nuclear and cell surface markers is being used.

Flow cytometry is the most widely used technique for immunophenotyping haematological malignancies. It has the major advantage that large number of cells can be analysed using a combination of several labelled antibodies and physical parameters related to cell size and granularity. The power of flow cytometry lies in the ability to readily identify populations of neoplastic cells within complex mixtures of cells such as blood and bone marrow. Increasingly, flow cytometry is also used as the method of first choice for the immunophenotypic analysis of cell suspensions derived from lymph node and other tissue biopsies.

Flow cytometric techniques continue to develop with improved instruments and the increasing numbers of antibodies available. Reagents that allow cells to be fixed and permeabilised have expanded the scope of diagnostic techniques by allowing combinations of cell surface, cytoplasmic and nuclear markers to be studied. Detailed analysis of the immunophenotypes of individual tumour types and the increasing number of fluorochromes available have led to an increasing sensitivity of detection of minimal residual disease at levels often comparable to those obtained by some PCR techniques [3, 4].

APPLICATIONS OF IMMUNOPHENOTYPING TO THE DIAGNOSIS OF LYMPHOPROLIFERATIVE DISORDERS

The extent of the literature on immunophenotyping is such that it is now impossible to provide a succinct review of all aspects of the use of immunological markers in the diagnosis of leukaemia and lymphoma. In order to illustrate the general principles and problems underlying the use of immunophenotyping, a number of the major diagnostic categories of the WHO classification are considered below. However, this is far from comprehensive, and space limitations have meant that several important categories, such as myeloma, acute leukaemia and T-cell lymphomas, could not be considered.

B-CELL CHRONIC LYMPHOCYTIC LEUKAEMIA AND MANTLE CELL LYMPHOMA

The diagnosis of B-CLL is now based primarily on the immunophenotype, with additional important prognostic information being provided by immunoglobulin heavy chain sequencing and molecular cytogenetics [5–8]. Morphological examination of a trephine biopsy may be helpful in assessing the extent of disease and response to therapy. The defining feature of B-CLL is the co-expression of CD5 and CD23. This has led to a considerable debate as to the cell of origin of B-CLL and comparison with the immunophenotype of mouse B1 cells. However, gene expression data and the presence of mutated immunoglobulin genes in most cases point to an origin in cells that have passed through a germinal centre prior to malignant transformation [9, 10]. CD5 is also found in other germinal-centre-derived lymphomas including follicular lymphoma and its pathogenic significance in this context remains uncertain [11, 12]. The other key diagnostic features of B-CLL are weak expression of the immunoglobulin/CD79 complex and weak expression of CD20. The combination of these four immunophenotypic features allows a confident diagnosis of B-CLL to be made in a large majority of cases [13]. Although these criteria are universally accepted, it should be remembered that they are empirically based and not rooted in an understanding of the pathogenesis of B-CLL. As such, they may eventually be superseded as a more detailed model of the oncogenesis of B-CLL emerges.

In specimens of bone marrow or lymph node involved by B-CLL, there is a much greater degree of cellular heterogeneity than is routinely found in the peripheral blood. This is due to the presence of proliferation centres which contain a population of large lymphoid blast cells. Particularly in lymph node specimens, proliferation centres can be a dominant morphological feature and it is important to recognise that they have a distinctive immunophenotype. The proliferating component shows strong expression of the nuclear transcription factor IRF-4, which is not found in the small lymphocytic component. There is also stronger expression of CD23, and the cell cycle marker Ki67 is almost exclusively confined to this blast cell population. Proliferation centres do not express other germinal centre markers such as CD10 and bcl-6. This is important in making a distinction from follicular lymphoma in cases with prominent proliferation centres. This is a surprisingly common diagnostic error when the diagnosis is based on morphology alone.

B-CLL is not a uniform entity in terms of prognosis. Some patients have indolent disease that may never require treatment. In contrast, other patients may progress rapidly and die of disease within a few years. The major prognostic factor that can be used to separate these groups is the degree of somatic hypermutation of the immunoglobulin heavy chain genes. To study this is a relatively expensive procedure and considerable efforts have been made to identify immunophenotypic correlates of mutation status. Early studies suggested that expression of CD38 could be used to identify poor-risk patients [6, 7]. However, more recent studies showed that the correlation with mutational status and prognosis was too weak to be an effective substitute for gene sequencing. The most promising marker to have emerged is Zap-70 [14–16]. This is a cell-signalling molecule that is mainly associated with the T-cell antigen receptor; it is rarely found in normal B cells. However, expression of this molecule is found on a significant proportion of B-CLL and its presence correlates with both non-mutated immunoglobulin genes and poor clinical outcome. Zap-70 can be demonstrated by flow cytometry and immunocytochemistry. The mRNA can be readily detected by reverse transcription PCR (RT-PCR). Differences in methods may account for the varying degree of correlation with adverse outcome that has been reported in different studies. The mechanisms that link clinical outcome with immunoglobulin mutation and Zap-70 remain poorly understood.

Although most cases of B-CLL have the immunophenotype described above, there are cases that do not conform to this pattern and this may lead to considerable problems in diagnosis. Most cases have weak expression of sIgM and sIgD; less commonly only one of these markers is present. In a small minority of cases of B-CLL, immunoglobulin class switching has occurred and the cells express sIgG [17, 18]. In a further group of cases, the tumour cells express sIgM/D but an IgG paraprotein is detectable in the serum and this can be shown to be derived from a class-switched tumour cell population [19]. The clinical significance of this finding remains poorly understood.

A wide variety of other phenotypic variants are commonly seen, but are poorly described in the literature. These include intermediate or strong expression of immunoglobulin or CD20 or the presence of CD38. However, the most important variant from the point of view of differential diagnosis are the cases with absent CD23 expression. This is often associated with other atypical morphological and immunophenotypic features. In these cases, it is important to consider the possibility of mantle cell lymphoma whether or not the patient has evidence of nodal or extranodal tumours. The gold standard for making this distinction is the demonstration of the t(11;14) using interphase FISH. However, the presence of bcl-1 expression in the context of a CD5+, CD23− phenotype has a very high correlation with the presence of the translocation. Absence of clearly defined proliferation centres in lymph nodes or bone marrow is also a feature that distinguishes CLL from mantle cell lymphoma, but at least in some cases IRF-4 expression may be widespread in mantle cells. Tumours with a CD5+, CD23− immunophenotype but which lack a t(11;14) are often classified as atypical B-CLL; however, it should not be assumed that these patients will have an indolent clinical course. Lack of immunoglobulin mutation and extensive disease may be more common in this group and the prognosis may be more like mantle cell lymphoma than typical B-CLL. Mantle cell lymphoma has a much poorer clinical outcome than typical CLL. Most patients have progressive disease that becomes refractory to therapy [20, 21]. Interestingly, a small minority of patients who fulfil the phenotypic criteria of mantle cell lymphoma may have an indolent clinical course but as yet there is no reliable immunophenotypic method of identifying these patients at presentation; there is some evidence that, like B-CLL, more indolent disease is associated with mutated immunoglobulin genes [22].

WALDENSTROM'S MACROGLOBULINAEMIA AND SYSTEMIC MARGINAL ZONE LYMPHOMA

The classification of Waldenstrom's macroglobulinaemia, splenic marginal zone lymphoma (SMZL) and lymphoplasmacytoid lymphoma has been the subject of considerable confusion. This group of tumours is characterised by predominately splenic and bone marrow involvement and frequent occurrence of an IgM paraprotein. In practice, a diagnostic label is often applied to these patients depending on their primary presentation and dominant clinical features [23]. There seems little merit in this approach and in clinical practice this is best regarded as a single entity. In this context, systemic marginal zone lymphoma (MZL) would seem to be an appropriate term pending a fuller understanding of the cellular origin of these tumours or until a clear pathological separation of discrete biological entities from within this group is established. Further characteristics of this group are the presence of immunoglobulin gene hypermutation with interclonal heterogeneity in almost every case and an absence of balanced translocations involving the immunoglobulin heavy chain locus. One of the reasons why this has proven to be a problematic diagnosis is that the immunophenotypic diagnosis is based mainly on exclusion of other entities [24]. Systemic MZL expresses pan B-cell markers but lacks evidence of germinal centre differentiation. Cells do not express CD10, CD23 or bcl-6 and IRF-4 is generally confined to cells with plasmacytoid features [25]. However, because of phenotypic heterogeneity in bone marrow tumour populations, the distinction between SMZL and follicular lymphoma requires exclusion of a t(14;18). The distinction between CLL, mantle cell lymphoma and MZL is based on the criteria described above. However, it should be noted that a minority of cases with the classical clinical features of MZL may express weak CD5 and this may be a diagnostic problem. This is best resolved by correlation of the immunophenotype with other clinical and morphological features.

LYMPHOMAS OF GERMINAL CENTRE ORIGIN – FOLLICULAR LYMPHOMA, BURKITT LYMPHOMA AND DIFFUSE LARGE B-CELL LYMPHOMA

This is the major group of nodal lymphomas and the immunophenotype is a key factor in both primary diagnosis and assessment of prognosis. Follicular lymphoma is the prototype of germinal-centre-derived tumours characterised by both follicle formation and cellular morphology that resembles the normal composition of the germinal centre. Almost all follicular lymphomas co-express CD10 and bcl-6 (Figure 2.1). Around half of all cases express

(a)   (b)

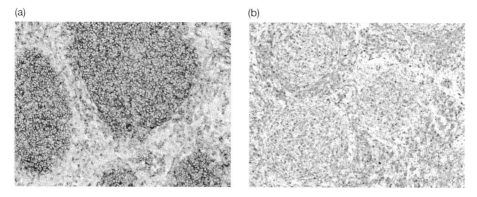

Figure 2.1 Follicular Lymphoma. Almost all cases of follicular lymphoma show strong expression of CD10 (a) and bcl-2 (b). In making this diagnosis it is important to establish that bcl-2 is present in cells with germinal centre morphology and phenotype because of the widespread expression of this protein by normal cells.

CD23 and a significant proportion have class-switched their immunoglobulin genes. Almost all cases have strong expression of CD20. Normal germinal centre cells do not express significant levels of bcl-2 and the presence of this molecule in the context of a germinal centre phenotype is almost invariably associated with a t(14;18). Problems in the diagnosis of follicular lymphoma may arise in cases that do not express bcl-2 or do not have a detectable translocation. This accounts for about 5% of cases and is probably more common in the heterogeneous grade 3 histological category. In these cases, the detection of monoclonality by light chain restriction, PCR or the presence of other translocations such as bcl-6 rearrangements, is essential for diagnosis [26, 27].

Diagnostic problems may arise because of phenotypic heterogeneity in follicular lymphoma. Tumour cells in the bone marrow, peripheral blood and even the interfollicular areas of nodes may differ from the classical phenotype found in neoplastic follicles. CD10 and bcl-6 expression may be much weaker or absent in these locations. The presence of CD23 or IgG, which are relatively rare in other lymphoproliferative disorders, may be a clue to the diagnosis but formal demonstration of t(14;18) by FISH or PCR is important in this context.

A proportion of diffuse large B-cell lymphoma (DLBCL) has an immunophenotype identical to follicular lymphoma. In some cases, these tumours may have arisen by transformation of an underlying follicular lymphoma, although this is not always the case. Recent gene expression microarray studies have shown that germinal-centre-type DLBCL has a better prognosis than the activated or post-germinal-centre type of tumour, although this needs to be qualified by the presence of specific genetic abnormalities, such as t(14;18) or bcl-6 rearrangements, which adversely affect prognosis [28–32] (Figure 2.2). The classification of DLBCL into these important prognostic groups can be readily carried out using immunophenotypic criteria. The germinal centre group includes the cases with a follicular lymphoma type phenotype and a group of cases that lack CD10 expression but have a variable expression of bcl-6 and IRF-4 [30, 31]. The activated B-cell group is characterised by absence of bcl-6 and CD10, although IRF-4 may be present. Many of these cases also express the transcription factor FOX-P1 and CD30[33]. In a small number of cases of DLBCL, overt plasma cell differentiation may be present. These are large cell, highly proliferative tumours, often, but not exclusively, HIV associated, which have a plasma cell immunophenotype including down-regulation of CD20, cytoplasmic immunoglobulin, loss of PAX-5 and surface CD138. Weak or absent CD45 may lead to diagnostic problems and some cases may be mis-

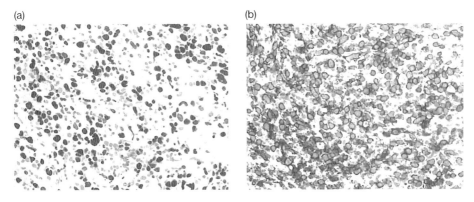

Figure 2.2 Germinal Centre Type Diffuse Large B-cell Lymphoma. The expression of bcl-6 protein in the nucleus of the tumour cells (**a**) is an important criterion in the sub-classification of DLBCL into germinal centre and activated B-cell types. It is important to demonstrate that bcl-6 is present in CD20 positive cells (**b**) with the appropriate morphology as bcl-6 may be expressed by a variety of normal cells including macrophages and activated endothelium.

diagnosed as non-haematopoetic tumours [34, 35]. A few cases have been described that have rearrangement of Alk-1 [36]. The distinction between plasmablastic lymphoma and disseminated myeloma is to some extent arbitrary and depends on the clinical features [37].

Burkitt lymphoma is a highly aggressive tumour that may be curable using intensive therapy [38, 39]. The defining feature is the presence of a rearrangement and abnormal activation of c-myc [40, 41]. This tumour is not reproducibly recognised by morphology and the immunophenotypic features are critical to the diagnosis. Abnormal activation of c-myc leads to a hyperproliferative state and this can be recognised by uniformly high expression of the cell cycle marker Ki67. In normal cells this would induce a compensatory high level of apoptosis through the p53 pathway [42]. Therefore, for c-myc to successfully induce the formation of tumour, this pathway must be blocked by inactivation of p53, usually through a combination of deletion and mutation. It is also known that the t(8;14) only occurs in cells with a germinal centre phenotype. From these principles, it is possible to deduce an immunophenotype that will predict the presence of the c-myc activation. This is a sensitive, but not entirely specific, technique and the diagnosis must be confirmed in all cases using interphase FISH or metaphase cytogenetic analysis.

HODGKIN'S LYMPHOMA

The nature of Hodgkin's lymphoma has been debated for many decades and it is only in the past few years that the relationship to peripheral B-cell lymphomas has been clarified. At the same time, it became apparent that Hodgkin's lymphoma itself could be divided into classical

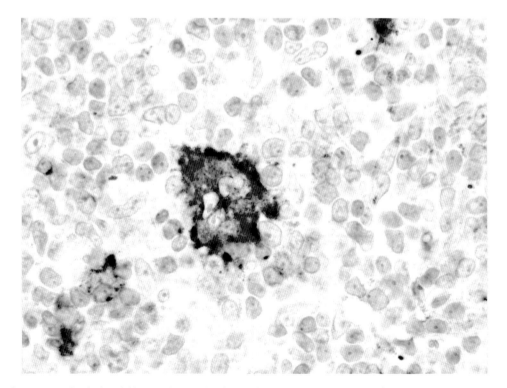

Figure 2.3   Classical Hodgkin Lymphoma. This figure shows the typical nuclear and cytoplasmic distribution of CD30 in classical type Reed Sternberg cells. The expression of CD30 is a key diagnostic feature of classical Hodgkin Lymphoma but is also found in both normal B and T-cells and close correlation with morphology and other markers is essential.

and lymphocyte predominant nodular types on the basis of immunophenotype and clinical behaviour. The relationship between classical Hodgkin's lymphoma and other B-cell malignancies has been highlighted by the similarity in gene expression profiles between Hodgkin's lymphoma and mediastinal B-cell lymphoma [43, 44]. The immunophenotype of classical Hodgkin's lymphoma includes expression of CD30 and IRF-4 with partial down-regulation of CD45. In most cases there is cytoplasmic expression of CD15 (Figure 2.3). In typical cases there is loss of B-cell characteristics including absence of CD20, CD79, immunoglobulin and PAX-5. Bob-1 and Oct-2, which are transcriptional activators of immunoglobulin, are usually absent or weakly expressed by comparison to normal B cells [45–47]. As yet there is no unifying mechanism to explain this abnormal pattern. Diagnostic problems arise when there is only partial down-regulation of the B-cell phenotype and some or all of the cells express CD20 or CD79 or bcl-6. In a few cases, there is no clear immunophenotypic distinction between Hodgkin's lymphoma and the activated type of DLBCL. In cases with strong CD20 expression, which some reports have suggested is a marker of poor prognosis, it could be argued that patients should be treated with CHOP-R rather than Hodgkin-type chemotherapy [48].

Lymphocyte predominant nodular Hodgkin's lymphoma (LPNHL) is now recognised as a separate disease entity. Most cases have an excellent outcome and there is debate as to the extent of treatment required [49]. In some cases, it may be difficult to distinguish this from the lymphocyte-rich variant of classical Hodgkin's lymphoma on morphological grounds. However, these entities are phenotypically distinct [47, 50, 51]. The immunophenotype of the tumour cells in LPNHL is almost the inverse of classical Hodgkin's lymphoma. The cells do not express CD30 or CD15 but have strong expression of CD20 and bcl-6. Oct-2 is present

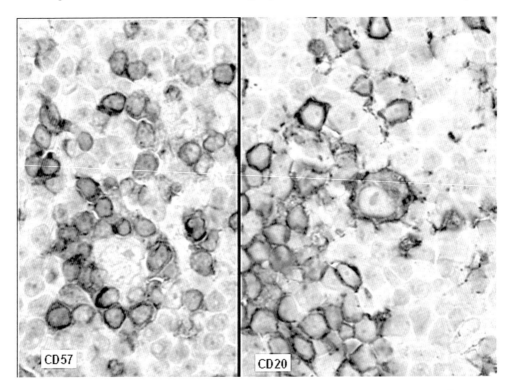

Figure 2.4 Lymphocyte Predominant Nodular Hodgkin Lymphoma. Unlike Classical Hodgkin Lymphoma, strong CD20 expression is a key feature of lymphocyte predominant nodular Hodgkin Lymphoma. A further distinctive feature is the tendency of the tumour cells to form rosettes with T-cells expressing CD57. This is a T-cell population normally found in germinal centres.

at very high levels and this is a useful aid to the identification of the tumour cells, which can be clearly demarcated from the B-cell background. A further useful feature is the presence of large number of CD4+, CD57+ T cells, which form rosettes around the tumour cells. The strong expression of CD20 by the tumour cells has led to trials of single-agent therapy with rituximab in patients with LPNHL [52] (Figure 2.4).

DETECTING CLONALITY IN LYMPHOPROLIFERATIVE DISORDERS

Monoclonality is a key feature of almost all malignancies. However, lymphomas are the only type of tumour where the demonstration of monoclonality is part of routine diagnosis. In B-cell malignancies, the presence of light chain restriction is taken to indicate that the cells are monoclonal. Where material is available for flow cytometric analysis, light chain restriction can be readily identified in almost all B-cell malignancies, provided a technique is used that allows accurate gating on the B-cell population. Problems may arise where there is a large non-neoplastic B-cell population present with a κ : λ ratio near the normal range or where multiple B-cell clones with different light chains are present. In each case, a clonal B-cell population may be missed. In the bone marrow, a population of precursor B cells with no detectable surface immunoglobulin expression is always present. However, in peripheral lymphoid tissue, the number of surface-immunoglobulin-negative B cells should be negligible and a significant number of these cells almost always implies that a neoplastic population is present.

In contrast to flow cytometry, the demonstration of light chain restriction by immuno-cytochemistry in fixed tissue sections is difficult. There is almost always a high background caused by free tissue immunoglobulin and in most cases it is not possible to demonstrate reliably surface light chain expression. This is less of a problem when attempting to demon-strate cytoplasmic light chain restriction in plasma cells, but again this is prone to artefact. Unfortunately, PCR-based techniques for the demonstration of clonality are less reliable when DNA is extracted from fixed tissues [53].

PCR is the technique of choice for the demonstration of T-cell monoclonality. However, an alternative approach is to use a panel of Vβ-family-specific antibodies. This is rarely used in routine diagnostic work because of the high cost and difficulty in interpreting the results where a mixture of normal and neoplastic T cell is present [54, 55].

SUMMARY

Flow cytometry and immunocytochemistry are core techniques in haematopathology. A morphological diagnosis that is not supported by appropriate immunophenotyping should no longer be acceptable in routine practice. To be fully effective it is important that immunological markers are applied systemically with panels chosen to provide an inde-pendent route to the diagnosis rather than simply confirming morphological impressions.

Diagnostic techniques are changing rapidly with new concepts and technologies becoming available. A key question is the extent to which gene expression microarrays will replace current diagnostic techniques. In principle, this is a feasible approach and it may become more attractive as costs decrease. However, there are a number of potential problems. Antibody-based approaches rely on the detection of protein and it is clear that mRNA and protein expression are not always closely related. It is also likely that in the near future the ability to characterise a protein's activation state with the use of specific antibodies or the interaction between proteins using fluorescence resonant energy trans-fer methods may become central to diagnosis as understanding of tumour pathogenesis increases. At a more practical level, the effectiveness of microarray approaches in analysing complex mixtures of cells, especially where the tumour cells are in a minority, remains to be demonstrated. The resolution of these questions will determine the future direction of haematopathology and will have a major influence on the development of targeted biological therapies.

REFERENCES

1. Harris NL, Jaffe ES, Stein H *et al*. A revised European-American classification of lymphoid neoplasms: a proposal from the International Lymphoma Study Group. *Blood* 1994; 84:1361–1392.
2. Marafioti T, Jones M, Facchetti F *et al*. Phenotype and genotype of interfollicular large B cells, a subpopulation of lymphocytes often with dendritic morphology. *Blood* 2003; 102:2868–2876.
3. Rawstron AC, Kennedy B, Evans PA *et al*. Quantitation of minimal disease levels in chronic lymphocytic leukemia using a sensitive flow cytometric assay improves the prediction of outcome and can be used to optimize therapy. *Blood* 2001; 98:29–35.
4. Rawstron AC, Davies FE, Dasgupta R *et al*. Flow cytometric disease monitoring in multiple myeloma: the relationship between normal and neoplastic plasma cells predicts outcome after transplantation. *Blood* 2002; 100:3095–3100.
5. Dohner H, Stilgenbauer S, Benner A *et al*. Genomic aberrations and survival in chronic lymphocytic leukemia. *N Engl J Med* 2000; 343:1910–1916.
6. Hamblin TJ, Orchard JA, Ibbotson RE *et al*. CD38 expression and immunoglobulin variable region mutations are independent prognostic variables in chronic lymphocytic leukemia, but CD38 expression may vary during the course of the disease. *Blood* 2002; 99:1023–1029.
7. Hamblin TJ, Orchard JA, Gardiner A *et al*. Immunoglobulin V genes and CD38 expression in CLL. *Blood* 2000; 95:2455–2457.
8. Garcia-Manero G. Chromosomal abnormalities in chronic lymphocytic leukemia. *N Engl J Med* 2001; 344:1254.
9. Haslinger C, Schweifer N, Stilgenbauer S *et al*. Microarray gene expression profiling of B-cell chronic lymphocytic leukemia subgroups defined by genomic aberrations and VH mutation status. *J Clin Oncol* 2004; 22:3937–3949.
10. Stratowa C, Loffler G, Lichter P *et al*. CDNA microarray gene expression analysis of B-cell chronic lymphocytic leukemia proposes potential new prognostic markers involved in lymphocyte trafficking. *Int J Cancer* 2001; 91:474–480.
11. Tiesinga JJ, Wu CD, Inghirami G. CD5+ follicle center lymphoma. Immunophenotyping detects a unique subset of 'floral' follicular lymphoma. *Am J Clin Pathol* 2000; 114:912–921.
12. Taniguchi M, Oka K, Hiasa A *et al*. De novo CD5+ diffuse large B-cell lymphomas express VH genes with somatic mutation. *Blood* 1998; 91:1145–1151.
13. Matutes E, Owusu-Ankomah K, Morilla R *et al*. The immunological profile of B-cell disorders and proposal of a scoring system for the diagnosis of CLL. *Leukemia* 1994; 8:1640–1645.
14. Rassenti LZ, Huynh L, Toy TL *et al*. ZAP-70 compared with immunoglobulin heavy-chain gene mutation status as a predictor of disease progression in chronic lymphocytic leukemia. *N Engl J Med* 2004; 351:893–901.
15. Crespo M, Bosch F, Villamor N *et al*. ZAP-70 expression as a surrogate for immunoglobulin-variable-region mutations in chronic lymphocytic leukemia. *N Engl J Med* 2003; 348:1764–1775.
16. Durig J, Nuckel H, Cremer M *et al*. ZAP-70 expression is a prognostic factor in chronic lymphocytic leukemia. *Leukemia* 2003; 17:2426–2434.
17. Fais F, Sellars B, Ghiotto F *et al*. Examples of *in vivo* isotype class switching in IgM+ chronic lymphocytic leukemia B cells. *J Clin Invest* 1996; 98:1659–1666.
18. Katayama Y, Sakai A, Katsutani S, Takimoto Y, Kimura A. Lack of allelic exclusion and isotype switching in B cell chronic lymphocytic leukemia. *Am J Hematol* 2001; 68:295–297.
19. Wakai M, Hashimoto S, Omata M *et al*. IgG+, CD5+ human chronic lymphocytic leukemia B cells. Production of IgG antibodies that exhibit diminished autoreactivity and IgG subclass skewing. *Autoimmunity* 1994; 19:39–48.
20. Kauh J, Baidas SM, Ozdemirli M, Cheson BD. Mantle cell lymphoma: clinicopathologic features and treatments. *Oncology (Huntingt)* 2003; 17:879–891, 896.

21. Hiddemann W, Dreyling M. Mantle cell lymphoma: therapeutic strategies are different from CLL. *Curr Treat Options Oncol* 2003; 4:219–226.
22. Orchard J, Garand R, Davis Z *et al*. A subset of t(11; 14) lymphoma with mantle cell features displays mutated IgVH genes and includes patients with good prognosis, nonnodal disease. *Blood* 2003; 101:4975–4981.
23. Owen RG, Parapia LA, Higginson J *et al*. Clinicopathological correlates of IgM paraproteinemias. *Clin Lymphoma* 2000; 1:39–43.
24. Owen RG, Barrans SL, Richards SJ *et al*. Waldenstrom macroglobulinemia. Development of diagnostic criteria and identification of prognostic factors. *Am J Clin Pathol* 2001; 116:420–428.
25. Dogan A, Isaacson PG. Splenic marginal zone lymphoma. *Semin Diagn Pathol* 2003; 20:121–127.
26. Bosga-Bouwer AG, van Imhoff GW, Boonstra R *et al*. Follicular lymphoma grade 3B includes 3 cytogenetically defined subgroups with primary t(14; 18), 3q27, or other translocations: t(14; 18) and 3q27 are mutually exclusive. *Blood* 2003; 101:1149–1154.
27. Ott G, Katzenberger T, Lohr A *et al*. Cytomorphologic, immunohistochemical, and cytogenetic profiles of follicular lymphoma: 2 types of follicular lymphoma grade 3. *Blood* 2002; 99:3806–3812.
28. Barrans SL, Evans PA, O'Connor SJ *et al*. The t(14; 18) is associated with germinal center-derived diffuse large B-cell lymphoma and is a strong predictor of outcome. *Clin Cancer Res* 2003; 9:2133–2139.
29. Barrans SL, O'Connor SJ, Evans PA *et al*. Rearrangement of the BCL6 locus at 3q27 is an independent poor prognostic factor in nodal diffuse large B-cell lymphoma. *Br J Haematol* 2002; 117:322–332.
30. Barrans SL, Carter I, Owen RG *et al*. Germinal center phenotype and bcl-2 expression combined with the International Prognostic Index improves patient risk stratification in diffuse large B-cell lymphoma. *Blood* 2002; 99:1136–1143.
31. Hans CP, Weisenburger DD, Greiner TC *et al*. Confirmation of the molecular classification of diffuse large B-cell lymphoma by immunohistochemistry using a tissue microarray. *Blood* 2004; 103:275–282.
32. Alizadeh AA, Eisen MB, Davis RE *et al*. Distinct types of diffuse large B-cell lymphoma identified by gene expression profiling. *Nature* 2000; 403:503–511.
33. Barrans SL, Fenton JA, Banham A, Owen RG, Jack AS. Strong expression of FOXP1 identifies a distinct subset of diffuse large B-Cell lymphoma patients with poor outcome. *Blood* 2004.
34. Brown RS, Campbell C, Lishman SC, Spittle MF, Miller RF. Plasmablastic lymphoma: a new subcategory of human immunodeficiency virus-related non-Hodgkin's lymphoma. *Clin Oncol (R Coll Radiol)* 1998; 10:327–329.
35. Chetty R, Hlatswayo N, Muc R, Sabaratnam R, Gatter K. Plasmablastic lymphoma in HIV+ patients: an expanding spectrum. *Histopathology* 2003; 42:605–609.
36. Onciu M, Behm FG, Downing JR *et al*. ALK-positive plasmablastic B-cell lymphoma with expression of the NPM-ALK fusion transcript: report of 2 cases. *Blood* 2003; 102:2642–2644.
37. Vega F, Chang CC, Medeiros LJ *et al*. Plasmablastic lymphomas and plasmablastic plasma cell myelomas have nearly identical immunophenotypic profiles. *Mod Pathol* 2004.
38. Cairo MS, Sposto R, Perkins SL *et al*. Burkitt's and Burkitt-like lymphoma in children and adolescents: a review of the Children's Cancer Group experience. *Br J Haematol* 2003; 120:660–670.
39. Mead GM, Sydes MR, Walewski J *et al*. An international evaluation of CODOX-M and CODOX-M alternating with IVAC in adult Burkitt's lymphoma: results of United Kingdom Lymphoma Group LY06 study. *Ann Oncol* 2002; 13:1264–1274.
40. Hecht JL, Aster JC. Molecular biology of Burkitt's lymphoma. *J Clin Oncol* 2000; 18:3707–3721.
41. Bishop PC, Rao VK, Wilson WH. Burkitt's lymphoma: molecular pathogenesis and treatment. *Cancer Invest* 2000; 18:574–583.
42. Klumb CE, De Resende LM, Tajara EH *et al*. p53 gene analysis in childhood B non-Hodgkin's lymphoma. *Sao Paulo Med J* 2001; 119:212–215.
43. Savage KJ, Monti S, Kutok JL *et al*. The molecular signature of mediastinal large B-cell lymphoma differs from that of other diffuse large B-cell lymphomas and shares features with classical Hodgkin lymphoma. *Blood* 2003; 102:3871–3879.
44. Rosenwald A, Wright G, Leroy K *et al*. Molecular diagnosis of primary mediastinal B cell lymphoma identifies a clinically favorable subgroup of diffuse large B cell lymphoma related to Hodgkin lymphoma. *J Exp Med* 2003; 198:851–862.
45. Browne P, Petrosyan K, Hernandez A, Chan JA. The B-cell transcription factors BSAP, Oct-2, and BOB.1 and the pan-B-cell markers CD20, CD22, and CD79a are useful in the differential diagnosis of classic Hodgkin lymphoma. *Am J Clin Pathol* 2003; 120:767–777.

46. Re D, Muschen M, Ahmadi T *et al*. Oct-2 and Bob-1 deficiency in Hodgkin and Reed Sternberg cells. *Cancer Res* 2001; 61:2080–2084.
47. Stein H, Marafioti T, Foss HD *et al*. Down-regulation of BOB.1/OBF.1 and Oct2 in classical Hodgkin disease but not in lymphocyte predominant Hodgkin disease correlates with immunoglobulin transcription. *Blood* 2001; 97:496–501.
48. Portlock CS, Donnelly GB, Qin J *et al*. Adverse prognostic significance of CD20 positive Reed-Sternberg cells in classical Hodgkin's disease. *Br J Haematol* 2004; 125:701–708.
49. Wilder RB, Schlembach PJ, Jones D *et al*. European Organization for Research and Treatment of Cancer and Groupe d'Etude des Lymphomes de l'Adulte very favorable and favorable, lymphocyte-predominant Hodgkin disease. *Cancer* 2002; 94:1731–1738.
50. Anagnostopoulos I, Hansmann ML, Franssila K *et al*. European Task Force on Lymphoma project on lymphocyte predominance Hodgkin disease: histologic and immunohistologic analysis of submitted cases reveals 2 types of Hodgkin disease with a nodular growth pattern and abundant lymphocytes. *Blood* 2000; 96:1889–1899.
51. Fan Z, Natkunam Y, Bair E, Tibshirani R, Warnke RA. Characterization of variant patterns of nodular lymphocyte predominant hodgkin lymphoma with immunohistologic and clinical correlation. *Am J Surg Pathol* 2003; 27:1346–1356.
52. Ekstrand BC, Lucas JB, Horwitz SM *et al*. Rituximab in lymphocyte-predominant Hodgkin disease: results of a phase 2 trial. *Blood* 2003; 101:4285–4289.
53. van Dongen JJ, Langerak AW, Bruggemann M *et al*. Design and standardization of PCR primers and protocols for detection of clonal immunoglobulin and T-cell receptor gene recombinations in suspect lymphoproliferations: report of the BIOMED-2 Concerted Action BMH4-CT98-3936. *Leukemia* 2003; 17:2257–2317.
54. Schwab C, Willers J, Niederer E *et al*. The use of anti-T-cell receptor-Vbeta antibodies for the estimation of treatment success and phenotypic characterization of clonal T-cell populations in cutaneous T-cell lymphomas. *Br J Haematol* 2002; 118:1019–1026.
55. Tissier F, Martinon F, Camilleri-Broet S *et al*. T-cell receptor Vbeta repertoire in nodal non-anaplastic peripheral T-cell lymphomas. *Pathol Res Pract* 2002; 198:389–395.

3

Diagnostic and prognostic markers of lymphoid malignancies; the latest genetic, cytogenetic and haematological parameters

T. J. Hamblin

INTRODUCTION

For most malignancies, diagnosis is the domain of the histopathologist, and prognosis the province of the clinician. However, the haematopathologist has something to contribute in distinguishing different forms of low-grade lymphoproliferative diseases, especially when these reside mainly in the blood and bone marrow, and, thanks to new techniques in molecular biology and cytogenetics, can override the prognostications of the physician, who can only determine how much disease is present.

DIAGNOSIS

At one time, excessive lymphocytes in blood signified lymphatic leukaemia, which was divided on morphological grounds into acute and chronic depending on whether the cells were blast-like or not.

CHRONIC LYMPHOCYTIC LEUKAEMIA

On the basis of the presence of immunoglobulin molecules on the cell surface or reactivity with anti-CD3, lymphoid malignancies are diagnosed as B cell or T cell, and the practice of calling chronic lymphocytic leukaemias (CLL) either B-CLL or T-CLL evolved. This should now be unnecessary as T-CLL has disappeared from classifications. All cases of CLL are B-CLL and the B has become superfluous. In the past, series of patients with CLL have included cases with other diagnoses. The most commonly mistaken alternative diagnoses are splenic marginal zone lymphoma (SMZL), mantle cell lymphoma (MCL), the CLL – prolymphocytic leukaemia (PLL) interface, and small cell versions of some T-cell leukaemias, notably T-PLL and Sezary syndrome.

The immunophenotypes of the different lymphoid tumours that often present with a lymphocytosis are shown in Table 3.1. CLL cells express surface immunoglobulin, usually IgM plus IgD. The number of immunoglobulin molecules is only about 10% of those on normal B cells, so the staining is usually weak to moderate. The immunoglobulin-associated molecule Igβ or CD79b is similarly reduced in quantity and is generally weak or absent.

Terry J. Hamblin DM, FRCP, FRCPath, FMedSci, Professor of Immunohaematology, University of Southampton, Department of Haematology, Royal Bournemouth Hospital, Bournemouth, UK.

Table 3.1 Typical immunophenotyping of the low and some intermediate grade B and T cell lymphoproliferative disorders

	CLL	CLL/PLL	B-PLL	HCL	HCLv	SLVL	MCL	FL	LGL-L T	LGL-L NK	T-PLL	ATLL
sIg	±	+	++	++	++	++	++	++	–	–	–	–
CD19	++	++	++	++	++	++	++	++	–	–	–	–
CD20	+	++	++	++	++	++	++	++	–	–	–	–
FMC7	–	±	++	++	++	++	++	++	–	–	–	–
CD5	++	+	+ or –	–	–	– or +	++	–	++	–	++	++
CD10	–	–	–	–	–	–	–	++	–	–	–	–
CD22	–	±	++	++	++	++	++	++	–	–	–	–
CD23	++	++	–	–	–	–	–	+	–	–	–	–
CD79b	±	±	++	++	++	++	++	++	–	–	–	–
CD25	++	++	–	++	–	–	–	–	–	–	–	++
CD103	–	–	–	++	–	–	–	–	–	–	–	–
CD2									++	++	++	++
CD3									++	–	++	++
CD4									–	–	++	++
CD8									++	++	–	–
CD16									++	++	–	–
CD56									–	++	–	–
CD57									++	–	–	–

This table gives the most common variants. Atypical cases of CLL have brighter sIg and CD20, and may be weakly positive for FMC7. About a third of PLL cases are CD5 positive as are 20% of cases of SLVL. In CLL CD22 is present in the cytoplasm but not on the surface of the cells.

Table 3.2 Royal Marsden scoring system for CLL and similar tumours

CD5	Pos	1 point	Neg	0 points
CD79b	Weak or neg	1 point	Pos	0 points
CD23	Pos	1 point	Neg	0 points
Surface Ig	Weak	1 point	Strong	0 points
FMC7	Neg	1 point	Pos	0 points

Most patients with CLL score 4 or 5. Most patients with mantle cell lymphoma or SMZL score 1 or 2

CD20 is present, but again the staining is weaker than on normal B cells. FMC7 is an antibody that detects an epitope of CD20 that is not exposed in CLL. FMC7 is usually weak or absent on CLL cells. The cells are CD19 positive, but unlike most B cell lymphomas they are also CD5 positive. CD22 is a ubiquitous B-cell antigen, but in CLL it tends to be present not on the cell surface, but only in the cytoplasm. Finally, CD23, the Fcε receptor, is expressed on CLL cells unlike other B-cell malignancies. In biology nothing is absolute, and cases of atypical CLL are fairly common. To help elucidate these difficulties, The Royal Marsden Hospital (Sutton, Surrey, UK) has introduced a scoring system [1] (Table 3.2).

There is no characteristic karyotype for CLL and classical cytogenetics are difficult to do. However, several abnormalities have been reported and confirmed by the use of fluorescent *in-situ* hybridisation (FISH) on interphase cells [2]. The commonest abnormality (between 50 and 80% of cases) is a deletion at 13q14. The search for a functional gene responsible for CLL in the minimally deleted region has uncovered two micro-RNA genes at 13q14, miR15 and miR16 [3]. Deletions at 13q are not confined to CLL, being a feature of myeloma and found in other haematological malignancies [4].

The next most common abnormality is trisomy 12, present in about 20% of cases. Again it is not confined to CLL but can be seen in other lymphoid tumours. CLL with trisomy 12 is often characterised by atypical morphology [5], often with increased numbers of prolymphocytes. The immunophenotype is slightly atypical, with rather denser surface immunoglobulin and a degree of positivity with FMC7.

Deletions at 11q23 are thought to involve the ataxia telangectasia mutated (ATM) gene, although this is still not fully established. It is found in 15–20% of cases and characteristically in younger patients with bulky lymphadenopathy [6]. Deletions at 17p13 are believed to involve the *p53* gene. This is rarely an early finding (<5%) but is one of the most common transforming events, occurring in >10% of patients [7]. It is often a feature of Richter's syndrome. Similarly, deletions at 6q21 are almost always secondary events. The gene involved is unknown.

Translocations at 14q32, the site of the gene encoding the immunoglobulin heavy chain gene, are important. The t(11;14)(q13;q32) translocation is a feature of MCL and an important investigation in the differential diagnosis (see below). The t(14;18)(q32;q21) translocation and the light chain variants t(2;18) and t(18;22) translocations, all of which result in the rearrangement of the BCL2 gene, are rare in CLL, being found in only 1–2% of cases [8]. Analysis of the BCL2 breakpoints shows that these are usually 5′ prime and distinct from the breakpoints associated with follicle centre cell lymphoma. The expression of BCL 2 protein is usually higher than that found in typical CLL but patients with BCL 2 rearrangements have no distinct clinical or morphological features.

The t(14;19)(q32;q13) translocation is another rare finding in CLL [9] occurring in 0.5% of cases. Lymphocyte morphology is frequently atypical and most patients have progressive disease. The breakpoint on chromosome 19 involves the BCL3 gene which encodes an I-κB-like protein.

B-PLL AND THE CLL/PLL INTERFACE

Prolymphocytes are large lymphocytes some 10–15 μm in diameter compared to 7–10 μm for CLL cells. They have round or indented nuclei with chromatin that is less dense than that of CLL cells, but more dense than that of lymphoblasts and they possess a single prominent nucleolus. The cytoplasm is more abundant than that of a typical CLL cell and in Romanowsky-stained specimens is pale blue and agranular. Although small numbers of prolymphocytes are usually found in CLL, there is a distinct B-cell PLL that is completely unrelated to CLL. First recognised by Galton and colleagues [10] in 1974, it occurs in the same age group as CLL with a similar male preponderance. Clinically, splenomegaly without lymphadenopathy is the rule, but it is defined by the presence of >55% circulating prolymphocytes [11].

B-PLL is an extremely rare disease, some experts doubting its existence. Certainly, it exists as a clinical entity, but when immunophenotyping and molecular markers are explored, the disease seems heterogeneous. Some cases seem to have transformed from CLL, some seem to be blastic variants of MCL [12], and some a distinct disease.

The surface immunoglobulin is much denser than in CLL [13]. Other pan-B cell markers, CD19, CD20, are positive. In most cases, the cells are CD23 negative [13]. They may be either CD5 positive or negative. Cases with clear evidence of having transformed from CLL and those with features of MCL are CD5 positive. The cells are usually surface CD22 and FMC7 positive [13].

Prolymphocytoid transformation of CLL or CLL/PLL was first reported by Galton's group in 1979 [14]. It was specifically noted that the cells retained the immunophenotype of CLL cells. In a series of papers [13, 15–17] the same group defined typical CLL as having <10% prolymphocytes and CLL/PLL as those cases with between 10 and 55% prolymphocytes. Although, as a group, patients with CLL/PLL had more surface immunoglobulin than those with typical CLL, there was no sudden transition from a lower density at an earlier stage of the disease, and the immunophenotype of small and large cells was indistinguishable.

A karyotypic abnormality is seen in about 60% of cases of B-PLL. No consistent abnormality has been found, but prominent amongst them have been translocations or deletions at 14q32, particularly t(11;14)(q14;q32), a t(6;12)(q15;p13) translocation, a t(2;3)(q35;q14) translocation and trisomy 12 [18]. The range of karyotypes of CLL/PLL is similar to that seen in CLL, but del13q14 is under-represented.

SPLENIC MARGINAL ZONE LYMPHOMA

A combination of splenomegaly, circulating atypical 'hairy' cells and a paraprotein was first described in 1979 [19]. A variety of different names have been used to describe this disorder and the term splenic lymphoma with villous lymphocytes (SLVL) was introduced by the group at the Royal Marsden Hospital in 1987 [20]. In the WHO classification, the name SMZL has been adopted [21], since the presence of villi on the cells is not constant, and is heavily dependent on the quality of blood film preparation. There are two other types of marginal zone lymphoma (nodal and extra-nodal marginal zone lymphomas) which are discrete from SMZL [21]. Most patients with SMZL have marked splenomegaly but lymphadenopathy is usually absent. Fifty to 70% of patients have a low level paraprotein which is usually IgM but sometimes IgG. The immunophenotype (Table 3.1) is not distinctive. In a minority of cases, CD5 and/or CD23 are expressed. An abnormal karyotype is found in the majority of cases and is frequently complex [22]. Recurring abnormalities include deletions or translocations of 7q particularly involving bands 7q22 to 7q36. The suggestion has been made that dysregulation of the cyclin-dependent kinase 6 (CDK6) gene contributes to the pathogenesis of SMZL [23]. The t(11;14) translocation is found in 15% of cases suggesting the possibility that pleomorphic MCL can appear in the guise of SMZL [24].

MANTLE CELL LYMPHOMA

MCL has been relatively recently defined and represents between 3 and 10% of adult non-Hodgkin's lymphomas [21]. However, peripheral blood involvement is found in about 25% of cases. In some cases this represents the appearance of advanced and pre-terminal disease, with bizarre and unusual morphology, but in others it is seen as a characteristic part of early disease. Since MCL is CD5 positive, and in some cases the cells are morphologically very similar to CLL cells, diagnosis can be difficult. Immunophenotyping and karyotyping make the distinction. The cells characteristically express CD5, CD19, CD20, CD79b, FMC7 and dense surface immunoglobulin. They are CD23 negative. The characteristic karyotype shows the t(11;14)(q14;q32) translocation, and the cells stain for nuclear cyclin D1(BCL1) [25].

Problems arise because MCL is pleomorphic and the tumour can masquerade as CLL, SMZL and PLL. The t(11;14) translocation can be found in multiple myeloma [26] as well as MCL.

HAIRY CELL LEUKAEMIA AND HAIRY CELL VARIANT

Hairy cell leukaemia (HCL) is rarer than SMZL but more common than B-PLL [21]. It comprises about 2% of lymphoid leukaemias. It has a male preponderance and is most commonly seen in late middle age. The leukaemic cells have a distinct morphology, and the tumour is mainly in the spleen and bone marrow with associated leucopaenia rather than a leucocytosis. Immunophenotyping is characteristic (Table 3.1).

Hairy cell variant (HCLv) is extremely rare and distinguished from HCL by morphology and immunophenotyping [21] (Table 3.1). Characteristically, the lymphocyte count is raised. No distinctive pattern of chromosomal abnormality has been reported in either HCL or HCLv.

T-CELL LEUKAEMIAS

The immunophenotypes of the low- and intermediate-grade T-cell leukaemias are given in Table 3.1. The commonest type of T-cell leukaemia is large granular lymphocytic leukaemia (LGL-L) which comprises 2–3% of the cases of small lymphocytic leukaemia [27]. Around 85% of cases have clonal T cells. Although a third of cases are asymptomatic, the characteristic blood count abnormality is neutropenia and the characteristic clinical feature is bacterial infection. Associated rheumatoid arthritis is found in 25% of cases, which must be distinguished from Felty's syndrome. About 15% of patients with LGL-L have a clonal expansion of natural killer (NK) cells. This tends to occur at a younger age and has an aggressive clinical course.

T-PLL comprises 1.5% of lymphoproliferative disorders with lymphocyte counts $>10 \times 10^9/l$ [21]. It is an aggressive and almost always fatal disorder. T-PLL almost invariably demonstrates inv(14)(q11;q32) or other 14q abnormalities [28]. The 14q11 breakpoint involves the T-cell receptor α and δ chain genes [29]. The breakpoints at 14q32 are not homogeneous and span a region of at least 300 kb not involving the immunoglobulin heavy chain gene [30].

Sezary Syndrome is the spillover form of mycosis fungoides (MF) and a rare, late and aggressive complication. When the cells are particularly small they occasionally resemble those of CLL. In such cases, the cerebreform appearance of the nucleus is revealed by transmission electron microscopy.

The cellular morphology adult T-cell leukaemia lymphoma (ATLL) is distinctive [21]. ATLL is endemic in Japan, the Caribbean and parts of Central Africa but is seen increasingly in Europe and America following immigration. The disease is linked to infection with HTLV-I, a virus usually acquired in infancy and spread by breast milk, blood and blood products. It presents at a median age of 55 with a gender ratio of 1.5:1. About 2.5% of HTLV-I carriers eventually develop ATLL. There are smouldering and acute variants with about 25% converting after a long latent period.

PROGNOSIS

Historically, prognosis in lymphoid malignancies has been estimated using clinical staging and a variety of scoring systems such as the International Prognostic Index [31]. Immunophenotyping and molecular studies have enhanced our prognostic ability.

IMMUNOGLOBULIN VARIABLE REGION GENES

In order to encompass every possible antibody response to the huge variety of possible pathogens, each B lymphocyte comes 'pre-fitted' with a bespoke set of genes encoding an immunoglobulin molecule. For the heavy chain alone there are over 8,000 possibilities made by choosing one of 51 variable region (V) genes, one of 27 diversity segment (D) genes and one of 6 junctional (J) genes. This number is increased enormously by imprecise joining at V-D and D-J, allowing for the possibility of three reading frames.

Refining the immune response to produce the best possible fit after the B lymphocyte has encountered the favoured antigen requires minor adjustments to the shape of the immunoglobulin molecule, and is achieved by random somatic mutations of the immunoglobulin genes followed by a Darwinian selection process. This process takes place in the germinal centre. Since the presence or absence of somatic mutations can be deter- mined by comparing the gene sequence with known germline sequences available from internet sites, such mutations can be used like a passport stamp to discover whether a cell has passed through a germinal centre.

For some tumours, such as follicular lymphoma and some diffuse large B-cell lymphomas, a series of subclones is usually found which can be arranged like a family tree. This indicates that the cell of origin is still subject to the mutational pressure within the germinal centre, possibly being held there by the acquisition of new N-glycosylation sites in the variable region [32]. Most other B-cell tumours can be located as pre- or post-germinal centre tumours based on whether somatic mutations are present.

CLL was traditionally regarded as a pre-germinal centre lymphoma on the basis of early studies, but a review of 76 patients in a series of small studies revealed that about half had somatic mutations [33]. In 1999, two papers published simultaneously demonstrated that not only did the majority of cases have somatic mutations, but the presence of these mutations indicated a sharp clinical and prognostic demarcation [34, 35]. Patients whose cells show somatic mutations had a median survival of 25 years, typical cellular morphology, non- diffuse bone marrow histology, del13q14 as a single chromosomal abnormality, low numbers of proliferation centres in lymph nodes and bone marrow, and a stable lymphocyte count. On the other hand, those whose cells lacked somatic mutations had a median survival of 8 years, were more likely to have increased numbers of prolymphocytes, diffuse bone marrow histology, 17p13 or 11q23 chromosomal deletions, higher numbers of proliferation centres and a progressively increasing lymphocyte count.

This observation has been confirmed in many subsequent publications [7, 36–38] (Figure 3.1), including one dealing with small lymphocytic lymphoma, the version of CLL where the tumour is confined to lymph nodes [39]. The demarcation line between mutated and unmutated is awkwardly set, with up to 2% of mutations being firmly in the unmu- tated camp. Originally, this was because slight variation in sequence might be attributed to as yet undiscovered polymorphisms, but in later studies simultaneous sequencing of genomic DNA showed this not to be the case [40], and that about 20% of those with 3% mutations also behaved as though unmutated [41].

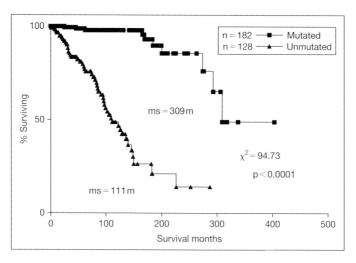

Figure 3.1 Actuarial survival curve for 310 patients with CLL comparing patients with mutated and unmutated IgVH genes. Censored for non-CLL related deaths.

The one major exception to the mutated/unmutated dichotomy is the tumour that makes use of the V_H3-21 gene segment, where all cases behave as though they are unmutated [37]. Closer scrutiny of this group of patients reveals that they predominantly use J_H6 with almost complete loss of the D segment gene, with the light chain often coded by $V_\lambda2$-14/$J_\lambda3$ genes [42]. This produces an antibody-binding site of specific configuration and strongly suggests that a particular antigen is implicated in the aetiology of the patient's CLL. Nor is this the only repeated configuration seen in CLL: cases using the γ constant region with V_H4-39, D6-13 and J_H5b with the $V_\kappa O12/2$ gene segments in germ line configuration [43] and others using V_H1-69, V_H1-02, V_H1-03, V_H1-18, V_H1-46, V_H4-34 and V_H5-51 have been reported [44], and together these suggest that perhaps 15% of cases of CLL show evidence of being antigen driven.

Two other tumour types have also shown the mutated/unmutated dichotomy: MCL and SMZL. In MCL, between 15 and 30% of cases have unmutated immunoglobulin variable region heavy chain (IgVH) genes, perhaps more in those cases without lymph node enlargement [12]. There is no evidence of a difference in prognosis between mutated and unmutated cases, though in one series, 5 out of 5 very long survivors had mutated IgVH genes [12]. There is evidence of antigenic drive with an increased use V_H3-21 and $V_\lambda3$-19, and such cases seem to have a better prognosis [45, 46].

In SMZL there have been fewer studies, but one series of 35 cases showed roughly half the cases with mutated and half with unmutated IgVH genes [47]. Cases with unmutated IgVH genes had a shorter survival and were more likely to show the 7q31 deletion. There was a biased use of the V_H1-02 gene.

In B-PLL, most cases, including those with MCL immunophenotype and karyotype, seem to have mutated IgVH genes [12] and this disease still resists categorisation. Contrary to the common perception, half of the cases of CLL/PLL showed a stable picture without a progressive increase in prolymphocytes [15]. The prognosis of this group was similar to that of stable CLL without prolymphocytes. In one third of cases the increase in prolymphocytes was unsustained and in only 18% was there a definite progression towards a more malignant phase of the disease. In a multivariate analysis of prognostic factors in CLL/PLL, only an absolute number of prolymphocytes and spleen size were of independent prognostic significance. The median survival for patients with prolymphocytes $>15 \times 10^9/l$ was 3 years [11].

EXPRESSION OF CD38

As sequencing IgVH genes was thought to be too difficult for the routine laboratory, a surrogate assay was sought. CD38 expression, which can be easily assayed using flow cytometry, seemed promising [35]. CD38 [48–50] is a type II transmembrane glycoprotein, the extracellular domain acting as an ectoenzyme, catalyzing the conversion of NAD+ into nicotinamide, ADP-ribose (ADPR) and cyclic ADPR. Its expression during B-cell ontogeny is tightly regulated: it appears on bone marrow precursor cells, but is lost on mature lymphocytes; on germinal centre cells it protects against apoptosis, but on leaving the germinal centre, memory cells lack the antigen; on terminally differentiated plasma cells it is one of the few surface antigens present.

Although CD38 expression is clearly an adverse prognostic factor in CLL, it was found to give discordant results to IgVH mutations in about 30% of cases [34]. Moreover, it was found to change during the course of the disease in about a quarter of cases [34]. Perhaps more remarkably, it was found to be better at predicting death rather than death from CLL (Figure 3.2). This seemed to imply that CD38 expression on the CLL cells could rise in response to a morbid condition elsewhere in the body, perhaps mediated through cytokines.

In MCL CD38 expression it is often absent in the non-nodal form, and this carries a good prognosis [12].

ZETA-ASSOCIATED PROTEIN 70 (ZAP-70)

Once the mutational status of the IgVH genes had so comprehensively separated B-CLL into two clinical types, the question was asked as to whether B-CLL was one or two diseases. One approach used to resolve this question was to look at the gene expression of mutated and unmutated CLL on cDNA microarrays. Rosenwald and colleagues [51] reported that B-CLL has a distinct gene expression profile, but in the expression of a small number of genes, the mutated and unmutated subtypes were different and identified zeta-associated protein with a molecular weight of 70 kD (ZAP-70) as the gene best able to distinguish the two subtypes.

ZAP-70 interacts with the T-cell receptor in T cells and transmits a signal to downstream pathways. It is not normally expressed in B cells, where the receptor signalling molecule is Syk, but in cases of CLL with unmutated IgVH genes, it seems to be drawn into the signalling reaction.

Antibodies to ZAP-70 are available and several assays have been developed. Immunohistochemistry is easy and effective, but only semi-quantitative; Western blotting requires prior T-cell depletion, which limits its use [52]. Flow cytometric assays have proved difficult, especially as ZAP-70 is an intracellular antigen so that the cells require permeabilisation, but three different methods have been reported [53–55]. The first two both used the Upstate antibody 2F3.2 in an indirect assay, differing mainly on where to set the zero, one using an isotype control and the other using the lower limit of the patient's own T cells. Not surprisingly, the two assays give different normal ranges. The third assay uses a directly labelled antibody. Directly labelled 2F3.2 seems to give too many false positives, and this group has therefore used a different antibody, 1E7.2, labelled with a new fluorochrome ALEXA 488.

Seen as surrogate assays for VH gene mutations, the first two assays perform similarly, with around 94% concordance (Figure 3.3), but with the newer conjugated antibody, the concordance with VH gene mutations was only 77%. On the other hand, in this study, ZAP-70 expression performed better than VH mutations in predicting treatment-free survival. Patients who were ZAP-70 positive, VH mutated had a worse survival than those who were ZAP-70 negative, VH unmutated. This rather surprising result has not yet been confirmed elsewhere and the population studied, which was drawn from many American specialist centres, had a median age of only 55. We must await further studies to find out which of

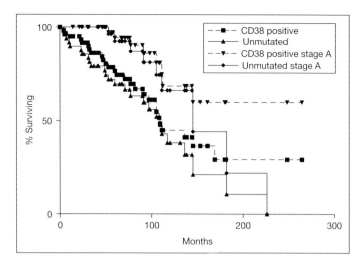

Figure 3.2 145 patients with CLL: comparison of survival curves between those with unmutated IgVH genes and those expressing CD38. Graphs are shown for all patients and for stage A patients dying of CLL. Note that CD38 positivity is almost as good as unmutated IgVH genes in predicting death, but not as good as IgVH gene mutations at predicting deaths from CLL in stage A patients.

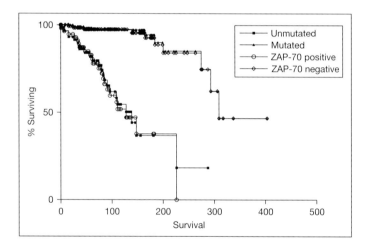

Figure 3.3 Actuarial survival curve for 180 patients with CLL comparing IgVH mutational status and ZAP-70 tested by flow cytometry according to the method of Orchard *et al.* [54].

these assays has the greatest utility, and until then the results of commercial assays already being marketed should be interpreted with caution.

FLUORESCENCE IN-SITU HYBRIDISATION (FISH)

Conventional metaphase cytogenetics yields only a small proportion of patients with CLL who have abnormalities. The principal reason for this is technical, in that the assay requires CLL cells to divide *in vitro*, which is difficult to achieve. However, the use of interphase

FISH allows the identification of chromosomal abnormalities in resting cells. FISH reveals recurrent cytogenetic abnormalities in approximately 80% of cases of CLL. In order of increasing severity, the important chromosomal aberrations in CLL are del 13q14, trisomy 12, del 11q23 and del 17p13 [7]. Del 13q14 is associated with a better than average survival, but this is only true if it is an isolated lesion. Of course, unless full karyotyping is done, which it rarely is, 13q14 deletion cannot be confirmed as an isolated lesion.

Trisomy 12 is associated with atypical morphology [5], particularly CLL/PLL. Survival outcome is average for CLL and depends on mutational status.

Del 11q23 is classically associated with younger patients with bulky lymphadenopathy and in many series carries a poor prognosis [7, 56]. However, not all cases fit this model, and in our series [57] there was no survival difference between those with del 11 and those with trisomy 12. Del 11 occurs in patients with mutated and unmutated VH genes. It is not clear whether ATM is the gene implicated in the deletion or another nearby. Studies with an *in vitro* assay that stresses the p53 pathway with X-irradiation may uncover the answer [58].

Del 17p13 or other assays that uncover a deleted or mutated *p53* gene carry a grave prognosis with an average survival of less than 3 years [7, 57]. It has been suggested that at least 20% of cells need to be affected to indicate such a poor prognosis [59]. Such cases are frequently drug resistant and deserve a different treatment strategy, perhaps using therapies which do not depend upon a functional p53 pathway for their activity, such as alemtuzumab [60] or high-dose methylprednisolone [61].

Deletions at 6q21 are usually secondary lesions in a poor prognosis group, but do not show an independent prognostic effect in multivariate analysis. It is important to include a probe for the immunoglobulin heavy chain locus in FISH testing, so as not to miss the CLL-like cases of MCL.

In other low-grade lymphoid malignancies, the same genetic abnormalities, deletions or mutations of ATM or p53 carry an adverse prognosis and a tendency to transform into an aggressive large cell lymphoma [62–64].

SUMMARY

As classifications of lymphoid malignancies have developed, immunophenotyping and molecular studies have assumed an increasing importance in the differential diagnosis. Formerly, large multi-centre series were contaminated by interlopers with incorrect diagnoses that distorted outcomes. This has been particularly true for CLL, where patients with MCL and SMZL were not uncommonly misdiagnosed. Immunophenotyping has enabled us to remove whole categories of disease such as T-CLL and to refine the diagnosis of LGL leukaemia.

Molecular studies have revealed two subtypes of CLL with widely differing prognoses, and helped us to understand the pathogenesis of the disease. Clinical trials using these markers to stratify patients are already underway and will shortly lead to patient-designed treatment protocols.

REFERENCES

1. Moreau EJ, Matutes E, A'Hern RP *et al*. Improvement of the chronic lymphocytic leukaemia scoring system with the monoclonal antibody SN8 (CD79b). *Am J Clin Pathol* 1997; 108:378.

2. Dohner H, Stilgenbauer S, Benner A *et al*. Genomic aberrations and survival in chronic lymphocytic leukemia. *N Engl J Med* 2000; 343:1910–1916.

3. Calin GA, Dumitru CD, Shimizu M *et al*. Frequent deletions and down regulation of micro-RNA genes miR15 and miR16 at 13q14 in chronic lymphocytic leukemia. *Proc Natl Acad Sci USA* 2002; 99:15524–15529.

4. Fitchett M, Griffiths MJ, Oscier DG *et al*. Chromosome abnormalities involving band 13q14 in hematologic malignancies. *Cancer Genet Cytogenet* 1987; 24:143–150.
5. Matutes E, Oscier D, Garcia-Marco-J *et al*. Trisomy 12 defines a group of CLL with atypical morphology: correlation between cytogenetic, clinical and laboratory features in 544 patients. *Br J Haematocl* 1996; 92:382–388.
6. Starostik P, Manshouri T, O'Brien S *et al*. Deficiency of the ATM protein expression defines an aggressive subgroup of B-cell chronic lymphocytic leukemia. *Cancer Res* 1998; 58:4552–4557.
7. Krober A, Seiler T, Benner A *et al*. V(H) mutation status, CD38 expression level, genomic aberrations, and survival in chronic lymphocytic leukemia. *Blood* 2002; 100:1410–1416.
8. Dyer MJS, Zani VJ, Lu WZ *et al*. *BCL2* translocations in leukemias of mature B cells. *Blood* 1994; 83:3682–3688.
9. Michaux L, Mecucci C, Stul M *et al*. BCL3 rearrangement and t(14;19)(q32;q13) in lymphoproliferative disorders. *Genes Chromosomes Cancer* 1996; 15:38–47.
10. Galton DAG, Goldman JM, Wiltshaw E *et al*. Prolymphocytic leukaemia. *Br J Haematol* 1974; 27:7–23.
11. Melo JV, Catovsky D, Galton DA. Chronic lymphocytic leukemia and prolymphocytic leukemia: a clinicopathological reappraisal. *Blood Cells* 1987; 12:339–353.
12. Orchard J, Garand R, Davis Z *et al*. A subset of t(11;14) lymphoma with mantle cell features displays mutated IgVH genes and includes patients with good prognosis, nonnodal disease. *Blood* 2003; 101:4975–4981.
13. Melo JV, Catovsky D, Galton DAG. The relationship between chronic lymphocytic leukaemia and prolymphocytic leukaemia. I. Clinical and laboratory features of 300 patients and characterisation of an intermediate group. *Br J Haematol* 1986; 63:377–387.
14. Enno A, Catovsky D, O'Brien M *et al*. 'Prolymphocytoid' transformation of chronic lymphocytic leukaemia. *Br J Haematol* 1979; 41:9–18.
15. Melo JV, Catovsky D, Galton DA. The relationship between chronic lymphocytic leukaemia and prolymphocytic leukaemia. II. Patterns of evolution of 'prolymphocytoid' transformation. *Br J Haematol* 1986; 64:77–86.
16. Melo JV, Wardle J, Chetty M *et al*. The relationship between chronic lymphocytic leukaemia and prolymphocytic leukaemia. III. Evaluation of cell size by morphology and volume measurements. *Br J Haematol* 1986; 64:469–478.
17. Melo JV, Catovsky D, Gregory WM *et al*. The relationship between chronic lymphocytic leukaemia and prolymphocytic leukaemia. IV. Analysis of survival and prognostic features. *Br J Haematol* 1987; 65:23–29.
18. Brito-Bapapulle V, Pittman S, Melo JV *et al*. Cytogenetic studies on prolymphocytic leukaemia. 1 B cell prolymphocytic leukaemia. *Hematol Pathol* 1987; 1:27–33.
19. Neiman RS, Sullivan AL, Jaffe R. Malignant lymphoma simulating leukaemic reticuloendotheliosis. A clinicopathologic study of ten cases. *Cancer* 1979; 43:329–342.
20. Melo JV, Robinson DSF, Gregory C *et al*. Splenic B cell lymphoma with 'villous' lymphocytes in the peripheral blood: a disorder distinct from hairy cell leukemia. *Leukemia* 1987; 1:294–299.
21. Jaffe ES, Harris NL, Stein H, Vardiman JW. Tumors of Haematopoietic and Lymphoid Tissues. OUP, Oxford; 2001.
22. Oscier DG, Matutes E, Gardiner E *et al*. Cytogenetic studies in splenic lymphoma with villous lymphocytes. *Br J Haematol* 1993; 85:487–491.
23. Corcoran MM, Mould SJ, Orchard JA *et al*. Dysregulation of cyclin dependent kinase 6 expression in splenic marginal zone lymphoma through chromosome 7q translocations. *Oncogene* 1999; 18:6271–6277.
24. Jadayel D, Matutes E, Dyer MJS *et al*. Splenic lymphoma with villous lymphocytes: analysis of BCL−1 rearrangements and expression of the cyclin D1 gene. *Blood* 1994; 83:3664–3671.
25. Leroux D, Le Marc'Hadour F, Gressin R *et al*. Non-Hodgkin's lymphomas with t(11;14)(q13;q32): a subset of mantle zone/intermediate lymphocytic lymphoma? *Br J Haematol* 1991; 77:346–353.
26. Tsujimoto Y, Jaffe E, Cossman J *et al*. Clustering of breakpoints on chromosome 11 in human B-cell neoplasms with the t(11;14) chromosome translocation. *Nature* 1985; 315:340–343.
27. Loughran TP, Jr. Clonal diseases of large granular lymphocytes. *Blood* 1993; 82:1–14.
28. Matutes E, Brito-Bapapulle V, Swansbury J *et al*. Clinical and laboratory features of T-prolymphocytic leukemia. *Blood* 1991; 78:3269–3274.
29. Croce CM, Isobe M, Polumbo A *et al*. Gene for alpha chain of human T cell receptor: location on chromosome 14 region involved in T cell neoplasms. *Science* 1985; 227:1044–1047.

30. Brito-Bapapulle V, Catovsky D. Inversions and tandem translocations involving chromosome 14q11 and 14q32 in T prolymphocytic leukemia and T cell leukemias in patients with ataxia telangectasia. *Cancer Genet Cytogenet* 1991; 55:1–9.

31. The Non-Hodgkin's Lymphoma Classification Project. A clinical evaluation of the International Lymphoma Study Group classification of non-Hodgkin's lymphoma. *Blood* 1997; 89:3909–3918.

32. Zhu D, McCarthy H, Ottensmeier CH *et al.* Acquisition of potential N-glycosylation sites in the immunoglobulin variable region by somatic mutation is a distinctive feature of follicular lymphoma. *Blood* 2002; 99:2562–2568.

33. Schroeder HW, Jr, Dighiero G. The pathogenesis of chronic lymphocytic leukemia: analysis of the antibody repertoire. *Immunol Today* 1994; 15:288–294.

34. Hamblin TJ, Davis Z, Gardiner A *et al.* Unmutated Ig V(H) genes are associated with a more aggressive form of chronic lymphocytic leukemia. *Blood* 1999; 94:1848–1854.

35. Damle RN, Wasil T, Fais F *et al.* Ig V gene mutation status and CD38 expression as novel prognostic indicators in chronic lymphocytic leukemia. *Blood* 1999; 94:1840–1847.

36. Maloum K, Davi F, Merle-Beral H *et al.* Expression of unmutated V_H genes is a detrimental prognostic factor in chronic lymphocytic leukemia. *Blood* 2000; 95:377–378.

37. Tobin G, Thunberg U, Johnson A *et al.* Somatically mutated IgV_H3-21 genes characterize a new subset of chronic lymphocytic leukemia. *Blood* 2002; 99:2262–2264.

38. Jelinek DF, Tschumper RC, Geyer SM *et al.* Analysis of clonal B-cell CD38 and immunoglobulin variable region sequence status in relation to clinical outcome for B-chronic lymphocytic leukaemia. *Br J Haematol* 2001; 115:854–861.

39. Bahler DW, Aguilera NS, Chen CC *et al.* Histological and immunoglobulin VH gene analysis of interfollicular small lymphocytic lymphoma provides evidence for two types. *Am J Pathol* 2000; 157:1063–1070.

40. Davis ZA, Orchard JA, Corcoran MM *et al.* Divergence from the germ-line sequence in unmutated chronic lymphocytic leukemia is due to somatic mutation rather than polymorphisms. *Blood* 2003; 102:3075.

41. Hamblin TJ, Orchard JA, Davies ZA *et al.* How many somatic mutations should we allow in chronic lymphocytic leukemia with unmutated IgVH genes? *Blood* 2004; 104:219a.

42. Tobin G, Thunberg U, Johnson A *et al.* Chronic lymphocytic leukemias utilizing the VH3–21 gene display highly restricted Vlambda2-14 gene use and homologous CDR3s: implicating recognition of a common antigen epitope. *Blood* 2003; 101:4952–4957.

43. Ghiotto F, Fais F, Valetto A *et al.* Remarkably similar antigen receptors among a subset of patients with chronic lymphocytic leukemia J Clin Invest 2004; 113:1008–1016.

44. Messmer BT, Albesiano E, Efremov DG *et al.* Multiple distinct sets of stereotyped antigen receptors indicate a role for antigen in promoting chronic lymphocytic leukemia. *J Exp Med* 2004; 200:519–525.

45. Walsh SH, Thorselius M, Johnson A *et al.* Mutated VH genes and preferential VH3-21 use define new subsets of mantle cell lymphoma. *Blood* 2003; 101:4047–4054.

46. Camacho FI, Algara P, Rodriguez A *et al.* Molecular heterogeneity in MCL defined by the use of specific VH genes and the frequency of somatic mutations. *Blood* 2003; 101:4042–4046.

47. Algara P, Mateo MS, Sanchez-Beato M *et al.* Analysis of the IgV_H somatic mutations in splenic marginal zone lymphoma defines a group of unmutated cases with frequent 7q deletion and adverse clinical course. *Blood* 2002; 99:1299–1304.

48. Howard M, Grimaldi JC, Bazan JF *et al.* Formation and hydrolysis of cyclic ADP-ribose catalysed by lymphocyte antigen CD38. *Science* 1993; 262:1056–1059.

49. Malavasi F, Funaro A, Roggero S, Horenstein A, Calosso L, Mehta K. Human CD38: a glycoprotein in search of a function. *Immunol Today* 1994; 15:95–97.

50. Deaglio S, Mehta K, Malavasi F. Human CD38: a (r)evolutionary story of enzymes and receptors. *Leuk Res* 2001; 25:1–12.

51. Rosenwald A, Alizadeh AA, Widhopf G *et al.* Relation of gene expression phenotype to immunoglobulin mutation genotype in B cell chronic lymphocytic leukemia. *J Exp Med* 2001; 194:1639–1647.

52. Wiestner A, Rosenwald A, Barry TS *et al.* ZAP-70 expression identifies a chronic lymphocytic leukemia subtype with unmutated immunoglobulin genes, inferior clinical outcome, and distinct gene expression profile. *Blood* 2003; 101:4944–4951.

53. Crespo M, Bosch F, Villamor N *et al.* ZAP-70 expression as a surrogate for immunoglobulin-variable-region mutations in chronic lymphocytic leukemia. *N Engl J Med* 2003; 348:1764–1775.

54. Orchard JA, Ibbotson RE, Davis Z *et al.* ZAP-70 expression and prognosis in chronic lymphocytic leukaemia. *Lancet* 2004; 363:105–111.
55. Rassenti LZ, Huynh L, Toy TL *et al.* ZAP-70 compared with immunoglobulin heavy-chain gene mutation status as a predictor of disease progression in chronic lymphocytic leukemia. *N Engl J Med* 2004; 351:893–901.
56. Dohner H, Stilgenbauer S, James MR *et al.* 11q deletions identify a new subset of B-cell chronic lymphocytic leukemia characterized by extensive nodal involvement and inferior prognosis. *Blood* 1997; 89:2516–2522.
57. Oscier DG, Gardiner AC, Mould SJ *et al.* Multivariate analysis of prognostic factors in CLL: clinical stage, V_H gene mutational status, and loss or mutation of the *p53* gene are independent prognostic factors. *Blood* 2002; 100:1177–1184.
58. Lin K, Sherrington P, Dennis M *et al.* Relationship between p53 dysfunction, CD38 expression, and *IgV$_H$* mutation in chronic lymphocytic leukemia. *Blood* 2002; 100:1404–1409.
59. Catovsky D, Richards S, Matutes E *et al.* Response to therapy and survival in CLL is influenced by genetic markers. Preliminary analysis from the LRF CLL4 trial. *Blood* 2004; 104:13a.
60. Lozanski G, Heerema NA, Flinn IW *et al.* Alemtuzumab is an effective therapy for chronic lymphocytic leukemia with p53 mutations and deletions. *Blood* 2004; 103:3278–3281.
61. Thornton PD, Matutes E, Bosanquet AG *et al.* High dose methylprednisolone can induce remissions in CLL patients with p53 abnormalities. *Ann Hematol* 2003; 82:759–765.
62. Camacho FI, Algara P, Rodriguez A *et al.* Molecular heterogeneity in MCL defined by the use of specific VH genes and the frequency of somatic mutations. *Blood* 2003; 101:4042–4046.
63. Gronbaek K, Worm J, Ralfkiaer E *et al.* ATM mutations are associated with inactivation of the ARF-TP53 tumor suppressor pathway in diffuse large B-cell lymphoma. *Blood* 2002; 100:1430–1437.
64. Camacho FI, Mollejo M, Mateo MS *et al.* Progression to large B-cell lymphoma in splenic marginal zone lymphoma: a description of a series of 12 cases. *Am J Surg Pathol* 2001; 25:1268–1276.

4

CD20: B-cell antigen and therapeutic target

P. McLaughlin, J. P. Deans

DISCOVERY OF THE CD20 ANTIGEN

CD20 was one of many lymphocyte surface antigens that were identified in a flurry of work in the 1970–1980s [1, 2]. The prototype antigen, B1, was found to be specific for B cells, and distinct from other B-cell markers such as surface immunoglobulin. Anti-B1 and other anti-CD20 antibodies promptly came into wide use as diagnostic agents and research tools. Only later was attention paid to the potential of CD20 as a therapeutic target.

CD20 AND OTHER GENE FAMILY MEMBERS

The gene that encodes CD20 is in the region of chromosome 11q12–q13.1 [3]. CD20 is a member of a family of proteins collectively described as the MS4A family (membrane-spanning 4-domain family, sub-family A). Besides CD20, the family members that are best characterised are the β chain of the high-affinity receptor for IgE (FcεRIβ), and HTm4 [4–7]. Both of these proteins are also encoded by genes in the same region of chromosome 11.

Besides structural similarity and limited (up to about 30%) amino acid sequence homology, many MS4A family members share functional features that in a general way relate to immune function. FcεRIβ is expressed by mast cells and basophils. HTm4 is expressed by haematopoietic cells of lymphoid and myeloid origin. Other family members are expressed mainly in lymphoid tissues including the thymus and spleen [5]. Some of them appear to function as components of a calcium channel.

ANATOMY OF CD20

CD20 is a 33 to 37-kDa non-glycosylated phosphoprotein with four transmembrane regions, a relatively short extracelluar loop of 43–44 amino acids, and cytoplasmic N- and C-terminal regions [8–11]. The molecule is phosphorylated at a basal level in resting B cells, and becomes heavily phosphorylated following activation in both normal and malignant B cells.

Peter McLaughlin, MD, Professor of Medicine, Department of Lymphoma/Myeloma, University of Texas MD Anderson Cancer Center, Houston, Texas, USA.

Julie P. Deans, PhD, Associate Professor, AHFMR Senior Scholar Chair, Immunology Research Group, Department of Biochemistry and Molecular Biology, University of Calgary, Calgary, Alberta, Canada.

Supported in part by NCI Core Grant CA16672 awarded to The University of Texas M.D. Anderson Cancer Center, Houston, Texas USA

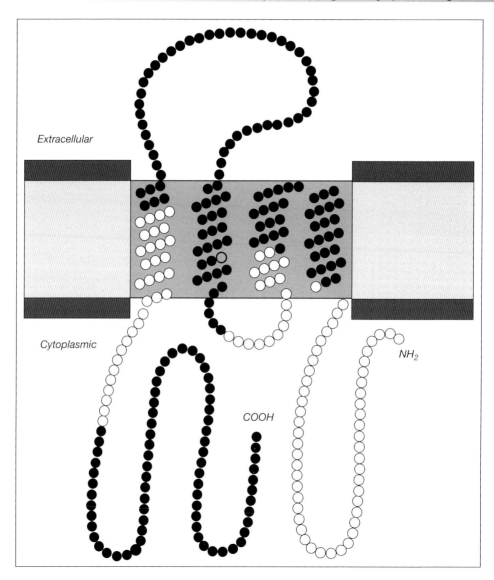

Figure 4.1 Schematic diagram of CD20. The extracellular portion (amino acid residues 142–184) is the site of attachment for most monoclonal antibodies. The alanine residue at 170 and proline at 172 are critical for anti-CD20 antibody binding. Adapted from [8].

Numerous antibodies have been developed that recognise different epitopes of CD20. Most recognise the extracellular portion of CD20, including B1 and other antibodies that were developed early, such as 1F5 and 2H7. Some anti-CD20 antibodies recognise only assembled multimeric complexes of CD20 [12]. The level of expression of the CD20 epitope recognised by the FMC7 antibody is dependent on the cell membrane cholesterol content [13].

The amino acids at positions 170 (alanine) and 172 (proline) of CD20 are critical determinants for binding of the anti-CD20 antibodies that recognise extracellular epitopes [12].

L26 is a notable anti-CD20 antibody because it recognises an intracellular epitope that is preserved even on paraffin-embedded tissue, and thus it is well suited for diagnostic haematopathology use [14].

Therapeutic anti-CD20 monoclonal antibodies recognise extracellular epitopes. Clinical trials first used unconjugated murine antibodies, including 1F5 [15]. Later, the murine antibodies B1 and 2B8 were developed as radioimmunoconjugates to deliver radioiodine (131-I tositumomab; Bexxar) and yttrium (90-Y ibritumomab tiuxetan; Zevalin), respectively [16–19]. The chimeric mouse–human monoclonal antibody rituximab was developed from the murine antibody 2B8 [20].

Although CD20 does not show much potential to modulate or shed [21], it does distribute on the cell surface, in membrane rafts, in the context of performance of its signalling functions [22, 23].

FUNCTION OF CD20

The normal function of CD20 is only partially understood. The identity of its natural ligand, if one exists, remains unknown. Evidence from *in vitro* antibody studies indicates that CD20 plays an important signalling function for B lymphocytes. Ligation of CD20 at different epitopes can induce a variety of responses, ranging from regulation of cell cycle progression (1F5) to inhibition of mitogen-induced immunoglobulin production (B1).

Antibody attachment to CD20 can induce [18, 22, 24–26] or in some circumstances suppress apoptosis [27]. Some antibodies, including B1, appear to be more effective in inducing apoptosis than others [28]. Down-regulation of interleukin (IL)-10 and subsequent decrease in the anti-apoptotic protein bcl-2 may be steps in this signalling pathway [29, 30].

CD20 probably participates in signalling in the context of a cell surface complex that can include dimers and tetramers of CD20, as well as co-localisation with CD40 and major histocompatibility complex (MHC) class II [31]. This cell surface complex appears to function as a calcium channel [32, 33]. Ectopic expression of CD20 conveys increased inward calcium conductance in response to membrane hyperpolarisation [32], and increased calcium entry following depletion of intracellular calcium stores [34]. Targeted small interfering RNA (siRNA)-mediated down-regulation of CD20 reduced calcium influx following B-cell receptor stimulation [34].

Despite the strong evidence for its physiological importance, CD20 appears not to be essential, suggesting that there is redundancy of the functions that CD20 performs. CD20-deficient mice thrive and have nearly normal B-cell function [35], although a reduction in cell surface IgM has been noted, as well as reduced transmembrane calcium influx after CD19 or IgM ligation [36].

EXPRESSION OF CD20

NORMAL CELLULAR EXPRESSION

CD20 is expressed on virtually all normal B cells, starting at the pre-B cell stage; expression is lost upon differentiation to the plasma cell stage. Cell surface CD20 is absent on stem cells.

EXPRESSION ON MALIGNANT CELLS

The density of CD20 on the cell surface varies among different B-cell malignancies . Only about half of childhood B-cell acute lymphoblastic leukaemia cases are positive for CD20 [2]. Among the mature B-cell malignancies, the lowest levels of CD20 expression are found in chronic lymphocytic leukaemia (CLL) and small lymphocytic lymphoma (SLL) [37, 38]. A very high level of CD20 expression is seen in hairy cell leukaemia.

Abundant expression is seen in most mature B-cell malignancies, including follicular lymphomas, mantle cell lymphoma, and marginal zone B-cell lymphoma. CD20 is expressed in including Waldenstrom's macroglobulinaemia [39, 40], but not in multiple myeloma [2].

PHYSIOLOGY OF CD20 AND ITS INTERACTION WITH ANTIBODY

MEMBRANE DYNAMICS

While CD20 does not appear to internalise or shed when bound by antibody, it is a dynamic molecule within the cell membrane. It is preferentially distributed on microvilli in membrane rafts, in proximity with the B-cell receptor [33, 41]. Most, but not all (notably B1), antibodies increase the affinity of CD20 for rafts. With B-cell activation, there is phosphorylation and clustering of CD20, and the formation of complexes that function in a variety of signalling processes.

UP-REGULATION

CD20 can be up-regulated, at least *in vitro*. In CLL cells, exposure to several cytokines, including granulocyte macrophage colony-stimulating factor (GM-CSF), tumour necrosis factor (TNF)-α and IL-4, can increase the expression of CD20 [42]. Plasma cells can be induced to express CD20 by gamma interferon [43]. However, an attempt to take one of these *in vitro* observations to the clinic was unsuccessful; Rossmann and co-workers [44] studied CD20 expression in CLL patients and normal volunteers who were treated with IL-4, and found no consistent increase in the expression of CD20 in the CLL patients.

ANTIGEN SHEDDING OR INTERNALISATION

Antibody-bound CD20 antigen does not usually shed, modulate or internalise [21], although internalisation can be induced by CD40 engagement [45]. In contrast to the CD20

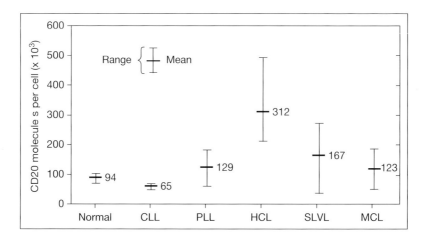

Figure 4.2 Levels of expression of cell surface CD20 in circulating B cells from normal subjects and several B-cell malignancies. CD20 expression is significantly lower in CLL than in normal subjects; conversely, CD20 expression is significantly higher than normal in all other tested B-cell malignancies. Adapted from [37]. CLL = Chronic lymphocytic leukaemia; PLL = prolymphocytic leukaemia; HCL = hairy cell leukaemia; SLVL = splenic lymphoma with villous lymphocytes; MCL = mantle cell lymphoma.

target, the efficacy of monoclonal antibody treatment directed at several other targets appeared to be limited when it was found that the target antigen was not stably expressed on the cell surface after antibody ligation. In the case of CD5, modulation occurred. In the case of anti-idiotype antibodies, sufficient shedding occurred that a cumbersome counter-measure, plasmapheresis, had to be incorporated, which was one of several logistic issues that ultimately led to the judgment that anti-idiotype antibody therapy was not practical, despite the theoretical elegance of this approach.

Circulating CD20 (cCD20) has been described in CLL and lymphoma patients [46, 47], and appears to be an indicator of adverse prognosis. However, the cCD20 is probably the full-length CD20 protein. The findings are consistent with the hypothesis that the cCD20 is located on a fragment of the cell membrane, related to cell breakdown or turnover, rather than representing shed antigen. Nonetheless, patients with high levels of cCD20 may have an impaired response to anti-CD20 antibody therapy. This observation may partly explain why CLL and SLL patients do not respond as well as other chronic lymphoproliferative disorders to conventional dose rituximab therapy.

THERAPEUTIC ANTI-CD20 ANTIBODIES

UNCONJUGATED ANTIBODIES: MURINE, CHIMERIC AND HUMANISED

The CD20 antigen target is the primary focus of this review. Several aspects of the success of the anti-CD20 antibody rituximab [48–50] are related more to the chimeric nature of the antibody than to the antigen. Although not directly related to the CD20 antigen, some of those issues are noteworthy enough to deserve brief discussion.

Prior to the development of the chimeric mouse–human monoclonal antibody rituximab (then known as IDEC C2B8), most monoclonal antibody trials had utilised murine antibodies. Lessons were learned, but results were mixed. In an early anti-CD20 monoclonal antibody clinical trial that utilised the murine antibody 1F5 [15], encouraging efficacy was observed, but it was mainly limited to elimination of circulating B cells. Little impact was seen on the marrow or on nodal disease, which was attributed to poor penetration of the antibody into those compartments. Some patients developed a human anti-murine antibody (HAMA) response, although perhaps less than expected from other murine monoclonal antibody trials. When HAMA occurs, it theoretically limits prospects for long-term therapy with that agent, or for future therapy with any other murine monoclonal antibody.

Antibody-related stumbling blocks with murine antibodies included more than the HAMA response. Murine antibodies have a short half-life in humans. In addition, the murine constant region of the antibody does not mediate effector functions optimally, including complement-dependent cytotoxicity (CDC) and antibody-dependent cellular cytotoxicity (ADCC). Rituximab, compared to its murine parent antibody IDEC-2B8, was much more capable of mediating CDC and ADCC in preclinical testing [20].

In addition to the chimeric antibody rituximab, other anti-CD20 antibodies have been developed that are fully humanised [51–53]. Teeling and colleagues [52] have reported preclinical experiments that identify antibodies that are superior to rituximab in terms of CDC. Hagenbeek and co-workers [53] have reported favourable early safety results in humans of another fully human anti-CD20 monoclonal antibody.

MODIFIED ANTIBODIES: FRAGMENTS; BI-SPECIFIC ANTIBODIES

Once the target is identified and the mechanism of the therapeutic effect of an antibody is defined, numerous refinements of the therapeutic antibody can be contemplated and engineered [54, 55]. For instance, if antibody penetration is an issue, the approach of using

Fab fragments can overcome the penetration problem. If recruitment of effector cells is considered desirable, a suitably constructed bi-specific antibody can recruit relevant effector cells to the vicinity of the targeted cells. The possibilities are numerous, but both scientific and practical stumbling blocks exist.

In the case of CD20, developing a better understanding of the normal function of CD20 is an obvious key to improving targeted therapy approaches. Closely related to that is the need for a better understanding of the mechanism(s) of action of, and resistance to, rituximab and other anti-CD20 antibodies. As insights in these areas point the way towards useful modifications of the anti-CD20 antibody (or other ligand), formidable practical/scientific issues would still loom, since new constructs would have to be developed and tested, as with any other new drug.

CONJUGATED ANTIBODIES: DELIVERY SYSTEMS

While toxin-antibody conjugates have been developed and approved against other targets, CD20 has been regarded as an unlikely candidate for such an approach because it does not internalise, but there may be exceptions. Law and colleagues [56] reported internalisation in the Ramos cell line after exposure to a conjugate of rituximab and monomethyl auristatin E (a synthetic anti-mitotic agent related to dolastatin 10, which targets cellular microtubules).

For radioimmunotherapy (RIT), CD20 has proven to be an excellent target. Two anti-CD20 RIT agents are available, one linked to ^{131}I and one to ^{90}Y. Both are murine antibodies, largely because the longer half-life of a chimeric or a humanised antibody delivery system would demand re-thinking of the dose-time issues related to the isotope. RIT strategies are being explored that may limit radiation to normal tissues and increase the dose of radionuclide delivered to tumours. Forero and colleagues [57] reported a phase I trial using a pre-targeting approach, first delivering an anti-CD20/streptavidin fusion protein, followed by delivery of ^{90}Y linked to biotin.

ANTIBODIES IN CONJUNCTION WITH CHEMOTHERAPY: SENSITISATION

The impact of rituximab in conjunction with chemotherapy appears to be more than additive. There appears to be sensitisation by rituximab to the effects of many chemotherapeutic agents. Efforts to elucidate this process suggest that sensitisation is related to signalling. In 2F7 and 10C9 cell lines (but not in Ramos or Daudi [29]), attachment by antibody to surface CD20 initiates a signalling cascade, in which down-regulation of IL-10 occurs, followed by a downstream decrease of bcl-2 [29, 30]. Since bcl-2 is an anti-apoptotic protein and is over-expressed in many lymphomas, this model fits well with numerous clinical observations of enhanced efficacy when rituximab is combined with numerous chemotherapeutic agents. Such a model also fits the converse observation that rituximab may not enhance the impact of chemotherapy in lymphomas which do not over-express bcl-2 [58, 59].

RESISTANCE TO RITUXIMAB

ANTIBODY-RELATED ISSUES

Many of the most promising insights concerning rituximab resistance are related more to the therapeutic antibody than to the CD20 antigen. Impairment of complement-mediated cytotoxicity may be related to complement inhibitory molecules [60, 61], and experimental models to overcome this problem are being explored. The relevance of these *in vitro* observations to clinical practice has been questioned [62]. The ADCC response of the host can be variable, in part related to polymorphisms of the IgG Fc receptor (FcγRIIIa) gene. Better rates of response to rituximab, an IgG1 antibody, have been noted in lymphoma patients with IgG Fc receptors that bind more strongly to IgG1 antibodies [63]. Clinical approaches to enhance the host ADCC response during rituximab therapy have been encouraging [64–68].

CD20 ANTIGEN-RELATED RESISTANCE ISSUES

Loss of CD20 expression has been reported, but is rare, and some of the existing reports may be artifactual [69], related to blocking of antibody binding sites by anti-CD20 antibody therapy.

As already noted, insufficiently dense CD20 expression is a concern in CLL and SLL. In myeloma, plasma cells typically do not express CD20. Efforts to up-regulate CD20 can be successful *in vitro*, but it is not clear yet if these observations can be translated to the clinic.

CD20 PEPTIDE SEQUENCES AS VACCINES

Peptides derived from CD20 can generate a T-cell response, although the resultant cytotoxic T-lymphocyte responses in healthy individuals and in patients with B-cell malignancies were of low avidity in one report [70]. With the identification and selection of highly immunogenic CD20 peptides, this strategy may merit further study [71]. In mice, vaccination with CD20 peptides can induce a specific immune response [72]. One concern about such a therapeutic strategy is the potential for prolonged suppression of normal B cells.

SUMMARY

The successful strategy of targeting CD20 with therapeutic monoclonal antibodies was an important milestone in cancer therapy. The development of rituximab involved thoughtful approaches to overcome stumbling blocks encountered in early monoclonal antibody trials, and has brought to fruition the labours of many investigators who pioneered the identification of surface antigens, and their targeting by monoclonal antibodies.

The success of therapeutic anti-CD20 monoclonal antibodies has drawn renewed attention to gaps in our knowledge, largely in two areas: (1) our evolving but still limited understanding of the normal function of CD20; and (2) our imprecise understanding of the predominant mechanisms through which anti-CD20 antibodies exert their effects. Ongoing research will hopefully lead to refinements in the current treatments directed against CD20, and to the development of additional ways to exploit this B-cell-specific target.

ACKNOWLEDGEMENTS

The authors thank Joyce Palmer-Brown for preparation of the manuscript, and Jan Gore for adaptation of the figures.

REFERENCES

1. Stashenko P, Nadler LM, Hardy R *et al*. Characterization of a human B lymphocyte-specific antigen. *J Immunol* 1980; 125:1678–1685.
2. Anderson KC, Bates MP, Slaughenhoupt BL *et al*. Expression of human B cell-associated antigens on leukemias and lymphomas: a model of human B cell differentiation. *Blood* 1984; 63:1424–1433.
3. Tedder TF, Disteche CM, Louie E *et al*. The gene that encodes the human CD20 (B1) differentiation antigen is located on chromosome 11 near the t(11;14)(q13;q32) translocation site. *J Immunol* 1989; 142:2555–2559.

4. Liang Y, Buckley TR, Tu L *et al*. Structural organization of the human MS4A gene cluster on chromosome 11q12. *Immunogenetics* 2001; 53:357–368.

5. Ishibashi K, Suzuki M, Sasaki S *et al*. Identification of a new multigene four-transmembrane family (MS4A) related to CD20, HTm4 and beta subunit of the high-affinity IgE receptor. *Gene* 2001; 264:87–93.

6. Liang Y, Tedder TF. Identification of a CD20-, FcεRIβ-, and HTm4-related gene family: sixteen new MS4A family members expressed in human and mouse. *Genomics* 2001; 72:119–127.

7. Gingras MC, Lapillonne H, Margolin JF. CFFM4: a new member of the CD20/FcepsilonRIbeta family. *Immunogenetics* 2001; 53:468–476.

8. Tedder TF, Klejman G, Schlossman SF *et al*. Structure of the gene encoding the human B lymphocyte differentiation antigen CD20 (B1). *J Immunol* 1989; 142:2560–2568.

9. Einfeld DA, Brown JP, Valentine MA *et al*. Molecular cloning of the human B cell CD20 receptor predicts a hydrophobic protein with multiple transmembrane domains. *EMBO J* 1988; 7:711–717.

10. Tedder TF. CD20. In: Mason DY, Andre P, Bensussan A *et al*. (eds) Leucocyte Typing VII: White Cell Differentiation Antigens. Oxford University Press, Oxford, 2002, p 766.

11. Macardle PJ, Nicholson IC. CD20. *J Biol Regul Homeost Agents* 2002; 16:136–138.

12. Polyak MJ, Deans JP. Alanine-170 and proline-172 are critical determinants for extracellular CD20 epitopes; heterogeneity in the fine specificity of CD20 monoclonal antibodies is defined by additional requirements imposed by both amino acid sequence and quaternary structure. *Blood* 2002; 99:3256–3262.

13. Polyak MJ, Ayer LM, Szczepek AJ *et al*. A cholesterol-dependent CD20 epitope detected by the FMC7 antibody. *Leukemia* 2003; 17:1384–1389.

14. Mason DY, Comans-Bitter WM, Cordell JL *et al*. Antibody L26 recognizes an intracellular epitope on the B-cell-associated CD20 antigen. *Am J Pathol* 1990; 136:1215–1222.

15. Press OW, Appelbaum F, Ledbetter JA *et al*. Monoclonal antibody 1F5 (anti-CD20) serotherapy of human B cell lymphomas. *Blood* 1987; 69:584–591.

16. Kaminski MS, Zelenetz AD, Press OW *et al*. Pivotal study of iodine I 131 tositumomab for chemotherapy-refractory low-grade or transformed low-grade B-cell non-Hodgkin's lymphomas. *J Clin Oncol* 2001; 19:3918–3928.

17. Witzig TE, Gordon LI, Cabanillas F *et al*. Randomized controlled trial of yttrium-90-labeled ibritumomab tiuxetan radioimmunotherapy versus rituximab immunotherapy for patients with relapsed or refractory low-grade, follicular, or transformed B-cell non-Hodgkin's lymphoma. *J Clin Oncol* 2002; 20:2453–2463.

18. Hernandez MC, Knox SJ. Radiobiology of radioimmunotherapy: targeting CD20 B-cell antigen in non-Hodgkin's lymphoma. *Int J Radiat Oncol Biol Phys* 2004; 59:1274–1287.

19. Macklis RM. How and why does radioimmunotherapy work? *Int J Radiat Oncol Biol Phys* 2004; 59:1269–1271.

20. Reff ME, Carner K, Chambers KS *et al*. Depletion of B cells *in vivo* by a chimeric mouse human monoclonal antibody to CD20. *Blood* 1994; 83:435–445.

21. Press OW, Farr AG, Borroz KI *et al*. Endocytosis and degradation of monoclonal antibodies targeting human B-cell malignancies. *Cancer Res* 1989; 49:4906–4912.

22. Deans JP, Li H, Polyak MJ. CD20-mediated apoptosis: signalling through lipid rafts. *Immunology* 2002; 107:176–182.

23. Semac I, Palomba C, Kulangara K *et al*. Anti-CD20 therapeutic antibody rituximab modifies the functional organization of rafts/microdomains of B lymphoma cells. *Cancer Res* 2003; 63:534–540.

24. Shan D, Ledbetter JA, Press OW. Signaling events involved in anti-CD20-induced apoptosis of malignant human B cells. *Cancer Immunol Immunother* 2000; 48:673–683.

25. Ghetie MA, Bright H, Vitetta ES. Homodimers but not monomers of Rituxan (chimeric anti-CD20) induce apoptosis in human B-lymphoma cells and synergize with a chemotherapeutic agent and an immunotoxin. *Blood* 2001; 97:1392–1398.

26. Maloney DG, Smith B, Appelbaum FR. The anti-tumor effect of monoclonal antibody CD20 therapy includes direct anti-proliferative activity and induction of apoptosis in CD20 positive non-Hodgkin's lymphoma cell lines. *Blood* 1996; 88(suppl 1):637a.

27. Holder M, Grafton G, MacDonald I *et al*. Engagement of CD20 suppresses apoptosis in germinal center B cells. *Eur J Immunol* 1995; 25:3160–3164.

28. Cragg MS, Asidipour A, O'Brien L *et al*. Opposing properties of CD20 mAb. In: Mason DY, Andre P, Bensussan A *et al*. (eds) Leucocyte Typing VII: White Cell Differentiation Antigens. Oxford University Press, Oxford, 2002, pp 95–97.

29. Alas S, Emmanouilides C, Bonavida B. Inhibition of interleukin 10 by rituximab results in down-regulation of bcl-2 and sensitization of B-cell non-Hodgkin's lymphoma to apoptosis. *Clin Cancer Res* 2001; 7:709–723.

30. Vega MI, Huerta-Yepaz S, Garban H *et al*. Rituximab inhibits p38 MAPK activity in 2F7 B NHL and decreases IL-10 transcription: pivotal role of p38 MAPK in drug resistance. *Oncogene* 2004; 23:3530–3540.

31. Leveille C, Al-Daccak R, Mourad W. CD20 is physically and functionally coupled to MHC class II and CD40 on human B cell lines. *Eur J Immunol* 1999; 29:65–74.

32. Bubien JK, Zhou LJ, Bell PD *et al*. Transfection of the CD20 cell surface molecule into ectopic cell types generates a Ca^{2+} conductance found constitutively in B lymphocytes. *J Cell Biol* 1993; 121:1121–1132.

33. Li H, Ayer LM, Polyak MJ *et al*. The CD20 calcium channel is localized to microvilli and constitutively associated with membrane rafts: antibody binding increases the affinity of the association through an epitope-dependent cross-linking-independent mechanism. *J Biol Chem* 2004; 279:19893–19901.

34. Li H, Ayer LM, Lytton J, Deans JP. Store-operated cation entry mediated by CD20 in membrane rafts. *J Biol Chem* 2003; 278:42427–42434.

35. O'Keefe TL, Williams GT, Davies SL *et al*. Mice carrying a CD20 gene disruption. *Immunogenetics* 1998; 48:125–132.

36. Uchida J, Lee Y, Hasegawa M *et al*. Mouse CD20 expression and function. *Int Immunol* 2004; 16:119–129.

37. Ginaldi L, De Martinis M, Matutes E *et al*. Levels of expression of CD19 and CD20 in chronic B cell leukaemias. *J Clin Pathol* 1998; 51:364–369.

38. Almasri NM, Duque RE, Iturraspe J *et al*. Reduced expression of CD20 antigen as a characteristic marker for chronic lymphocytic leukemia. *Am J Hematol* 1992; 40:259–263.

39. Dimopoulos MA, Panayiotidis P, Moulopoulos LA *et al*. Waldenstrom's macroglobulinemia: clinical features, complications, and management. *J Clin Oncol* 2000; 18:214–226.

40. Weber DM, Gavino M, Huh Y *et al*. Phenotypic and clinical evidence supports rituximab for Waldenstrom's macroglobulinemia. *Blood* 1999; 94 (suppl 1):125a.

41. Petrie RJ, Deans JP. Colocalization of the B cell receptor and CD20 followed by activation-dependent dissociation in distinct lipid rafts. *J Immunol* 2002; 169:2886–2891.

42. Venugopal P, Sivaraman S, Huang XK *et al*. Effects of cytokines on CD20 antigen expression on tumor cells from patients with chronic lymphocytic leukemia. *Leuk Res* 2000; 24:411–415.

43. Treon SP, Pilarski LM, Belch AR *et al*. CD20-directed serotherapy in patients with multiple myeloma: biologic considerations and therapeutic applications. *J Immunother* 2002; 25:72–81.

44. Rossmann ED, Lundin J, Lenkei R *et al*. Variability in B-cell antigen expression: implications for the treatment of B-cell lymphomas and leukemias with monoclonal antibodies. *Hematol J* 2001; 2:300–306.

45. Anolik J, Looney RJ, Bottaro A *et al*. Down-regulation of CD20 on B cells upon CD40 activation. *Eur J Immunol* 2003; 33:2398–2409.

46. Manshouri T, Do KA, Wang X *et al*. Circulating CD20 is detectable in the plasma of patients with chronic lymphocytic leukemia and is of prognostic significance. *Blood* 2003; 101:2507–2513.

47. Giles FJ, Vose JM, Do KA *et al*. Circulating CD20 and CD52 in patients with non-Hodgkin's lymphoma or Hodgkin's disease. *Br J Haematol* 2003; 123:850–857.

48. McLaughlin P. Rituximab: perspective on single agent experience, and future directions in combination trials. *Crit Rev Oncol Hematol* 2001; 40:3–16.

49. von Schilling C. Immunotherapy with anti-CD20 compounds. *Semin Cancer Biol* 2003; 13:211–222.

50. Johnson PWM, Glennie MJ. Rituximab: mechanisms and applications. *Br J Cancer* 2001; 85:1619–1623.

51. Stein R, Qu Z, Chen S *et al*. Characterization of a new humanized anti-CD20 monoclonal antibody, IMMU-106, and its use in combination with the humanized anti-CD22 antibody, epratuzumab, for the therapy of non-Hodgkin's lymphoma. *Clin Cancer Res* 2004; 10:2868–2878.

52. Teeling JL, French RR, Cragg MS *et al*. Characterization of new human CD20 monoclonal antibodies with potent cytolytic activity against non-Hodgkin lymphomas. *Blood* 2004; 104:1793–1800.

53. Hagenbeek A, Plesner T, Walewski J *et al*. HuMax-CD20 fully human monoclonal antibody in follicular lymphoma. First human exposure: early results of an ongoing phase I/II trial. *Blood* 2004; 104(suppl 1):393a.

54. Reff ME, Hariharan K, Braslawsky G. Future of monoclonal antibodies in the treatment of hematologic malignancies. *Cancer Control* 2002; 9:152–166.

55. Presta L. Antibody engineering for therapeutics. *Curr Opin Struct Biol* 2003; 13:519–525.

56. Law CL, Cerveny CG, Gordon KA *et al.* Efficient elimination of B-lineage lymphomas by anti-CD20-auristatin conjugates. *Clin Cancer Res* 2004; 10:7842–7851.

57. Forero A, Weiden PL, Vose JM *et al.* Phase 1 trial of a novel anti-CD20 fusion protein in pretargeted radioimmunotherapy for B-cell non-Hodgkin lymphoma. *Blood* 2004; 104:227–236.

58. Wilson WH, Pittaluga S, O'Connor P *et al.* Rituximab may overcome Bcl-2-associated chemotherapy resistance in untreated diffuse large B-cell lymphoma. *Blood* 2001; 98(suppl 1):343a.

59. Mounier N, Briere J, Gisselbrecht C *et al.* Rituximab plus CHOP (R-CHOP) overcomes bcl-2-associated resistance to chemotherapy in elderly patients with diffuse large B-cell lymphoma (DLBCL). *Blood* 2003; 101:4279–4284.

60. Golay J, Lazzari M, Facchinetti V *et al.* CD20 levels determine the *in vitro* susceptibility to rituximab and complement of B-cell chronic lymphocytic leukemia: further regulation by CD55 and CD59. *Blood* 2001; 98:3383–3389.

61. Treon SP, Mitsiades C, Mitsiades N *et al.* Tumor cell expression of CD59 is associated with resistance to CD20 serotherapy in patients with B-cell malignancies. *J Immunother* 2001; 24:263–271.

62. Weng WK, Levy R. Expression of complement inhibitors CD46, CD55, and CD59 on tumor cells does not predict clinical outcome after rituximab treatment in follicular non-Hodgkin lymphoma. *Blood* 2001; 98:1352–1357.

63. Cartron G, Dacheux L, Salles G *et al.* Therapeutic activity of humanized anti-CD20 monoclonal antibody and polymorphism in IgG Fc receptor FcγRIIIa gene. *Blood* 2002; 99:754–758.

64. Liu NS, Grimm E, Poindexter N *et al.* Antibody dependent cellular cytotoxicity and natural killer cell activity in patients with recurrent indolent lymphoma receiving rituximab in combination with GM-CSF. *Blood* 2003; 102(suppl 1):411a.

65. Sacchi S, Federico M, Vitolo U *et al.* Clinical activity and safety of combination immunotherapy with interferon-alpha 2a and rituximab in patients with relapsed low grade non-Hodgkin's lymphoma. *Haematologica* 2001; 86:951–958.

66. Ansell SM, Witzig TE, Kurtin PJ *et al.* Phase 1 study of interleukin-12 in combination with rituximab in patients with B-cell non-Hodgkin lymphoma. *Blood* 2002; 99:67–74.

67. van der Kolk LE, Grillo-Lopez AJ, Baars JW *et al.* Treatment of relapsed B-cell non-Hodgkin's lymphoma with a combination of chimeric anti-CD20 monoclonal antibodies (rituximab) and G-CSF: final report on safety and efficacy. *Leukemia* 2003; 17:1658–1664.

68. Friedberg JW, Neuberg D, Gribben JG *et al.* Combination immunotherapy with rituximab and interleukin 2 in patients with relapsed or refractory follicular non-Hodgkin's lymphoma. *Br J Haematol* 2002; 117:828–834.

69. Lee R, Braylan RC. Regarding the loss of CD20 after rituximab therapy. *Br J Haematol* 2002; 118:927.

70. Grube M, Rezvani K, Wiestner A *et al.* Autoreactive, cytotoxic T lymphocytes specific for peptides derived from normal B-cell differentiation antigens in healthy individuals and patients with B-cell malignancies. *Clin Cancer Res* 2004; 10:1047–1056.

71. Bae J, Martinson JA, Klingemann HG. Identification of CD19 and CD20 peptides for induction of antigen-specific CTLs against B-cell malignancies. *Clin Cancer Res* 2005; 11:1629–1638.

72. Roberts WK, Livingston PO, Agus DB *et al.* Vaccination with CD20 peptides induces a biologically active, specific immune response in mice. *Blood* 2002; 99:3748–3755.

5

Rituximab and chemotherapy for non-Hodgkin's lymphomas: improved response and survival

F. J. Hernandez-Ilizaliturri, M. S. Czuczman

INTRODUCTION

According to last year's published cancer statistics, approximately 54,370 new cases were diagnosed and 19,410 patients died from lymphoma despite currently available treatment [1]. Non-Hodgkin's lymphomas (NHL) are the fifth most common cancer in the United States and the sixth most common cause of cancer-related death in the United States [1].

Recent advances in immunology, genetics, and molecular biology have provided a large and diverse body of information that has changed the management of patients with human immunodeficiency virus (HIV) infection, leukaemia and lymphoma [2–7]. Increasing use of laboratory tools such as polymerase chain reaction (PCR) amplification of DNA/RNA, Southern blotting, and fluorescent *in situ* hybridisation for chromosomal analysis has led to a better understanding not only of the biological process of lymphoid maturation, but also the pathophysiology of NHL.

NHL is a heterogeneous group of malignancies with diverse biology, clinical behaviour, and prognosis. In the past, treatment modalities depended primarily on the histological type/stage of NHL and ranged from watchful waiting, radiotherapy, single-agent chemotherapy, combination chemotherapy, and high-dose chemotherapy with autologous or allogeneic stem cell rescue.

The development of target-specific therapies such as monoclonal antibodies (mAbs i.e. rituximab) has emerged in response to the need to develop novel treatments with increased efficacy and decreased toxicity than that associated with existing treatment regimens.

Rituximab has been evaluated worldwide in multiple clinical trials as a single agent or in combination with systemic chemotherapy in patients with various subtypes of B-cell neoplasms. The information obtained from these clinical trials has significantly changed the treatment paradigm for, and the outcome of, patients with B-cell lymphomas. In this chapter we present an overview of the evolution of rituximab-based therapies for B-cell NHL and how the incorporation of rituximab into chemotherapy regimens has resulted in an improvement in time-to-progression (TTP) and overall survival (OS) in various subtypes of B-cell lymphoma.

Francisco J. Hernandez-Ilizaliturri, MD, Assistant Professor of Medicine, Department of Medical Oncology. Member of the Tumor Immunology Program, Department of Immunology, Roswell Park Cancer Institute, Buffalo, New York, USA.

Myron Stefan Czuczman, MD, Head, Lymphoma/Myeloma Service, Associate Professor of Medicine, Division of Medical Oncology, Roswell Park Cancer Institute, Buffalo, New York, USA.

RITUXIMAB

The concept of using mAbs to treat lymphoma was initially tested in the early 1980s when two independent groups of investigators reported the first cases of lymphoma patients responding to a mouse anti-idiotype antibody [8–9]. However, subsequent early clinical studies were disappointing. Several factors contributed to poor outcomes: (1) suboptimal antigen selection (i.e. modulation of the antibody-antigen complex or antigen shedding), (2) rapid clearance of antibody, and (3) development of xenograft immune reaction to the mAb (production of human anti-mouse antibodies by the host) [10–11]. Advances in molecular biotechnology and tumour immunology lead to the development of chimeric or humanised mAbs with increased biological anti-tumour activity, longer half-lives, and decreased immunogenicity. Results from recent clinical trials have confirmed the improved anti-tumour activity of these newer mAbs, particularly rituximab [12–14].

Rituximab is an IgGκ chimeric mAb directed against the CD20 antigen expressed on normal B cells and the majority of B-cell NHL [15]. Four weekly doses of rituximab are well tolerated and results in clinically meaningful responses in up to 50% of previously treated indolent NHL patients [13, 14]. Based on its clinical efficacy and excellent toxicity profile, rituximab became the first mAb to be approved by the FDA to treat patients with relapsed/recurrent low-grade B-cell lymphoma [12]. However, in ~50% of indolent NHL patients treated with rituximab, little or no clinical benefit was demonstrated. Augmentation of rituximab's anti-tumour activity requires a better understanding of its mechanisms of action and the biology of CD20.

Several biological effects have been postulated as being responsible for rituximab's primary mechanisms of anti-tumour activity, including: antibody-dependent cellular cytotoxicity (ADCC), complement-mediated cytotoxicity (CMC), and induction of apoptosis/anti-proliferation (Figure 5.1). A major area of research is the study of intracellular signals that result in apoptosis of lymphoma cells following binding of rituximab to its CD20 antigen and factors associated with activation of the innate immune system [16–27]. The function of CD20 has yet to be defined. Previous CD20 knockout mouse studies failed to show a normal murine phenotype [28]. Exposure of lymphoma cells to rituximab results in the activation of the Src-family of protein tyrosine kinases, leading to phosphorylation of PLCγ2 and increased cytoplasmic Ca^{2+} [17–23]. These early signal transduction events activate caspase 3 to promote apoptotic cell death of NHL B cells [21]. In addition, *in vitro* exposure of lymphoma cell lines to rituximab is associated with a sustained phosphorylation of p38-MAP, JNK, and ERK kinases [22]. Signalling had been demonstrated in lymphoma cells primarily following cross-linking of rituximab with a secondary antibody (usually a goat anti-mouse or mouse anti-human) or by Fc-receptor-bearing accessory cells [23]. We have recently demonstrated that neutrophils are necessary for optimal anti-tumour activity of rituximab, corroborating findings reported by other investigators [26, 27]. Re-organisation of the CD20 receptor into lipid raft domains occurs following rituximab binding and precedes the aforementioned signalling events [29, 30]. Structural changes in CD20 antigen may affect cellular responses to rituximab. Specific mutations and deletions in the intracellular domain of CD20 were transfected into Molt-4 lymphoblastic T cells and resulted in a significant decrease in CD20 re-organisation into lipid raft domains and reduction in signalling events, without affecting the extracellular binding of rituximab [30].

Preclinical studies demonstrated significant interactions between rituximab and chemotherapy agents [31–32]. Inhibition of interleukin-10 by rituximab resulted in down-regulation of bcl-2 and sensitisation of NHL cells to chemotherapy-induced apoptosis [31]. In addition, another group of investigators demonstrated that pre-treatment of B-cell lymphoma cell lines with fludarabine resulted in down-regulation of CD59, a complement inhibitory protein, and an increased sensitivity to rituximab-induced CMC [32]. The

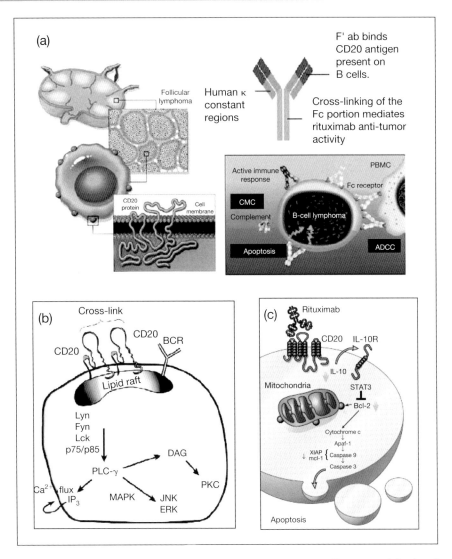

Figure 5.1 (a) Proposed mechanisms of action of rituximab. (b and c) Signalling events following rituximab binding to CD20. Recruitment of CD20 into lipid raft domains followed by activation of the Src-family of protein tyrosine kinases, leading to phosphorylation of PLC-γ2 and increased cytoplasmic Ca^{2+}. Cleavage of caspase 3 promotes apoptosis of NHL B cells. (b) Phosphorylation of p38-MAP and ERK kinases occurs. (c) Inhibition of interleukin-10 with subsequent down-regulation of bcl-2 has been demonstrated. ADCC = Antibody-dependent cellular cytotoxicity; CMC = complement-mediated cytotoxicity; PBMC = peripheral blood mononuclear cell; IL = interleukin; NHL = non-Hodgkin's lymphoma; PKC = protein kinase C; PLC = phospholipase C; ERK = extracellular-signal-regulated kinase; MAPK = mitogen-activated protein kinase; DAG = diacylglycerol; BCR = B-cell receptor; IP$_3$ = inositol triphosphate; XIAP = X chromosome-linked inhibitor-of-apoptosis protein.

clinical efficacy observed in clinical studies with single-agent rituximab, in addition to its excellent toxicity profile and encouraging results from *in vitro* studies, supported the evaluation of rituximab in combination with chemotherapy in patients with B-cell lymphomas.

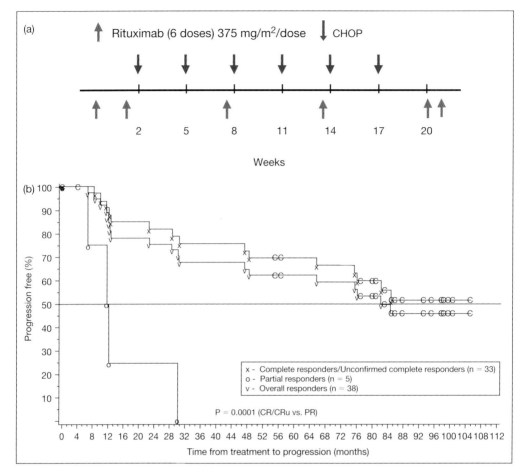

Figure 5.2 Rituximab in combination with CHOP chemotherapy for indolent lymphoma. (a) Treatment schedule consisted in 6 doses of rituximab administered before, during, and at completion of systemic chemotherapy. (b) The addition of rituximab to CHOP resulted in an improvement in time-to-progression. The median time to progression after 9 years of follow-up was 82.3 months. The 16 (42%) of 38 patients in continuous long-term remission (77.3+ to 105.6+ months) all achieved a CR. CHOP = cyclophosphamide, doxorobucin, vincristine, prednisone. C = censored; CR = complete response; CRu = unconfirmed complete response.

RITUXIMAB IN COMBINATION WITH CHEMOTHERAPY FOR FOLLICULAR LYMPHOMAS

The first study evaluating rituximab in combination with standard doses of chemotherapy (i.e. CHOP = cyclophosphamide, doxorubicin, vincristine, and prednisone) was reported by Czuczman and co-workers [33, 34]. The study was a multi-institutional phase II clinical trial that evaluated the safety and efficacy of rituximab in combination with CHOP and enrolled 40 patients with either newly diagnosed or previously treated low-grade or follicular B-cell NHL expressing CD20 [33]. Thirty-eight patients completed 6 courses of rituximab and 6 courses of CHOP chemotherapy administered as shown in Figure 5.2a. The median age of the patients was 49 years (29–77 years). According to the International Working Formulation (IWF) classification, 8 (21%) of the 38 treated patients had IWF A disease, 16 (42%) had IWF B, and 13 (34%) had IWF C. Twenty-four percent of patients were previously treated, 24% were considered poor risk according to the Follicular Lymphoma

International Prognostic Index (FLIPI) and, 26% were in the intermediate/high or high International Prognostic Index (IPI) risk groups. The vast majority (i.e. 90%) of patients have advanced-stage (i.e. Stage III/IV) disease at diagnosis. In addition, 13% of the patients had more than five nodal sites and 68% of the patients had extranodal disease (18 patients with bone marrow or splenic involvement and 7 patients with visceral disease).

The results of the study were equally impressive when initially reported in 1999 and when recently updated after a 9-year treatment follow-up period [33–34]. The initial over-all response rate (ORR) reported was 95% with 22 patients (55%) achieving a complete response (CR) and 16 patients (40%) a partial response (PR). In the subsequent and final analysis of the study, responses were updated using the International Workshop Response Criteria (IWRC) developed for NHL as described by Cheson and colleagues [35]. According to the IWRC, the updated ORR was 100%, with 87% of the patients achieving a CR or unconfirmed complete response (CRu) and 13% a PR. The median TTP in all patients was 82.3 months (range 4.5+ to 105.6+ months) and the median duration of response was 83.5 months (range, 3.1+ to 105.1+ months). At the time of the final analysis, 42% of the patients continue to be on long-term remission (Figure 5.2b). This first rituximab plus CHOP (R-CHOP) study demonstrated an approximate doubling of progression-free survival (PFS) when compared to historical data of upfront CHOP therapy of follicular lymphoma (FL) patients from numerous South West Oncology Group (SWOG) trials that demonstrated a 4-year PFS of 46% [36]. The toxicity profile of the combination was comparable to that observed with CHOP alone. Moreover, the addition of rituximab to CHOP did not com-promise the CHOP dose intensity or density [33–34].

Subsequent clinical studies evaluated concurrent or sequential rituximab in combination with CHOP or other chemotherapy regimens as outlined in Table 5.1. An Italian multi-centre clinical trial evaluated the biological effect of rituximab administered in patients failing to achieve molecular remission after induction chemotherapy with either CHOP or fludarabine/mitoxantrone (FM) combination [37]. The study reported by Zinzani and co-workers [37] enrolled previously untreated patients with FL grade 1 and 2 according to Revised European American Lymphoma (REAL) classification expressing CD20, with detectable bcl-2/Ig gene re-arrangement by PCR in either peripheral blood or bone mar-row. On completion of the clinical and molecular re-staging (6 weeks after the last cycle of CHOP or FM), only responding patients that did not achieve a molecular CR subsequently received 4 weekly doses of rituximab at $375 \, mg/m^2$.

The study enrolled 151 patients, of whom 140 were randomised to CHOP (68 patients) or FM (72 patients). The overall clinical response was similar between the two arms. However, the CR rate was higher in patients receiving FM (68%) than CHOP-treated patients (42%) (p = 0.003). The rate of molecular and CRs was also higher in the FM arm (39%) than in the CHOP arm (19%) (p = 0.001). In accordance with the protocol, 95 patients (41 from the FM arm and 54 from the CHOP arm) received rituximab. In the overall study population, ritux-imab led to a significant improvement in terms of both CR rate (from 57 to 86%) and com-bined clinical and molecular response rate (from 29 to 61%; p < 0.001).

Czuczman and colleagues [38] conducted a phase II study evaluating the safety and effi-cacy of rituximab in combination with fludarabine in patients with untreated or previously treated low grade FL [38]. Eligible patients received 6 cycles of fludarabine at $25 \, mg/m^2$ for 5 days repeated every 28 days and 7 courses of concurrent rituximab administered at $375 \, mg/m^2$. Two infusions of rituximab were administered 4 days apart before and also at the end of the chemotherapy. Three infusions of rituximab were administered 72 h prior to cycles 2, 4 and 6 of fludarabine. After the initial analysis of the first 10 enrolled patients demon-strated unexpected haematological toxicity, the protocol was amended to reduce the dose of fludarabine by 40% in cases of prolonged cytopaenia, to discontinue the use of prophylactic trimethoprim-sulfamethoxazole and to limit the use of growth factor support during active therapy [38]. The study accrued a total of 40 patients, 38 evaluable for response. All patients

Table 5.1 Clinical studies with Rituximab in Combination with systemic chemotherapy in indolent lymphomas

Investigator	Phase	Induction regimen	Consolidation regimen	Disease	Response rate	Time to progression (median)	Overall survival (median)
Czuczman et al.	II	R-CHOP	None	Untreated and relapsed indolent NHL (n = 40)	ORR = 100% CR/CRu = 87%	82.3 months	NR
Czuczman et al.	II	R-F	None	Untreated and relapsed indolent NHL (n = 40)	ORR = 90%	NR at 44 months	NR at 44 motnhs
Zinzani et al.	III	CHOP vs. FM	Observation (MCR) Rituximab x 4 (<MCR or ≥PR)	Previously Untreated FL (n = 151)	CR = 68% (FM) vs. 42% (CHOP) p = 0.003	Estimated 3-year RFS rate FM = 71% vs. CHOP = 54% (p = 0.20)	94% at 3 years for the entire group
Forstpointner et al. on Behalf of the GLSG	III	FCM vs. R-FCM	None	Relapsed FL or MCL (n = 147)	ORR R-FCM = 79% vs. FCM = 58% (p = 0.01)	R-FCM = 16 months vs. FCM = 10 months (p = 0.003)	R-FCM = NR vs. FCM = 24 months (p = 0.003)
Marcus et al.	III	CVP vs. R-CVP	None	Untreated FL (n = 321)	CRR R-CVP = 81% vs. CVP 41% (p<0.001)	R-CVP = 27 months vs. CVP = 15 months (p < 0.001)	No difference observed at 3 years
Hiddemann et al. on behalf of the GLSG	III	CHOP vs. R-CHOP	<60 years ASCT vs. INF >60 years high-dose INF vs. low-dose INF	Untreated FL or MCL (n = 789)	ORR FL R-CHOP (97%)vs. CHOP (91%) (P = 0.005) ORR MCL R-CHOP = 93% vs. CHOP = 76% (p = 0.015)	FL R-CHOP not reached at 4 years vs. CHOP = 2.6 years (p < 0.001) MCL R-CHOP = 2 years vs. CHOP = 1 year (p = 0.0032)	No differences at observed 4 years of follow-up

FL = Follicular lymphoma. MCL = mantle cell lymphoma; NHL = non-Hodgkin's lymphoma; R = rituximab; CHOP = cyclophosphamide, doxorubucin, vincristine and prednisone; FCM = fludarabine, cyclophosphamide and mitoxantrone; F = fludarabine; FM = fludarabine and mitoxantrone; CVP = cyclophosphamide, vincristine and prednisone; ASCT = autologous stem cell transplant; INF = interferon; GLSG = German Lymphoma Study Group; ORR = overall response rate; CRR = complete response rate; CR = complete response; CRu = unconfirmed complete response; PR = partial response; MCR = molecular complete remission; RFS = relapse-free survival; NR = not reached.

had advanced stage (III, IV) disease and the majority were previously untreated (68%). The majority of patients (65%) were IWF B. The median patient age was 53 years (range: 40–77 years). The most frequent extranodal site of disease was bone marrow (65%). Half the patients had IPI scores of 0 or 1, and the others had IPI scores of ≥ 2. Efficacy data was analysed on two subsets of patients: subgroup 1 (included the first 10 patients) and subgroup 2 (the next 30 patients following changes in the study design described above) [38]. The ORR (CR and PR) was 90% (95% CI: 76–97%); with an 80% CR rate. No significant differences were noted between the two subgroups of patients. Only 2 patients in the entire sample had progressive disease secondary to transformed lymphoma before completion of therapy. For the whole group, the median duration of response, TTP and OS have not been reached after a median follow-up time of 44 months (range: 15–66 months). At last follow-up, 22 of 36 (61%) patients had ongoing responses.

The toxicity profile of the combination was acceptable, especially after the protocol was amended. The majority of the toxicity was haematological, with most of the patients experiencing grade 1 or 2 anaemia or thrombocytopaenia. Notably, 76% of the entire cohort developed grade 3 or 4 neutropaenia. Overall, Grade 3 or 4 neutropaenia was transient and reversible in subgroup 2 patients. Whereas 70% of patients in subgroup 1 required granulocyte colony-stimulating factor (G-CSF) support, only 24% of the patients in subgroup 2 received G-CSF support. Infectious complications and/or hospitalisations were limited to: staphylococcal or culture-negative mediport infections (n = 3); neutropaenic fever requiring hospitalisation (n = 4); primary or secondary Herpes simplex/zoster skin infections (n = 6); recurrent UTI (n = 1). Overall, infectious complications [especially of *pneumocystis carinii* pneumonia (PCP) or other serious opportunistic infection] seen in the intent-to-treat group appeared to be similar to that expected in a similar population treated with fludarabine alone. However, acyclovir prophylaxis was subsequently prescribed to all treated patients for 12 months post-completion of therapy because of the relatively high incidence of herpes infections (6 of 40 patients; 15%) believed to be secondary to T-cell depletion from fludarabine. No patient on acyclovir prophylaxis developed a herpes infection.

Data from randomised clinical studies has demonstrated the superiority of rituximab in combination with chemotherapy vs. chemotherapy alone in terms of response rates, TTP and OS [39–41] in patients with indolent lymphomas. The German Low Grade Lymphoma Study Group (GLSG) conducted a prospective, randomised trial comparing fludarabine, cyclophosphamide and mitoxantrone (FCM) vs. rituximab in combination with FCM (R-FCM) in patients with relapsed follicular or mantle cell lymphoma (MCL). The FCM regimen consisted of fludarabine at $25\,mg/m^2/day$ on days 1–3, cyclophosphamide $200\,mg/m^2/day$ on days 1–3 and mitoxantrone $8\,mg/m^2$ on day 1. Chemotherapy was repeated every 4 weeks for a total of 4 cycles. Patients randomised, to the R-FCM arm received the addition of rituximab at $375\,mg/m^2$ 72 h prior to each cycle of chemotherapy [39]. A total of 147 patients were randomised, of which 128 were evaluable for study end points; 62 were randomised, for FCM and 66 for R-FCM. R-FCM-treated patients had a higher ORR of 79% (33.3% CR, 45.45% PR) as compared with patients treated with FCM alone who achieved an ORR of 58% (13% CR, 45% PR; p = 0.01), with similar results in a subgroup analysis of FL (94 vs. 70%) and MCL (58 vs. 46%). In the total group, the R-FCM arm was significantly superior concerning PFS (p = 0.0381) and OS (p = 0.0030). In FL, PFS was significantly longer in the R-FCM arm (p = 0.0139), whereas in MCL a significantly longer OS was observed (p = 0.0042). There were no differences in clinically relevant side-effects between the two study arms. This study is one of the first prospectively randomised clinical studies demonstrating that the addition of rituximab to systemic chemotherapy significantly improves the outcome of relapsed or refractory FL and MCL.

Another randomised study evaluated the effect of rituximab in combination with cyclophosphamide, vincristine and prednisone (CVP) vs. CVP alone. The study as reported by Marcus and colleagues [40] enrolled patients with previously untreated CD20 expressing stage III/IV FL. Eligible patients were randomised to R-CVP or CVP alone. Systemic chemotherapy consisted of a combination of cyclophosphamide at $750\,mg/m^2$ on day 1, vincristine at $1.4\,mg/m^2$ up to a maximal dose of $2\,mg$ on day 1, and prednisone at $40\,mg/m^2$ daily for days 1–5. Patients randomised to R-CVP, also received rituximab at $375\,mg/m^2$ on day 1 of each cycle. The treatments were administered every 21 days in both groups for a maximum of 8 cycles. No crossover between the two arms was planned. A total of 321 eligible patients were randomised to R-CVP (162 patients) or CVP (159 patients). The overall and CR rates were 81 and 41% in the R-CVP arm vs. 57 and 10% in the CVP arm ($p < 0.001$), respectively. After a median follow-up of 30 months, the TTP was statistically longer in patients receiving R-CVP (27 months) than patients treated with CVP (15 months) ($p < 0.001$). No differences in toxicity profiles were observed between treatment arms. The OS was not significantly different between treatment arms at 3 years. Despite these encouraging results, a concern raised from the data analysis was that the doses of cyclophosphamide used in this study were lower than those used in CVP regimens by other groups of investigators and may have caused a diminution in ORR, CR rate, and PFS in both arms of this study.

Hiddemann and co-workers [41] have presented the preliminary results from a randomised study comparing R-CHOP vs. CHOP alone in patients with untreated FL. Despite the impact that 'secondary' therapy (i.e. second randomisation to interferon or autologous stem cell transplantation; ASCT) has upon data analysis, the median ORR, time-to-treatment failure, and response duration was superior in patients receiving induction R-CHOP compared to that achieved by CHOP alone [41].

In summary, over the last decade there has been a significant amount of information obtained from clinical trials that supports the addition of rituximab to front-line chemotherapy for patients with indolent lymphomas. The beneficial effect of rituximab in combination with chemotherapy has been measured by TTP, median duration of response, time-to-treatment failure, response rates, time-to-next-treatment, or OS and have been increased, not only resulting in a better quality of life in patients with indolent lymphomas (i.e. longer periods of time off active therapy) but possibly to a 'cure' in a subset of patients. Ongoing clinical studies seek to evaluate additional novel strategies to improve the anti-tumour activity of rituximab-based regimens such as the extension of rituximab administration or the incorporation of the use of other target-specific therapies (i.e. other mAbs, bcl-2 antisense, proteasome inhibition, etc.) to induction immunochemotherapy.

DIFFUSE LARGE CELL B-CELL LYMPHOMA (DLBCL)

Since 1976 and until 2002, the CHOP regimen was considered the 'gold standard' for DLBCL therapy. Despite responses observed in approximately 80% of DLBCL patients, long-term survival was observed only in 35–40% of the patients treated with CHOP. Initial attempts to improve treatment outcomes consisted in utilising more aggressive chemotherapy regimens that resulted in increased toxicity without improvement in OS compared to CHOP alone as reported by the SWOG [42]. Following the results reported by Czuczman and colleagues in patients with FL, a phase II study evaluating the combination of rituximab and CHOP was conducted and subsequently reported and recently updated by Vose and co-workers [43, 44]. In that clinical study, 33 patients with previously untreated aggressive B-cell lymphoma received rituximab on day 1 of each cycle in combination with CHOP chemotherapy on day 3 administered every 21 days for 6 cycles. The ORR was 94% with 20 patients achieving a CR. At the time of the updated publication, and after a median follow-up time of 63 months (range 34–82 months), the Kaplan-Meier 5-year PFS rate was 82% (95% CI: 64%, 93%) and the Kaplan-Meier 5-year survival rate was 88% (95% CI: 72%, 97%). The median survival time has not been reached. In common with studies conducted in low-grade lymphomas, the addition of rituximab did not result in increased toxicity or compromise the dose or dose-density of CHOP chemotherapy [44].

Concurrent with the Phase II R-CHOP trial by Vose and colleagues was the confirmation of the superiority of R-CHOP to CHOP in DLBCL in a Phase III trial conducted by The Groupe d'Etude des Lymphomes de l'Adulte (GELA) (Table 5.2) [45]. Coiffier and co-workers conducted the first prospectively randomised trial in elderly patients with previously untreated DLBCL lymphomas, in which 197 patients received CHOP and 202 patients received R-CHOP. Rituximab was administered at $375\,mg/m^2$ on day 1 of each cycle of CHOP. Treatment was repeated every 21 days for a total of 8 cycles in both groups. The initial results, published after a median follow-up of 2 years, demonstrated that R-CHOP chemoimmunotherapy was superior. The addition of rituximab to CHOP resulted in a higher CR rate (76 vs. 63%, $p = 0.005$), disease-free survival ($p < 0.001$), and longer OS ($p = 0.007$) in this subgroup of NHL patients (Figure 5.3). Importantly, a significant benefit of combined R-CHOP over CHOP alone was observed among patients with low-risk disease (IPI score 0 or 1) as well as in those with high-risk disease (IPI score 2 or 3). Long-term follow-up data have been recently reported at the 2004 Annual Meeting of the American Society of Hematology and these confirmed the superiority of R-CHOP when compared to CHOP at 5-year follow-up [46]. The results of this particular study have firmly established R-CHOP as the new standard of treatment for elderly patients with untreated DLBCL [45–46].

Preliminary data from Eastern Cooperative Oncology Group (ECOG) study 4494 were recently reported. In this particular study, elderly patients with previously untreated DLBCL were initially randomised to R-CHOP vs. CHOP, and then only in responders to subsequent observation vs. rituximab maintenance. The results of the ECOG 4494 study demonstrated that the addition of rituximab to chemotherapy either during induction therapy or during a maintenance phase (but not both) improved the TTF (time to treatment failure) when compared with patients treated with CHOP chemotherapy alone [47].

The exciting preliminary results of the GELA clinical trial triggered conduction of the Mabthera International Trial (MinT) study comparing R-CHOP (or CHOP-like regimens) to CHOP (or CHOP-like regimens) alone in the management of DLBCL in patients aged 18–60 years [48]. The first planned interim analysis of data was presented at the 2004 Annual Meeting of the American Society of Hematology. A total of 823 patients with DLBCL and IPI score of 0/1 were randomised to receive either CHOP (or CHOP-like regimens) (410 patients) alone vs. rituximab in combination with CHOP/CHOP-like regimens (413 patients). The choice of induction chemotherapy was left to the discretion of the treating institution, with 50% of the patients receiving CHOP-etoposide (CHOEP) and 40% of the patients receiving CHOP. Patients with bulky disease received external beam radiation therapy at the completion of the chemotherapy. The addition of rituximab to induction chemotherapy in young patients with DLBCL resulted in an improvement in CR rates (81% for R-CHOP/R-CHOEP vs. 67% for CHOP/CHOEP; $p < 0.001$); time to treatment failure (76 vs. 60%; $p < 0.001$); and OS at 2 years of follow-up (94 vs. 87%; $p < 0.001$).

Additional clinical trials have explored the combination of rituximab with other chemotherapy regimens. Wilson and colleagues [49] from the National Cancer Institute have studied a dose-adjusted infusional regimen comprising etoposide, vincristine, and doxorubicin and bolus cyclophosphamide (DA-EPOCH) in combination with rituximab in previously untreated DLBCL. In this particular regimen the doses of etoposide, cyclophosphamide and doxorubicin are adjusted with each cycle to achieve an absolute neutrophil count nadir of 500/ml. Preliminary results are encouraging and demonstrate excellent PFS and OS to date.

Other clinical studies had evaluated the addition of rituximab to (1) salvage chemotherapy such as ifosfamide, etoposide and carboplatin (ICE), (2) infusional chemotherapy consisting of cyclophosphamide, doxorubicin, and etoposide (CDE) in HIV-lymphomas, or (3) high-dose (i.e. Hyper-CVAD) regimens in Burkitt's lymphomas [50–52]. While the

Table 5.2 Clinical studies with rituximab in combination with systemic chemotherapy in diffuse large B-cell lymphomas

Investigator	Phase	Induction regimen	Consolidation regimen	Disease	Response rate	Time to progression (median)	Overall survival (OS) (median)
Vose et al.	II	R-CHOP	None	Untreated DLBCL (n = 33)	ORR = 94% CR/CRu = 60%	Not reached at 26 months	80% at 40 months
Coiffier et al. on behalf of the GELA group	III	R-CHOP vs. CHOP	None	Untreated elderly DLBCL patients (n = 399)	CRR R-CHOP (76%) vs. CHOP (63%) (p = 0.005)	Not reported at 5 years	R-CHOP = NR vs. CHOP = 3.1 years (p < 0.001)
Habermann et al. on behalf of the ECOG	III	R-CHOP vs. CHOP	Observation vs. rituximab maintenance (R weekly × 4q6 months × 2 years)	Previously untreated elderly DLBCL patients (n = 632)	CR/PR = 78% (R-CHOP) vs. 77% (CHOP) p = 0.68	Estimated 2-year FFSrate R-CHOP/RM (79%) R-CHOP (77%) CHOP/RM (74%) CHOP (45%)	Estimated 2-year OS rate R-CHOP/RM (87%) R-CHOP (85%) CHOP/RM (83%) CHOP (72%)
Pfreundschuh et al. on Behalf of the MinT Group	III	R-CHOP or R-CHOEP vs. CHOP or CHOEP	None	Previously untreated young DLBCL patients (n = 823)	CRR R-CHOP = 86% vs. CHOP = 68% (p < 0.001)	Estimated 2-year FFS rate R-CHOP (80%) vs. CHOP (61%) (p < 0.001)	Estimated 2-year OS rate R-CHOP (95%) vs. CHOP (86%) (p = 0.002)
Wilson et al.	II	R-DA-EPOCH	None	untreated DLBCL (n = 77)	CR = 94% PR = 5%	At median follow-up of 28 months = 82%	At median follow-up of 28 months = 83%

DLBCL= Diffuse large B-cell lymphoma; R = rituximab; CHOP = cyclophosphamide, doxorubicin, vincristine, and prednisone; CHOEP = cyclophosphamide, doxorubicin, vincristine, etoposide, and prednisone; DA-EPOCH = Dose-adjusted-etoposide, prednisone, vincristine, cyclophosphamide, and doxorubicin; RM = rituximab maintenance; GELA = Groupe d'Etude des Lymphomes de l'Adulte; ECOG: Eastern Cooperative Oncology Group; MinT = Mabthera International Trial; ORR = overall response rate; CRR = complete response rate; CR = complete response; CRu = unconfirmed complete response; PR = partial response; FFS = failure-free survival; OS = overall survival; NR = not reached.

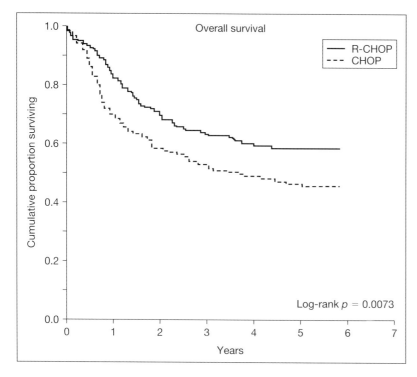

Figure 5.3 R-CHOP vs. CHOP in elderly patients with diffuse large B-cell lymphoma: five-year survival.

preliminary results from these studies appear promising with regard to anti-tumour efficacy, mature data await publication.

MANTLE CELL LYMPHOMA

MCL is a well-recognised type of lymphoma characterised by chemotherapy resistance and a very poor prognosis. Despite the significant progress observed in other histological subtypes of NHL, the treatment of MCL continues to be a challenge for the oncologist [53–54]. Rituximab in combination with systemic chemotherapy has been evaluated in clinical trials against MCL. In general, while an increase in response rates was observed, no significant improvement in OS or TTP was seen over chemotherapy alone [55–57].

ASCT following the achievement of first remission appears to be a current treatment approach that can potentially improve the clinical outcome of patients with MCL [58–60]. Recently, the MD Anderson group reported the results of a phase II study evaluating the efficacy and toxicity of rituximab in combination with alternating Hyper-CVAD and high-dose cytarabine/methotrexate (AraC-MTX) in previously untreated MCL patients aged less than 66 years. The investigators recently updated their results based on 97 patients. The CR rate of the cohort was 87%. The 3-year failure-free survival and OS were 67 and 81%, respectively. While the authors reported equivalent outcomes between R-Hyper-CVAD/AraC-MTX and their prior experience with Hyper-CVAD/AraC-MTX follow by ASCT, a significant number of treatment-related deaths (8 patients) were observed in MCL patients treated with R-Hyper-CVAD/AraC-MTX [61–62]. A series of novel target-specific agents have been designed based on the progress gained in the understanding of MCL biology (e.g. proteasome inhibitors) and are undergoing evaluation in clinical trials [63]. The results of their efficacy and safety are eagerly awaited.

SUMMARY

Over the last decade, mAb therapies have dramatically changed the treatment paradigms for lymphoma patients. Rituximab has validated the use of serotherapy against
cancer and justified the investigation of other biologically active mAbs against lymphomas and other neoplasms. Significant progress and information gained from
preclinical and clinical trials has allowed us to incorporate rituximab into front-line
therapy in combination with conventional/standard chemotherapy against B-cell lymphomas. Moreover, chemoimmunotherapy is being increasingly used in the treatment
of other malignancies (e.g. Herceptin in breast carcinoma, etc.).

Despite the progress achieved, a significant number of patients do not respond to rituximab-chemotherapy and a significant number relapse after an initial response. It is
conceivable that in the foreseeable future we will be able to accurately identify patients,
at a molecular level, for whom a standard treatment is unlikely to be beneficial and therefore alternative therapies should be utilised. In addition, development of rituximab resistance may potentially became a major healthcare issue in the near future, secondary to
the increasing use of rituximab in the treatment of B-cell neoplasms, not only as front-line
therapy, but also as 'maintenance' immunotherapy by many clinicians in an attempt to
prolong remission. Thus, current clinical and basic research efforts should not only be
aimed at optimising the dose and schedule of rituximab used as monotherapy or in combination immunochemotherapy, but also in understanding and developing ways to limit
or reverse mechanisms associated with rituximab resistance [64–65].

REFERENCES

1. Jemal J, Tiwar RC, Murray T *et al*. Cancer Statistics: 2004 *CA Cancer J Clin* 2004; 54:8–29.
2. Mrozek K, Heinonen K, de la Chapelle A *et al*. Clinical significance of cytogenetics in acute myeloid
    leukemia. *Semin Oncol* 1997; 24:17–31.
3. Druker BJ, Lydon NB. Lessons learned from the development of an Abl tyrosine kinase inhibitor for
    chronic myelogenous leukemia. *J Clin Invest* 2000; 105:3–7.
4. Roederer M. Getting HAART of T cell dynamics. *Nat Med* 1998; 4:145–146.
5. Gorochov G, Neumann AU, Kereveur A *et al*. Perturbation of CD4+ and CD8+ T-cell repertoires
    during progression to AIDS and regulation of the CD4+ repertoire during antiviral therapy. *Nat Med*
    1998; 4:215–221.
6. Shipp M, Ross KN, Tamayo P *et al*. Diffuse large B-cell lymphoma outcome prediction by gene
    expression profiling and supervised machine learning. *Nat Med* 2002; 8:68–74.
7. Alizadeh AA, Eisen MB, Davis RE *et al*. Distinct types of diffuse large B-cell lymphoma identified by
    gene expression profiling. *Nature* 2000; 403:503–511.
8. Nadler LM, Stashenko P, Hardy R *et al*. Serotherapy of a patient with a monoclonal antibody directed
    against a human lymphoma-associated antigen. *Cancer Res* 1980; 40:3147–3154.
9. Miller RA, Maloney DG, Warnke R, Levy R. Treatment of B-cell lymphoma with monoclonal anti-
    idiotype antibody. *N Engl J Med* 1982; 306:517–522.
10. Kohler G, Milstein C. Continuous cultures of fused cells secreting antibody of predefined specificity.
    Nature, 1975; 256:495–497.
11. Barinaga M. From bench top to bedside. *Science* 1997; 278:1036–1039.
12. Leget GA, Czuczman MS Use of rituximab, the new FDA-approved antibody. *Curr Opin Oncol* 1998;
    10:548–551.
13. Piro LD, White CA, Grillo-Lopez AJ *et al*. Extended Rituximab (anti-CD20 monoclonal antibody) therapy
    for relapsed or refractory low-grade or follicular non-Hodgkin's lymphoma. *Ann Oncol* 1999; 10:655–661.
14. McLaughlin P, Grillo-Lopez AJ, Link BK *et al*. Chimeric Anti-CD20 monoclonal antibody therapy for
    relapsed indolent lymphoma: half of patients respond to a 4-dose, 22-day treatment program. *J Clin
    Oncol* 1998; 16:2825–2833.
15. Bertram HC, Check IJ, Milano MA. Immunophenotyping large B-cell lymphomas. Flow cytometric
    pitfalls and pathologic correlation. *Am J Clin Pathol* 2001; 116:191–203.

16. Deans JP, Schieven GL, Shu GL *et al*. Association of tyrosine and serine kinases with B cell surface antigen CD20. *J Immunol* 1993; 151:4494–4504.

17. Shan D, Ledbetter JA, Press OW. Apoptosis of Malignant human B cell by ligation of CD20 with monoclonal antibodies. *Blood* 1998; 91:1644–1652.

18. Shan D, Ledbetter JA, Press OW. Signaling events involved in anti-CD20-induced apoptosis of malignant human B-cells. *Cancer Immunol Immunother* 2000; 48:673–683.

19. Popoff IJ, Savage JA, Blake J *et al*. The association between CD20 and Src-family tyrosine kinases requires an additional factor. *Mol Immunol* 1998; 35:207–214.

20. Taji H, Kagami Y, Okada Y *et al*. Growth inhibition of CD20-positive B lymphoma cell lines by IDEC-C2B8 anti-CD20 monoclonal antibody. *Jpn J Cancer Res* 1998; 89:748–756.

21. Holder M, Grafton G, MacDonald I *et al*. Engagement of CD20 suppresses apoptosis in germinal center B cells. *Eur J Immunol* 1995; 25:3160–3164.

22. Mathas S, Rickers A, Bommert K *et al*. Anti-CD20 and B-cell receptor-mediated apoptosis: evidence for shared intracellular signaling pathways. *Cancer Res* 2000; 60:7170–7176.

23. Hofmeister JK, Cooney D, Coggeshall KM. Clustered CD20 induced apoptosis: Src-family kinase, the proximal regulator of tyrosine phosphorylation, calcium influx, and caspase 3-dependent apoptosis. *Blood Cells Mol Dis* 2000; 26:133–143.

24. Harjunpaa A, Junnikkala S, Meri S. Rituximab (Anti-CD20) therapy of B-cell lymphomas: Direct complement killing is superior to cellular effector mechanisms. *Scand J Immunol* 2000; 51: 634–641.

25. Cragg MS, French RR, Glennie MJ. Signaling antibodies in cancer therapy. *Curr Opin Immunol* 1999; 11:541–547.

26. Hernandez-Ilizaliturri FJ, Jupudy V, Oflazoglu E *et al*. Neutrophils contribute to the biological anti-tumor activity of rituximab in a non-Hodgkin's lymphoma severe combined immunodeficiency (SCID) mouse model. *Clin Cancer Res* 2003; 9:5866–5873.

27. Clynes RA, Towers TL, Presta LG, Ravetch JV. Inhibitory Fc receptors modulate *in vivo* cytotoxicity against tumor targets. *Nat Med* 2000; 4:443–446.

28. O'Keefe TL, Williams GT, Davies SL, Neuberger MS. Mice carrying a CD20 gene disruption. *Immunogenetics* 1998; 48:125–132.

29. Semac I, Palomba C, Kulangara K *et al*. Anti-CD20 therapeutic antibody rituximab modifies the functional organization of rafts/microdomains of B lymphoma cells. *Cancer Res* 2003; 63:534–540.

30. Polyak M, Tailor SH, Deans JP. Identification of a cytoplasmic region of CD20 required for its distribution to a detergent-insoluble membrane compartment. *J Immunol* 1998; 161:3242–3248.

31. Alas S, Emmanouilides, Bonavida B. Inhibition of interleukin 10 by rituximab results in down-regulation of Bcl-2 and sensitization of B-cell non-Hodgkin's lymphoma to apoptosis. *Clin Cancer Res* 2001; 7:709–723.

32. Di Gaetano N, Xiao Y, Erba E *et al*. Synergism between fludarabine and rituximab revealed in a follicular lymphoma cell line resistant to the cytotoxic activity of either drug alone. *Br J Haematol* 2001; 114:800–809.

33. Czuczman MS, Grillo-Lopez AJ, White CA, *et al*. The treatment of patients with low-grade B-cell lymphoma with the combination of chimeric anti-CD20 monoclonal antibody (Rituxan, Rituximab) and CHOP chemotherapy. *J Clin Oncol* 1999; 17:268–276.

34. Czuczman MS, Weaver R, Alkuzweny B *et al*. Prolonged clinical and molecular remission in patients with low-grade or follicular non-Hodgkin's lymphoma treated with rituximab plus CHOP chemotherapy: 9-year follow-up. *J Clin Oncol* 2004; 22:4659–4664.

35. Cheson BD, Horning SJ, Coiffier B, *et al*. Report of an international workshop to standardize response criteria for non-Hodgkin's lymphoma. *J Clin Oncol* 1999; 17:1244–1253.

36. Fisher R, LeBlanc M, Press OW *et al*. New treatment options have changed the natural history of follicular lymphoma. *Blood* 2004; 104:583a.

37. Zinzani PL, Pulsoni A, Perrotti A *et al*. Fludarabine plus mitoxantrone with and without rituximab versus CHOP with and without rituximab as front-line treatment for patients with follicular lymphoma. *J Clin Oncol* 2004; 22:2654–2661.

38. Czuczman MS, Koryzna A, Mohr A *et al*. Rituximab in combination with fludarabine chemotherapy in low-grade or follicular lymphoma. *J Clin Oncol* 2005; *in press*.

39. Forstpointner R, Dreyling M, Repp R *et al*. The addition of rituximab to a combination of fludarabine, cyclophosphamide, mitoxantrone (FCM) significantly increases the response rate and prolongs survival as compared with FCM alone in patients with relapsed and refractory follicular and mantle

cell lymphomas: results of a prospective randomized study of the German Low-Grade Lymphoma Study Group. *Blood* 2004; 104:3064–3071.

40. Marcus R, Imrie K, Belch A *et al*. CVP chemotherapy plus Rituximab compared with CVP as first-line treatment for advanced follicular lymphoma. *Blood* 2005; *Epub ahead of print*.

41. Hiddemann W, Forstpointner R, Kneba M *et al*. The addition of rituximab to combination chemotherapy with CHOP has a long lasting impact on subsequent treatment in remission in follicular lymhoma but not in mantle cell lymphoma: results of two prospective randomized studies of the German Low Grade Lymphoma Study Group (GLSG). *Blood* 2004; 104:161a.

42. Fisher RI, Gaynor ER, Dahlberg S *et al*. Comparison of a standard regimen (CHOP) with three intensive chemotherapy regimens for advanced non-Hodgkin's lymphoma. *N Engl J Med*. 1993; 328:1002–1006.

43. Vose JM, Link BK, Grossbard ML *et al*. Phase II study of rituximab in combination with CHOP chemotherapy in patients with previously untreated, aggressive non-Hodgkin's lymphoma. *J Clin Oncol* 2001; 19:389–397.

44. Vose JM, Link BK, Grossbard ML *et al*. Long-term update of a Phase II study of rituximab in combination with CHOP chemotherapy in patients with previously untreated, aggressive non-Hodgkin's lymphoma. *J Clin Oncol* 2005; in press.

45. Coiffier B, Lepage E, Briére J *et al*. CHOP chemotherapy plus rituximab compared with CHOP alone in elderly patients with diffuse large B-cell lymphoma. *N Engl J Med* 2002; 346:235–242.

46. Coiffier B, Feugier P, Sebban C *et al*. Long term results of the GELA Study, R-CHOP vs. CHOP in elderly patients with diffuse large B-cell lymphoma. *Blood* 2004; 104:1383a.

47. Habermann TM, Weller EA, Morrison VA *et al*. Phase III trial of rituximab-CHOP (R-CHOP) vs. CHOP with a second randomization to maintenance rituximab (MR) or observation in patients 60 years of age and older with diffuse large B-cell lymphoma (DLBCL). *Blood* 2003; 102:6a.

48. Pfreundschuh M, Truemper L, Gill D *et al*. First analysis of the completed Mabthera International (MInT) Trial in young patients with low-risk diffuse large B-cell lymphoma (DLBCL): addition of rituximab to a CHOP-like regimen significantly improves outcome of all patients with the identification of a very favorable subgroup with IPI = O and no bulky disease. *Blood* 2004; 104:157a.

49. Wilson W, Dunleavy K, Pittaluga S *et al*. Dose-adjusted EPOCH-rituximab is highly effective in the GCB and ABC subtypes of untreated diffuse large B-cell lymphoma. *Blood* 2004; 104:159a.

50. Kewalramani T, Zelenetz AD, Nimer SD *et al*. Rituximab and ICE as second-line therapy before autologous stem cell transplantation for relapsed or primary refractory diffuse large B-cell lymphoma. *Blood* 2004; 103:3684–3688.

51. Tirelli U, Sparano JA, Hopkins U, Spina M, Vaccher E. Pilot trial of infusional cyclophosphamide, doxorubicin, and etoposide (CDE) plus the anti-CD20 monoclonal antibody rituximab in HIV-associated non-Hodgkin's lymphoma (NHL). *Proc Am Soc Clin Oncol* 2000; 19:170a.

52. Thomas D, Cortes J, Giles F *et al*. Rituximab and Hyper-CVAD for adult Burkitt's or Burkitt's-like leukemia or lymphoma. *Blood* 2001; 98:804a.

53. Bertoni F, Zucca E, Cavalli F. Mantle cell lymphoma. *Curr Opin Hematol* 2004; 11:411–418.

54. Hagemeister F. Mantle cell lymphoma: non-myeloablative versus dose intensive therapy. *Leuk Lymphoma* 2003; 44:S69-S75.

55. Howard OM, Gribben JG, Neuberg DS *et al*. Rituximab and CHOP induction therapy for newly diagnosed mantle-cell lymphoma: molecular complete responses are not predictive of progression-free survival. *J Clin Oncol* 2002; 20:1288–1294.

56. Herold M, Dolken G, Fiedler F *et al*. Randomized phase III study for the treatment of advanced indolent non-Hodgkin's lymphomas (NHL) and mantle cell lymphoma: chemotherapy versus chemotherapy plus rituximab. *Ann Hematol* 2003; 82:77–79.

57. Hiddemann W, Unterhalt M, Dreyling M *et al*. The addition of rituximab (R) to combination chemotherapy (CT) significantly improves the treatment of mantle cell lymphomas (MCL): results of two prospective randomized studies by the German Low Grade Lymphoma Study Group (GLSG). *Blood* 2002; 100:339a.

58. Andersen NS, Pedersen L, Elonen E *et al*. Primary treatment with autologous stem cell transplantation in mantle cell lymphoma: outcome related to remission pretransplant. *Eur J Haematol* 2003; 71:73–80.

59. Jacobsen E, Freedman A. An update on the role of high-dose therapy with autologous or allogeneic stem cell transplantation in mantle cell lymphoma. *Curr Opin Oncol* 2004; 16:106–113.

60. Vandenberghe E, Ruiz de Elvira C, Loberiza FR *et al*. Outcome of autologous transplantation for mantle cell lymphoma: a study by the European Blood and Bone Marrow Transplant and Autologous Blood and Marrow Transplant Registries. *Br J Haematol* 2003; 120:793–800.

61. Romaguera J, Cabanillas F, Dang N *et al*. Mantle cell lymphoma (MCL)-update on results after R-HCVAD without stem cell transplant (SCT). *Ann Oncol* 2002; 13(suppl 2):8.

62. Romaguera JE, Fayad L, Rodriguez MA *et al*. Rituximab plus hypercvad (R-HCVAD) alternating with rituximab plus high-dose methotrexate-cytarabine (R-M/A) in untreated mantle cell lymphoma (MCL): prolonged follow-up confirms high rates of failure-free survival (FFS) and overall survival (OS). *Blood* 2004; 104:128a.

63. Bertoni F, Ghielmini M, Cavalli F *et al*. Mantle cell lymphoma: new treatments targeted to the biology. *Clin Lymphoma* 2002; 3:90–96.

64. Czuczman MS, Olejniczak S, Gowda A *et al*. Acquirement of rituximab resistance in lymphoma cell lines is associated with structural changes in the internal domain of CD20 regulated at the post-transcriptional level. *Blood* 2004; 104:2280a.

65. Olejniczak S, Czuczman MS, Hernandez-Ilizaliturri FJ. Acquirement of rituximab resistance is associated with the development of chemotherapy resistance in B-cell lymphoma cells: evidence of shared pathways of resistance between chemotherapeutic agents and biological therapies. *Blood* 2004; 104:2297a.

6

Rituximab and chemotherapy in elderly patients with lymphomas

B. Coiffier

Lymphoma in elderly patients needs special attention because elderly patients represent half of all cases (the median age for all lymphomas is around 60–65 years) and because elderly patients usually require a different management compared to younger patients. Indeed, such patients usually have one or more other diseases diagnosed before the lymphoma; diseases that may alter their capacity to tolerate lymphoma treatment [1]. Moreover, the incidence of lymphoma in elderly patients has recently increased, probably more than that of young patients, and although recent results showed a trend to stabilisation, this will not occur for the elderly simply because they are living longer and the number of elderly patients will therefore increase [2, 3]. Few differences have been described in morphology and clinical presentation between young and elderly patients with lymphoma [4]. However, the prognosis for elderly patients with lymphoma is worse, particularly for those with aggressive subtypes, because of the difficulties encountered during treatment: difficulties related to the presence of other diseases, diminished organ function, and altered drug metabolism [1, 5, 6]. Recent studies have concluded that the best way to improve the survival of elderly patients with lymphoma was to treat them correctly, that is, with an optimal chemotherapy regimen [3, 7–9].

Treatment of lymphoma patients has completely changed during the last 5 years with the use of monoclonal antibodies, particularly rituximab [10, 11]. Rituximab, an unconjugated anti-CD20 chimeric monoclonal antibody, was the first monoclonal antibody to be used and the only one that has demonstrated activity in randomised studies [12]. Rituximab may be used alone, particularly in patients with follicular lymphoma, [13, 14] but its major activity has been demonstrated in combination with chemotherapy [11, 15, 16]. Rituximab does not add any toxicity to standard chemotherapy regimens and may thus be used safely in elderly patients without compromising their quality of life.

AGE AS A PROGNOSTIC FACTOR

Several studies have reported that older age correlated with shorter disease-free and overall survivals. In a study of 307 patients treated with CHOP (cyclophosphamide, adriamycin, vincristine, prednisone), the disease-free survival rates fell from 65% at 96 months for subjects less than 40 years old to 50% at 36 months for those older than 65 years [17]. A Scottish study demonstrated that stage and histology are comparable in patients under and over age 60, though the elderly have a significantly poorer survival [18]. Advancing age has also been associated with increased treatment-related death rates.

Bertrand Coiffier, MD, Professor of Haematology, Depertment of Haematology, Hospices Civils de Lyon and University, Lyon, France

Table 6.1 Response to treatment and survival according to age at diagnosis.
Adapted from Coiffier et al [4]

Treatment outcome	Number of patients	Percentages of patients				
		<35	35–49	50–59	60–69	≥70
Response to treatment						
Complete response	686	68	64	64	56	45
Partial response	313	21	18	27	32	30
No response	119	8	12	6	9	13
Not precise	65	3	6	3	3	12
Progression at time of analysis						
Yes	595	38	49	49	51	43
No	688	62	51	51	49	57
Relapse from CR	253	20	41	40	42	36
Event-free survival						
3-year	–	59	54	55	50	47
5-year	–	59	48	44	43	41
Median	–	NR	4.0	3.9	3.4	2.4
Overall survival						
3-year	–	65	70	70	61	44
5-year	–	61	66	62	51	34
Median	–	NR	NR	7.9	5.5	2.2

NR = Not reached.

Elderly patients usually have a more severe level of disease than young and middle-aged patients: complete remission rates decline steadily with age, from 68% in the young to 45% in the elderly [4]. Median event-free and overall survivals also decline with age (Table 6.1). All published studies show shorter survival in the elderly compared with younger patients matched for lymphoma and clinical characteristics [19]. This difference persists after correction for non-lymphoma-related deaths. The shorter survival has been ascribed to two main causes: a tendency by physicians to administer weaker, 'better-tolerated' (and hence less effective) treatment in the elderly [9] and poor drug toleration in the elderly, largely due to the presence of concomitant disease [20]. As in young patients, therapy in the elderly must be based on the type of lymphoma and the presence/absence of adverse prognostic factors.

Several studies have demonstrated that elderly patients treated with the appropriate therapy and effective management of putative toxicities may have a survival comparable to that observed in younger patients [21, 22]. Once a complete response (CR) has been obtained, disease-free survival in elderly patients may be comparable to that of younger patients, even if the initial chemotherapy regimen was less aggressive [23]. The major difficulty for physicians treating elderly lymphoma patients is thus to succeed in administering the chemotherapy required by the lymphoma without adverse toxicities and to reach a high complete remission rate. With the use of granulocyte colony stimulating factor (G-CSF), all studies have shown that full-dose standard chemotherapy can be safely administrated to elderly patients [24, 25].

TREATMENT OF DIFFUSE LARGE B-CELL LYMPHOMAS IN ELDERLY

Given their age and the presence of concomitant disease, the elderly have sometimes been considered ineligible for treatment with regimens that are potentially curative in the young. Two approaches have been proposed: the first prioritises the possibility of cure and uses the same regimens as in the young, provided there is no severe concomitant disease contraindicating their use; the second prioritises quality of life, and uses specific treatment regimens tailored to the elderly, which are reputedly less toxic but also less effective [8]. The debate has essentially centred on the treatment of diffuse large B-cell lymphoma (DLBCL), since it is potentially curable with proper treatment, CHOP being the reference therapy [26]. When CHOP is used at lower doses in the elderly, the remission rate declines and survival shortens compared with patients aged less than 60 years [17]. The standard CHOP regimen, on the other hand, achieves similar progression-free survival to that in younger patients, but carries a much higher risk of severe toxicity or death: 15–30% in different retrospective series. Several recent randomised studies have compared results obtained with standard CHOP therapy to those obtained using less intensive therapy in elderly patients with DLBCL [8].

A recent German trial showed that therapeutic results may be improved if the dose intensity of the CHOP regimen is increased, that is, CHOP given every 2 weeks (CHOP-14) instead of the more normal 3 weeks (CHOP-21) in patients over 60 years of age [27]. In a multivariate analysis, giving chemotherapy every 2 weeks was associated with a longer event-free survival. In both cases, survival was not statistically different. This increase in dose intensity was not associated with an increase of severe complications. However, the median age of the patients included in this study was only 65 years and only 20% of the patients were older than 70 years. The conclusion of all of these trials is that CHOP should be recommended for the treatment of elderly patients with DLBCL, except for patients with a formal cardiac contraindication to doxorubicin.

FIRST STUDIES WITH RITUXIMAB IN AGGRESSIVE B-CELL LYMPHOMAS

The first studies evaluating the response rate in patients with aggressive lymphoma [DLBCL or mantle cell lymphoma (MCL)] were conducted in Europe 6 years ago [28, 29]. The first study showed that more aggressive lymphomas than follicular lymphoma may respond to rituximab therapy, and it opened up the development of rituximab for all types of B-cell lymphomas.

PHASE II STUDIES COMBINING RITUXIMAB AND CHEMOTHERAPY

The first phase II study of a combination of chemotherapy (CHOP) and rituximab was presented by Czuczman and colleagues [30] in patients with untreated follicular lymphoma. The median time to progression and duration of response were 82 and 83 months, respectively. Even in a selected group of patients, these results were quite impressive. In previously untreated MCL, CHOP plus rituximab (R-CHOP) was associated with a very good response [48% of CR and 48% of partial response (PR)] and half of the patients reached a molecular response [31]. However, the duration of response was not improved in patients with a molecular response and seemed no longer than that usually observed with CHOP chemotherapy alone.

The first phase II study of the treatment of aggressive B-cell lymphomas with the combination of CHOP and rituximab has been presented by Vose and colleagues [32]. The overall response rate was 94% (31 of 33 patients), with 61% CR. The median duration of response and time to progression had not been reached after a median observation of 26 months, 29 of the responding patients remaining in remission, including 15 of 16 patients with an International Prognostic Index (IPI) score greater than 2. These studies have included few patients over 60 years of age but efficacy and safety levels did not seem to be different from those observed in younger patients.

RANDOMISED TRIALS COMBINING CHEMOTHERAPY AND RITUXIMAB

Two randomised studies and one population-based study have demonstrated the benefit of the combination of rituximab with a chemotherapy (CHOP) regimen.

THE GROUPE D'ETUDE DES LYMPHOMES DE L'ADULTE (GELA) STUDY

The GELA study presented in 2001 and published in 2002, presented the results of a study in elderly patients with DLBCL comparing 8 cycles of CHOP to 8 cycles of R-CHOP [15, 16]. Standard doses of CHOP were given every 3 weeks and rituximab was given at the dose of 375 mg/m^2 on the same day of the CHOP. G-CSF may be added if patients had febrile neutropaenia or infection during the previous cycle and it was given in 50% of the patients. Three hundred and ninety-nine newly diagnosed elderly patients were included in this trial, 197 in the CHOP arm and 202 in the R-CHOP arm. Patients were 60–80 years old, were stratified for age-adjusted IPI scores (0–1 vs. 2–3) [33], had a performance status (PS) ≤2, and no contraindication to doxorubicin. The primary end point was event-free survival, with events defined as disease progression or relapse, death, or initiation of new alternative treatment. The median age of patients was 70 years. Adverse prognostic parameters were equally distributed between arms: 64% of the patients had stage IV disease, 20% had a PS > 1, 38% had B symptoms, 66% had elevated lactate dehydrogenase (LDH), 28% had bone marrow involvement, 31% had bulky tumours, 28% had greater than one extranodal disease sites, and 60% had an IPI of 2 or 3. No major difference between the two arms was observed regarding the toxicity.

At the end of treatment, 75% of the patients had reached a CR or an undocumented CR (CRu) in the R-CHOP arm compared to 63% in the CHOP arm (p = 0.005). Twenty-two percent of the patients treated with CHOP had a progression during treatment compared with 9.5% in the R-CHOP arm. With a median follow-up of 5 years, 142 events (72%) were observed in the CHOP arm and 106 (52.5%) in the R-CHOP arm, most of them being a progression during or after treatment (p < 0.001). The higher response and lower progression rate observed with the combination of CHOP and rituximab translated into statistically longer event-free survival, progression-free survival, disease-free survival, and overall survival [16]. As patients were stratified for the age-adjusted IPI [33], an analysis for low- and high-risk patients was possible and it showed that the benefit was observed in both groups but more importantly, in patients with low-risk disease, the improvement over CHOP alone at 2 years was greater than 50% (71% of the patients were event-free compared with 45%) (Figure 6.1). This study demonstrated that the addition of rituximab to CHOP chemotherapy led to significant prolongation of event-free survival and overall survival in elderly patients with DLBCL, without significant additional toxicity.

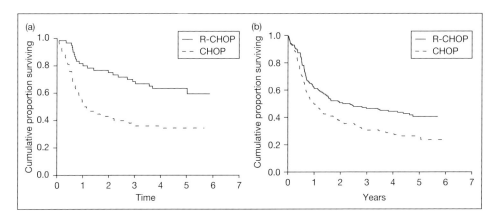

Figure 6.1   Event-free survival with a median follow-up of 5 years of patients treated with R-CHOP and CHOP according to the age-adjusted International Prognostic Index score at diagnosis: (a) low-risk patients (scores 0 and 1); (b) high-risk patients (scores 2 and 3). P values are 0.00085 and 0.0037, respectively. Edited from [16].

THE INTERGROUP STUDY FROM ECOG, CALGB, AND SWOG

This study with a double randomisation compared CHOP vs. R-CHOP, then, for responding patients, maintenance with rituximab alone; 4 infusions every 6 months for 2 years, vs. no more treatment [34]. This study has several differences with the GELA study: (1) rituximab was given only every 2 cycles of CHOP, so that patients received half of the dose of rituximab compared to GELA patients; (2) patients received 6–8 cycles of CHOP according to the response observed after 4 cycles; and (3) half of responding patients received maintenance with rituximab. Because rituximab was given both as induction (in combination with CHOP) and as maintenance, results must be analysed for the whole study and the benefit of R-CHOP vs. CHOP as induction was almost impossible to analyse. CHOP chemotherapy doses were the same as in the GELA study.

Patients had approximately the same characteristics as those in the GELA study; elderly patients (older than 60 years old) had a median age of 69 years, but only 25% of the patients had high-risk scores according to the IPI. Only 95 and 75% of the 632 included patients were available for induction and maintenance analyses, respectively. Median follow-up at the time of presentation was 3.5 years. The overall response rates were 79% for R-CHOP and 76% for CHOP but CR rates were not analysed. Contrary to the GELA study, rituximab treatment did not influence response rates and disease progression. The exact reason of this discrepancy is not known, but the lower doses of rituximab in the Intergroup study might have influenced these results.

Time to treatment failure was longer in the R-CHOP arm: 53% at 3 years compared to 46% for CHOP ($p = 0.04$) with no difference in overall survival. Patients receiving rituximab maintenance had a statistically longer time to treatment failure than those without rituximab ($p = 0.009$) without an additional impact on overall survival. This benefit was observed in patients who received CHOP only as induction but not in patients treated with R-CHOP. Even if this study was not designed to directly compare CHOP to R-CHOP, the following conclusions may be drawn: (a) in contrast to the GELA study, the addition of rituximab to CHOP did not seem to influence the response rate or early progression; (b) rituximab given as maintenance in patients treated with R-CHOP did not decrease the relapse rate; (c) rituximab given as maintenance in patients treated with CHOP alone improved the time to treatment failure; (d) rituximab given in induction concomitantly with CHOP and rituximab maintenance subsequent to CHOP both improved time to treatment failure in a relatively comparable fashion; (e) the median follow-up is currently too short to make any conclusions about overall survival.

THE POPULATION-BASED CANADIAN STUDY

Although this study is not a randomised study but a sequential historical comparison, the fact that it was based on the whole population of one Canadian province, British Columbia (BC), gives it an important weight in the interpretation of the effect of rituximab addition to CHOP in the treatment of DLBCL [35]. After the GELA had presented its data with R-CHOP combination, the BC Cancer Agency decided to modify the provincial policy for the treatment of patients with DLBCL: the recommended treatment for all centres of this province changed from CHOP to R-CHOP on March 1st, 2001. The investigators presented a retrospective analysis based on the whole population of patients with advanced DLBCL treated curatively with a CHOP-like combination during the 18 months prior to (pre-rituximab era or pre-R) and the 18 months following (post-rituximab era or post-R) this policy change. Clinical characteristics of the patients were identical in both groups: median age 63 years; IPI scores identical (52% with high-intermediate or high risk); elevated LDH in 65%, and bulky disease in 42%.

Median follow-up was 34 months for the pre-R patients and 17 months for post-R patients. This difference in follow-up is probably the only bias in this retrospective analysis. At 2

Table 6.2 Results of the retrospective population-based Canadian analysis showing progression-free survival (PFS) and overall survival (OS) at 2 years [35]

		Pre-rituximab era (%)	Post-rituximab era (%)	p value
All patients	2-year PFS	52	71	0.0009
(n = 294)	2-year OS	53	77	0.0001
Age ≥60	2-year PFS	44	73	0.0018
(n = 167)	2-year OS	40	67	0.0033
Age <60	2-year PFS	60	70	0.18
(n = 127)	2-year OS	69	87	0.018

years, both progression-free survival and overall survival showed a statistically significant difference in favour of the post-R group: 71 vs. 52% and 77 vs. 53%, respectively (Table 6.2). This retrospective analysis reflects the real life, day-to-day experience of patients. It clearly shows the improvement reached by the addition of rituximab to CHOP chemotherapy in the treatment of DLBCL patients; this being for young and elderly patients.

THERAPEUTIC STRATEGIES FOR OTHER LYMPHOMA SUBTYPES

If the therapeutic strategies have begun to be settled for the treatment of elderly patients with DLBCL, very few propositions have been made for the treatment of other lymphoma subtypes. Burkitt's lymphoma is a problem because of the poor results obtained with 'classical' CHOP and the near impossibility of increasing the dose intensity, except in young elderly patients, 60–65 or 68 years. R-CHOP is recommended and if patients fail on this therapy, palliative treatment is certainly the best option.

For patients with indolent lymphomas, there are no data to show that the conclusions drawn for DLBCL may not be applied, i.e. that they can be treated as younger patients.

SUMMARY

Age has been described as an adverse prognostic factor for the survival of patients with DLBCL, especially when co-morbid conditions are present. These poorer results in the elderly may reflect, at least partially, the use of lower doses of chemotherapeutic agents. As R-CHOP is a very well-tolerated regimen, and should be recommended for the treatment of these patients, decreasing dosage in the hope of achieving better tolerance only decreases the benefit associated with chemotherapy. Treatment with less toxicity must be reserved for patients with a contraindication to doxorubicin. Inclusion of growth factors in the therapeutic protocol can offset the risk of neutropaenia, neutropaenic infection, and higher treatment-related death rate, and these must certainly be used in the management of these elderly patients, particularly patients with a poor PS at diagnosis, where the risk of treatment-related death is the highest.

Questions that remain to be settled are: how many cycles of CHOP and infusions of rituximab are optimal? Is there any indication for a prolonged treatment with rituximab to decrease the relapse rate? Will maintenance with rituximab further improve the results? Will increasing the dose intensity by giving R-CHOP every 2 weeks increase the efficacy without increasing the toxicity? Currently, no randomised study has shown that 6 cycles of CHOP do the same as the standard 8 cycles. Decreasing the number of rituximab infusions may decrease the cost of this regimen but may also decrease the efficacy.

REFERENCES

1. Rao AV, Seo PH, Cohen HJ. Geriatric assessment and comorbidity. *Semin Oncol* 2004; 31:149–159.
2. Howe HL, Wingo PA, Thun MJ *et al*. Annual report to the nation on the status of cancer (1973 through 1998), featuring cancers with recent increasing trends. *J Natl Cancer Inst* 2001; 93:824–842.
3. Westin EH, Longo DL. Lymphoma and myeloma in older patients. Semin Oncol 2004; 31:198–205.
4. The NHL Classification Project. Effect of age on the characteristics and clinical behavior of non-Hodgkin's lymphoma patients. *Ann Oncol* 1997; 8:973–978.
5. Armitage JO, Potter JF. Aggressive chemotherapy for diffuse histiocytic lymphoma in the elderly: increased complications with advancing age. *J Am Geriatr Soc* 1984; 32:269–273.
6. Balducci L, Ballester OF. Non-Hodgkin's lymphoma in the elderly. *Cancer Control* 1996; 3(suppl 1):5–14.
7. Peters FPJ, Ten Haaft MA, Schouten HC. Intermediate and high grade non-Hodgkin's lymphoma in the elderly. *Leuk Lymphoma* 1999; 33:243–252.
8. Kouroukis CT, Browman GP, Esmail R, Meyer RM. Chemotherapy for older patients with newly diagnosed, advanced-stage, aggressive-histology non-Hodgkin lymphoma: a systematic review. *Ann Intern Med* 2002; 136:144–152.
9. Lyman GH, Dale DC, Friedberg J, Crawford J, Fisher RI. Incidence and predictors of low chemotherapy dose-intensity in aggressive non-Hodgkin's lymphoma: a nationwide study. *J Clin Oncol* 2004; 22:4302–4311.
10. Grillo-Lopez AJ, White CA, Varns C *et al*. Overview of the clinical development of rituximab: First monoclonal antibody approved for the treatment of lymphoma. *Semin Oncol* 1999; 26(suppl 14):66–73.
11. Coiffier B. Monoclonal antibodies combined to chemotherapy for the treatment of patients with lymphoma. *Blood Rev* 2003; 17:25–31.
12. Coiffier B. Monoclonal antibodies in the management of newly diagnosed, aggressive B-cell lymphoma. *Curr Hematol Rep* 2003; 2:23–29.
13. McLaughlin P, Grillolopez AJ, Link BK *et al*. Rituximab Chimeric anti-Cd20 monoclonal antibody therapy for relapsed indolent lymphoma – half of patients respond to a four-dose treatment program. *J Clin Oncol* 1998; 16:2825–2833.
14. Coiffier B. Monoclonal antibodies in the treatment of indolent lymphomas. *Best Pract Res Clin Haematol* 2005; 18:69–80.
15. Coiffier B, Lepage E, Briere J *et al*. CHOP chemotherapy plus rituximab compared with CHOP alone in elderly patients with diffuse large-B-cell lymphoma. *N Engl J Med* 2002; 346:235–242.
16. Feugier P, Hoof AV, Sebban C *et al*. Long-term results of the R-CHOP study in the treatment of elderly patients with diffuse large B-cell lymphoma. *J Clin Oncol* 2005; 23: in press.
17. Dixon DO, Neilan B, Jones SE *et al*. Effect of age on therapeutic outcome in advanced diffuse histiocytic lymphoma: the Southwest Oncology Group experience. *J Clin Oncol* 1986; 4:295–305.
18. Neilly IJ, Ogston M, Bennett B, Dawson AA. High grade non-Hodgkin's lymphoma in the elderly – 12 year experience in the Grampian region of Scotland. *Hematol Oncol* 1995; 13:99–106.
19. d'Amore F, Brincker H, Christensen BE *et al*. Non-Hodgkin's lymphoma in the elderly. A study of 602 patients aged 70 or older from a Danish population-based registry. *Ann Oncol* 1992; 3:379–386.
20. Vose JM, Armitage JO, Weisenburger DD *et al*. The importance of age in survival of patients treated with chemotherapy for aggressive non-Hodgkin's lymphoma. *J Clin Oncol* 1988; 6:1838–1844.
21. Zinzani PL, Storti S, Zaccaria A *et al*. Elderly aggressive-histology non-Hodgkin's lymphoma: first-line VNCOP-B regimen experience on 350 patients. *Blood* 1999; 94:33–38.
22. Tirelli U, Carbone A, Monfardini S, Zagonel V. A 20-year experience on malignant lymphomas in patients aged 70 and older at a single institute. *Crit Rev Oncol Hematol* 2001; 37:153–158.
23. Bastion YB, Blay JY, Divine M *et al*. Elderly patients with aggressive non-Hodgkin's lymphoma: disease presentation, response to treatment, and survival. A Groupe d'Etude des Lymphomes de l'Adulte study on 453 patients older than 69 years. *J Clin Oncol* 1997; 15:2945–2953.
24. Guerci A, Lederlin P, Reyes F *et al*. Effect of granulocyte colony-stimulating factor administration in elderly patients with aggressive non-Hodgkin's lymphoma treated with a pirarubicin-combination chemotherapy regimen. *Ann Oncol* 1996; 7:966–969.
25. Jacobson JO, Grossbard M, Shulman LN, Neuberg D. CHOP chemotherapy with preemptive granulocyte colony-stimulating factor in elderly patients with aggressive non-Hodgkin's lymphoma: a dose-intensity analysis. *Clin Lymphoma* 2000; 1:211–217; discussion 8.
26. Fisher RI, Gaynor ER, Dahlberg S *et al*. Comparison of a standard regimen (CHOP) with three intensive chemotherapy regimens for advanced non-Hodgkin's lymphoma. *N Engl J Med* 1993; 328:1002–1006.

27. Pfreundschuh M, Trumper L, Kloess M *et al*. Two-weekly or 3-weekly CHOP chemotherapy with or without etoposide for the treatment of elderly patients with aggressive lymphomas: results of the NHL-B2 trial of the DSHNHL. *Blood* 2004; 104:634–641.

28. Coiffier B, Haioun C, Ketterer N *et al*. Rituximab (anti-CD20 monoclonal antibody) for the treatment of patients with relapsing or refractory aggressive lymphoma: a multicenter phase II study. *Blood* 1998; 92:1927–1932.

29. Foran JM, Rohatiner AZS, Cunningham D *et al*. European phase II study of rituximab (chimeric anti-CD20 monoclonal antibody) for patients with newly diagnosed mantle-cell lymphoma and previously treated mantle-cell lymphoma, immunocytoma, and small B-cell lymphocytic lymphoma. *J Clin Oncol* 2000; 18:317–324.

30. Czuczman MS, Weaver R, Alkuzweny B, Berlfein J, Grillo-Lopez AJ. Prolonged clinical and molecular remission in patients with low-grade or follicular non-Hodgkin's lymphoma treated with rituximab plus CHOP chemotherapy: 9-year follow-up. *J Clin Oncol* 2005; 2:4711–4716. *Erratum in J Clin Oncol* 2005; 23:248. DOI: 10.1200/JCO.2004.04.020.

31. Howard OM, Gribben JG, Neuberg DS *et al*. Rituximab and CHOP induction therapy for newly diagnosed mantle-cell lymphoma: Molecular complete responses are not predictive of progression-free survival. *J Clin Oncol* 2002; 20:1288–1294.

32. Vose JM, Link BK, Grossbard ML *et al*. Phase II study of rituximab in combination with CHOP chemotherapy in patients with previously untreated, aggressive non-Hodgkin's lymphoma. *J Clin Oncol* 2001; 19:389–397.

33. The International Non-Hodgkin's Lymphoma Prognostic Factors Project. A predictive model for aggressive non-Hodgkin's lymphoma. *N Engl J Med* 1993; 329:987–994.

34. Habermann TM, Weller E, Morrison VA *et al*. Rituximab-CHOP versus CHOP with or without maintenance rituximab in patients 60 years of age or older with diffuse large B-cell lymphoma (DLBCL): an update. Blood 2004; 104:40a. Abstract 127. American Society of Hematology meeting, San Diego, CA, 2004.

35. Sehn LH, Donaldson J, Chhanabhai M *et al*. Introduction of combined CHOP-rituximab therapy dramatically improved outcome of diffuse large B-cell lymphoma (DLBC) in British Columbia (BC). *Blood* 2003; 102(suppl 1):29a.

7

Maintenance therapy with rituximab

B. D. Cheson, B. H. Mavromatis

INTRODUCTION

Rituximab has completely revolutionised our therapeutic paradigms for patients with B-cell malignancies. The results of a pivotal trial including 166 patients previously treated with chemotherapy demonstrated a response rate of 48% including 6% complete remissions (CRs) and a median duration of response of about a year [1]. These data led to the approval of rituximab by regulatory agencies such as the U.S. Food and Drug Administration, beginning in 1997. This level of activity, along with a favourable safety profile, encouraged investigators to identify ways to improve on the potential benefit of this important new agent. The most logical approaches to pursue included using the drug earlier in the course of the disease, or as maintenance following an induction regimen. The data from early studies suggested that the response rate to rituximab was higher in less heavily pre-treated patients [1]. Therefore, several groups studied this agent as initial treatment, primarily for indolent B-cell malignancies. Colombat and colleagues [2] reported their experience with 50 patients designated as having low tumour burden, CD20+ follicular non-Hodgkin's lymphoma (NHL), characterised by the absence of B symptoms, no tumour mass >7 cm, a normal serum lactate dehydrogenase (LDH) and β_2-microglobulin, no splenomegaly or organ compression, and no ascites or pleural effusion. Nevertheless, 46 had stage II or IV disease and two thirds had bone marrow involvement that was low in 45%, intermediate in 41%, and high in 14%. Patients received 4 weekly infusions of rituximab at a dose of 375 mg/m^2. The response rate one month after treatment (day 50) was 73%, with 10 patients in CR, 3 patients in complete remission/unconfirmed (CRu), and 23 patients in partial remission; 10 patients had stable disease, and 3 experienced disease progression. One of 13 (8%) patients in CR, 9 of 23 (39%) patients in partial remission, and 5 of 10 (50%) patients with stable disease exhibited disease progression during the first year. There were 32 patients who were initially positive for polymerase chain reaction (PCR) data on bcl-2-J(H) rearrangement. On day 50, 17 of 30 patients (57%) were negative for bcl-2-J(H) rearrangement in peripheral blood, and 9 of 29 (31%) were negative in bone marrow; a significant association was observed between molecular and clinical responses (p < 0.0001). After 12 months, 16 of 26 patients (62%) were PCR negative in the peripheral blood. These results indicate that early molecular responses can be sustained for up to 12 months and that this response is highly correlated with progression-free survival. Thus, rituximab had a high level of clinical activity and a low level of toxicity with a high complete molecular response rate in patients with follicular lymphoma and a low

Bruce D. Cheson, MD, Professor of Medicine, Division of Hematology/Oncology, Georgetown University, Lombardi Comprehensive Cancer Center, Washington, DC, USA.

Blanche H. Mavromatis, MD, Assistant Professor of Medicine, Lombardi Comprehensive Cancer Center, Washington, DC, USA.

tumour burden. In a recent long-term follow-up update (median 60 months), the overall response rate was 80% with 49% CR/CRu. The median progression-free survival was only 18 months, with a relapse-free survival of 27 months. There was no significant correlation between conversion to bcl-2 negative and relapse-free survival. This lack of durability of the responses in most patients is somewhat disappointing.

In another trial, Witzig and co-workers [3] treated 37 newly diagnosed patients with advanced stage follicular NHL using 4 weekly infusions of rituximab. Patients were considered to be at low risk, with no B symptoms; 39% were considered low risk by the International Prognostic Index, 44% low-intermediate, and only 17% high-intermediate. The overall response rate was 72% with 36% CRs. The median time to progression was 2.2 years and 18 patients required subsequent treatment with chemotherapy. Patients with an elevated LDH had a poor prognosis with a median time to progression of only 6 months. Grade 3 or worse adverse events occurred in 15% of patients. Based on these studies, it appears that a 4-week course of rituximab as initial treatment is active and well tolerated. However, the durability of responses requires considerable improvement.

The decision to consider the currently recommended dose and schedule of rituximab was somewhat empiric. Therefore, whether 4 weekly infusions of rituximab were optimal remains to be determined. In the first attempt to prolong the duration of therapy, Piro and colleagues [4] explored the possibility that 8 weekly infusions during induction might be more effective. They studied 37 patients, almost exclusively with advanced stages of follicular NHL who had failed prior therapies. Extending the duration of treatment resulted in higher peak post-infusion levels of antibody beyond the fourth infusion. However, the additional 4 infusions did not clearly increase the efficacy. The CR rate of 14% and overall response rate of 57% were not clearly superior to what was attainable with 4 infusions, neither were the median duration of response of 13 months nor the median time to progression for responders of 19.4+ months.

Maintenance rituximab therapy, defined as prolonged administration of rituximab beyond an induction phase, has also been evaluated in an attempt to prolong the time to disease progression and, possibly, survival [5–8] (Table 7.1). In an intergroup phase III study [8], 461 patients with relapsed or refractory follicular NHL who had failed up to 2 prior anthracycline-based regimens were randomised to CHOP (cyclophosphamide, adriamycin, vincristine, and prednisone) or R-CHOP both with or without maintenance rituximab (Table 7.2). The CR rate was superior in the chemoimmunotherapy arm (30.4 vs. 18.1%), and the 1- and 3-year progression-free survival demonstrated an advantage over maintenance; therapy (54.9 and 31.2% in the observation arm and 80.2 and 67.7% in patients who received maintenance, p = 0.0001). However, to date, no demonstrable survival benefit has been shown.

A chemotherapy regimen such as chlorambucil, CVP (cyclophosphamide, vincristine, and prednisone), or CHOP has been the standard initial approach for patients who require treatment for indolent NHL. Several trials have recently evaluated the potential benefit of maintenance rituximab following initial treatment with a chemotherapy regimen. Investigators in the Eastern Cooperative Oncology Group (ECOG) and Cancer and Leukaemia Group B (CALGB) [7] treated 516 patients with advanced-stage follicular NHL. The initial study design had included a randomisation during induction between CVP ($1,000\,mg/m^2$ with prednisone $100\,mg/m^2$ every 3 weeks for 6–8 cycles, determined by the rapidity of the response) and fludarabine plus cyclophosphamide; however, the latter arm was discontinued because of excessive toxicity. There were 322 assessable patients who were subsequently randomised to either observation or rituximab maintenance using a schedule of $375\,mg/m^2$ weekly for 4 doses every 6 months for 2 years. The study was terminated early because of the significant difference in progression-free survival that favoured the rituximab-CVP (R-CVP) arm at 2 and 4 years (74 vs. 42% and 58 vs. 34%, respectively). At the time of the presentation, there was a trend towards a survival advantage for the chemoimmunotherapy arm (p = 0.06) which will hopefully become significant with longer follow-up. In another study, 461 patients with relapsed or refractory follicular

Table 7.1 Rituximab maintenance results

Study (Ref)	Patients	Disease	Previous treatment	Rituximab maintenance schedule	Response rate (%) ORR (CR) (after induction)	Response rate(%) ORR(CR) (after maintenance)	Progression-free survival	Overall survival
Hainsworth et al. 2002 [5]	62	FL (61%) SLL (39%)	No	Weekly × 4q6m × 2 years	FL 76(NR) SLL 70(NR)	NR	MPFS 32 m FL 52 m	NR
Ghielmini et al. 2004 [6]	185 (78 maint. 73 obs.)	FL	64 No 136 Yes	Q2m × 4 vs. observation	Untreated: 67(9) Treated: 46(8)	All patients: 75(38) vs. 77(31)NS Untreated: 92(52) vs. 81(31)NS	All patients: 23 vs. 12 m Untreated: 36 vs. 19 m (p = 0.009)	NR
Hainsworth et al. 2005 [13]	90 (44 maint. 46 at progression)	FL (67%) SLL (23%)	Yes	Weekly × 4 q6m × 2 years vs. same at progression	39(1)	(52(10)	31.3 m maintenance vs. observation	72% maintenance vs. 68% observation at 3 years
RESORT	Ongoing	FL	No	Weekly × 1 q12 weeks or at progression	Ongoing	–	–	–
Gordon et al. 2005 [15]	29 23 (maint.)	CD20+ (excluding CLL/SLL)	Yes	Based on rituximab serum level, one dose q3–4m	59(27) Low grade NHL 63 (36) Aggressive HNL 43(0)	73(37) MPFS for low grade NHL not reached	19 m	NR
Hainsworth et al. 2003 [20]	44	CLL/SLL	No	Weekly × 4 q6m × 2 years	51(4)	58(9)	18.6 m MPFS 62% at 1 year MPFS 49% at 2 years	NR
Ghielmini et al. 2005 [30]	104	MCL	38 No 66 Yes	Q2m × 4vs. observation	All patients: 27(2) Untreated: 44(3) Treated: 28(2) NS	All patients: 9% maintenance vs. 15% observation at 2 years	All patients: EFS 12 m maintenance vs. 6 m observation (NS) Treated: EFS 5 m maintenance vs. 1 m observation p = 0.04.	NR

MPFS = Median progression-free survival; OS = overall survival; NR = not reached; NS = not significant; EFS = event-free survival.
CLL = Chronic lymphocytic leukaemia; FL = Follicular lymphoma; NHL = non-Hodgkin's lymphoma; MCL = mantle cell lymphoma; SLL = small lymphocytic lymphoma;
Maint. = maintenance; obs. = observed.
m = month.

Table 7.2 Chemotherapy with or without maintenance Rituximab

Study (Ref)	Patients	Disease	Previous treatment	Chemotherapy	Schedule	Response rate (%) ORR(CR)	Progression-free survival	Time to treatment failure	Overall survival
Hochster et al. 2004 [7]	322 (154 maint. 149 obs.)	FL	No	CVP	Weekly × 4 q6m × 2 years vs. observation	Post-induction: 14% CR Post-maintenance: 30 vs. 22%	74 vs. 42% at 2 years	NR	96% for maintenance vs. 86% for observation
Habermann et al. 2004 [28]	632 (174 maint. 178 obs.)	DLBCL	No	CHOP vs. R-CHOP	Weekly × 4 q6m × 2 years vs. observation	CHOP ORR 76% R-CHOP ORR $p = 0.76$	NR	CHOP 46% R-CHOP 53% $p = 0.04$	NR
Van Oers et al. 2004 [8]	369 (136 maint. 132 obs.)	FL	Yes No	CHOP vs. R-CHOP	Weekly × 4 q6m until relapse vs. observation	Post-chemo: 71(18) vs. 82(30)	CHOP 55% at 1 year 31% at 3 years R-CHOP 80% at 1 year 67% at 3 years $p < 0.0001$	NR	NR

MPFS = Median progression-free survival; OS = overall survival; NR = not reached; NS = not significant; FL = follicular lymphoma; DLBCL = diffuse large B-cell lymphoma; obs. = observation; Maint. = maintenance.

NHL were randomised to CHOP or R-CHOP as induction therapy followed by observation or rituximab maintenance every 3 months until relapse or 2 years, whichever came first [8]. In the 369 patients considered evaluable for response, R-CHOP was associated with a significantly higher CR rate (30.4 vs. 18.1%). There was also an advantage from the antibody in 1- and 3-year progression-free survival (80.2 and 67.7%) compared with observation (54.9 and 31.2%).

Based on the promising results with rituximab as initial treatment for follicular and low-grade NHL, rituximab has been studied in a number of trials as a single agent for induction followed by maintenance with the same antibody. The first study to examine the role of a maintenance strategy was published by Hainsworth and colleagues [5] who treated 62 patients with follicular lymphoma and chronic lymphocytic leukaemia/small lymphocytic lymphoma (CLL/SLL) with initial 4 weekly doses of rituximab at $375\,mg/m^2$. The response rate was 76% for the former patients, and 70% for the latter. Patients who did not progress were treated with an additional 4 weekly infusions every 6 months for a total of 2 years. These results are superior to what has been reported with induction rituximab alone [2]. The time to progression of 32 months was also longer than expected. In a follow-up report [9] these investigators confirmed this impression with a median time to progression in the patients with a follicular histology of 52.1 months. The median time to progression in the patients with CLL/SLL was significantly shorter at 30.6 months.

In another, larger randomised trial, Ghielmini and co-workers [6] from the SAKK Group evaluated the potential benefits of extended rituximab treatment in a study comparing the standard schedule with prolonged treatment in 202 patients with newly diagnosed or refractory/relapsed follicular lymphoma. All patients received rituximab treatment ($375\,mg/m^2$ weekly $\times$ 4). In 185 evaluable patients, the overall response rate was 67% in chemotherapy-naïve patients and 46% in pre-treated cases ($p < 0.01$). The 151 patients responding, or with stable disease at week 12, were randomised to no further treatment or prolonged rituximab administration ($375\,mg/m^2$ every 2 months $\times$ 4). At a median follow-up of 35 months, the median event-free survival (EFS) was 12 months in the no further treatment arm vs. 23 months in the prolonged treatment arm ($p = 0.02$), the difference being particularly notable in chemotherapy-naïve patients (19 vs. 36 months; $p = 0.009$) and in patients responding to induction treatment (16 vs. 36 months; $p = 0.004$). The number of t(14;18)-positive cells in peripheral blood ($p = 0.0035$) and in bone marrow ($p = 0.0052$) at baseline was predictive for clinical response. Circulating normal B lymphocytes and immunoglobulin M (IgM) plasma levels decreased for a significantly longer time after prolonged treatment, but the incidence of adverse events was not increased.

The role of maintenance therapy is confounded by the observation that re-treatment with rituximab may be an effective therapy [10, 11]. Davis and colleagues [10] reported on a series of 57 assessable patients who had first received a chemotherapy regimen and, upon relapse, were treated with rituximab. Those who previously responded to rituximab and then relapsed at least 6 months following therapy were re-treated with the antibody using the same dose and schedule. The overall response rate was 40% of patients, including 11% CRs. Responses were still ongoing in 6 of 23 patients at the time of the publication. In contrast to what would be expected with repeated courses of similar chemotherapy regimens, the data suggested that the second responses were at least as long as the first [12]. The median duration of response from the initial rituximab therapy was 9.8 months compared with 16.3 months with re-treatment, and the time to progression was 12.4 vs. 17.8 months, respectively. All patients remained CD20+ and none developed a human anti-chimeric antibody (HACA). Other reports have confirmed the potential efficacy of re-treatment [11].

Thus, an important remaining question is whether it is preferable to use one of the maintenance strategies or to re-treat patients upon relapse. In an attempt to address this issue, Hainsworth and co-workers [13] accrued 114 previously treated patients with follicular lymphoma or SLL and treated them with 4 weekly infusions of the antibody. Those who did not progress were randomised to either maintenance with 4 weekly infusions every 6 months for 2 years, or re-treatment upon relapse. Although the response rate improved in the maintenance arm (from 39 to 52%), with more patients in CR (10 vs. 1 in the re-treatment arm), and, at a median follow-up of 41 months, progression-free survival favouring the maintenance arm (31.3 vs. 7.4 months), the time until which a treatment other than rituximab was required was similar in the two treatment groups (31.3 vs. 27.4 months) as was the 3-year survival (72 vs. 68% for maintenance and re-treatment, respectively). The ongoing ECOG 'RESORT' (Rituximab Extended Therapy Or ReTreatment) trial is comparing continuous treatment with rituximab every 12 weeks until relapse with re-treatment at the time of recurrence in previously untreated patients with follicular NHL. Therefore, at the present time, the preferred approach is not clear.

To date, the strategies for maintenance rituximab therapy have been empiric: including a single dose of the antibody every 2 months [6], 4 weekly doses every 6 months [5, 7], or a single dose every 12 weeks as administered in the RESORT trial. A more rational approach to the selection of regimens would be welcome. An important observation was that, following its administration, rituximab can still be detected in the blood for as long as 6 months. In addition, data suggest a correlation between the blood level of this antibody and patient response [14]. Therefore, Gordon and colleagues [15] conducted a trial in which patients with CD20+ lymphoid malignancies (excluding CLL/SLL) were first treated with 4 weekly infusions of rituximab. The overall response rate was 59% with 27% CR. There were 22 of 29 possible patients available for maintenance based on the pharmacokinetics (PK) of the antibody. Blood levels of the antibody were measured monthly for up to a year, and patients were re-dosed in an individualised fashion with a single infusion of $375 \, mg/m^2$ on the basis of their rituximab blood levels to maintain what was considered to be a therapeutic level ($\geq 25 \, \mu g/ml$). Of the 29 patients, 23 went on to receive at least one dose of maintenance therapy. The median progression-free survival was 19 months at a median follow-up of 24.5 months. Responding patients tended to have higher blood levels. During maintenance, the quality of response improved in 3 patients; 2 from a partial remission to a CR, and one from stable disease to a partial response. They authors concluded that the optimal maintenance strategy would be to re-dose every 3–4 months.

CHRONIC LYMPHOCYTIC LEUKAEMIA

The activity of rituximab has been limited in patients with relapsed or refractory CLL/SLL [1, 4, 16–19]. However, when used as initial therapy in patients with CLL/SLL, there appears to be much more promising activity [5, 20]. Hainsworth and co-workers [20] reported on 44 previously untreated patients with stage III or IV CLL who required therapy and who were treated with single-agent rituximab at the standard dose and schedule. The initial response rate was 51% with 4% CRs. Patients with stable disease received an additional 4 weeks of the antibody every 6 months for 2 years. There was essentially no change in the response rate at 58% and 9% CRs. The median progression-free survival at a median follow-up of 20 months was 18.6 months, with 1- and 2-year PFS rates of 62 and 49%, respectively.

DIFFUSE LARGE B-CELL NHL

For decades, CHOP has remained the standard regimen for patients with diffuse large B-cell NHL (DLBCL). Using this relatively well-tolerated regimen, about 40% of patients were cured with prolonged follow-up. More intensive and aggressive regimens failed to demonstrate an advantage in randomised trials [21, 22]. Rituximab as a single agent was shown to have a response rate of 33% leading to interest in combining this antibody with chemotherapy. In the initial studies by Vose and co-workers [23, 24] the complete and overall response rates to R-CHOP were higher than would be expected with CHOP alone, with a suggestion of a possible survival benefit on longer follow-up [24, 25]. A marked paradigm shift followed the 2002 publication by the GELA group of their randomised trial in 399 patients between the ages of 60–80 years with DLBCL who received either CHOP alone or with rituximab given on day 1 of each cycle. The complete response rate (76 vs. 63%) as well as EFS and overall survival significantly favoured the combination arm [26]. This benefit from rituximab was subsequently confirmed by the MINT trial [27] in younger patients, as well as by a population-based study from the British Columbia Cancer Agency [28]. An ECOG, CALGB, and SWOG intergroup study compared CHOP with R-CHOP in 632 patients with DLBCL over the age of 60 years [29], but with a secondary randomisation in responding patients to rituximab maintenance (n = 174) or observation (n = 178). In contrast to the previously published GELA study, there were no differences in response rates. With a median follow-up of 3.5 years, time to treatment failure (TTF) favoured the R-CHOP arm (53 vs. 46%; p = 0.04). There was no significant difference in survival based on the induction therapy. An unplanned, secondary analysis performed to remove the confounding effect of rituximab maintenance suggested a benefit for rituximab when given either during induction or as maintenance; there was, however, no value to delivering the antibody during both portions of the treatment. The authors concluded that these observations demonstrated an additive rather than a synergistic effect of chemotherapy and rituximab.

MANTLE CELL LYMPHOMA

Mantle cell lymphoma (MCL) represents one of the most therapeutically challenging lymphomas. It usually behaves in an aggressive fashion, yet is incurable with currently available therapies. Since R-CHOP demonstrated a survival benefit in DLBCL, it was a natural response to explore this regimen in MCL as well. To date, the data have been somewhat discouraging [30]. Despite high overall and complete response rates, with many patients becoming PCR-negative, the median duration of response remains relatively brief. Recently, Ghielmini and colleagues [31] conducted a trial evaluating the role of rituximab as initial treatment and maintenance therapy in 104 patients with newly diagnosed or relapsed/refractory MCL. The single-agent response rate was only 27% with 2% CR, and was similar in the two arms. The median EFS was only 6 months in the observation arm and 12 months in the maintenance arm; however, this difference was not significant. There was a suggestion of an improvement in EFS with maintenance (5 vs. 11 months; p = 0.04). The frequency of grade 3–4 toxicity was similar in the two arms.

SUMMARY

Patients with B-cell NHL and CLL are increasingly being treated with rituximab-based combinations as their initial treatment. With some exceptions [29], this approach has improved complete and overall response rates. However, the effect on progression-free survival and overall survival has been inconsistent and has varied among histologies. Maintenance therapy with rituximab is being increasingly studied in clinical trials to improve on the durability of responses in B-cell malignancies. A number of important issues remain unresolved. Firstly, the optimal dose and schedule of administration have yet to be defined. While maintaining a therapeutic blood level seems to be a rational approach, it is not practical [15]. Whether it is preferable to combine rituximab with chemotherapy, use it as maintenance, or to deliver both is unresolved. However, current data would suggest that maintenance does not add to the benefit of using rituximab as part of initial treatment, at least in DLBCL [29]. The data suggesting a comparable outcome between maintenance and re-treatment must be considered carefully as to whether there is increased benefit, cost-effectiveness, and quality of life advantage for one approach compared with another. Although maintenance therapy with single-agent rituximab does not appear to improve outcome in MCL [31], combinations with other active agents may be more efficacious. While maintenance rituximab is a promising approach, its role is still being defined. Patients should be encouraged to participate in clinical trials exploring strategies that incorporate maintenance therapy leading to a lower likelihood of relapse, and an enhanced possibility of cure.

REFERENCES

1. McLaughlin P, Grillo-López AJ, Link BK, Levy R, Czuczman MS, Williams ME *et al*. Rituximab chimeric anti-CD20 monoclonal antibody therapy of relapsed indolent lymphoma: half of patients respond to a four-dose treatment program. *J Clin Oncol* 1998; 16:2825–2833.
2. Colombat P, Salles G, Brousse N, Eftekhari P, Soubeyran P, Delwail V *et al*. Rituximab (anti-CD20 monoclonal antibody) as single first-line therapy for patients with follicular lymphoma with a low tumor burden: clinical and molecular evaluation. *Blood* 2001; 97:101–106.
3. Witzig TE, Vukov AM, Habermann T, Geyer S, Kurtin P, Friedenberg WR *et al*. Rituximab therapy for patients with newly diagnosed, advanced-stage follicular grade I non-Hodgkin's lymphoma: a phase II trial in the North Central Cancer Treatment Group. *J Clin Oncol* 2005; in press.
4. Piro LD, White CA, Grillo-López AJ, Janakiraman N, Saven A, Beck TM *et al*. Extended rituximab (anti-CD20 monoclonal antibody) therapy for relapsed or refractory low-grade or follicular non-Hodgkin's lymphoma. *Ann Oncol* 1999; 10:655–661.
5. Hainsworth JD, Litchy S, Burris HA, 3rd, Scullin DC, Jr, Corso SW, Yardley DA *et al*. Rituximab as first-line and maintenance therapy for patients with indolent non-Hodgkin's lymphoma. *J Clin Oncol* 2002; 20:4261–4267.
6. Ghielmini M, Schmitz SF, Cogliatti SB, Pichert G, Hummerjohann J, Walzer U *et al*. Prolonged treatment with rituximab in patients with follicular lymphoma significantly increases event-free survival and response duration compared with weekly × 4 schedule. *Blood* 2004; 103:4416–4423.
7. Hochster HS, Weller E, Ryan T, Habermann TM, Gascoyne R, Frankel SR *et al*. Results of E1496: a phase III trial of CVP with or without maintenance rituximab in advanced indolent lymphoma (NHL). *Proc Am Soc Clin Oncol* 2004; 22(14S):558s (abstract 6502).
8. Van Oers MHJ, Van Glebbeke M, Teodorovic I, Rozewicz C, Klasa R, Marcus RE *et al*. Chimeric anti-CD20 monoclonal antibody (Rituximab; Mabthera) in remission induction and maintenance treatment of relapsed/resistant follicular non-Hodgkin's lymphoma: a phase III randomized intergroup clinical trial. *Blood* 2004; 104(suppl 1):169a (abstract 586).
9. Hainsworth JD, Litchy S, Morrissey L, Yardley DA, Greco FA. Rituximab as first-line and maintenance therapy for indolent non-Hodgkin's lymphoma (NHL): long-term follow-up of a Minnie Pearl Cancer Research Network phase II trial. *Blood* 2003; 102(suppl 1):411a (abstract 1496).
10. Davis TA, Grillo-López AJ, White CA, McLaughlin P, Czuczman MS, Link BK *et al*. Final report on the safety and efficacy of retreatment with rituximab for patients with non-Hodgkin's lymphoma. *Blood* 1999; 94(suppl 1):88a (abstract 385).
11. Igarashi T, Ohtsu T, Fujii H, Sasaki Y, Morishima Y, Ogura M *et al*. Re-treatment of relapsed indolent B-cell lymphoma with rituximab. *Int J Hematol* 2001; 73:213–221.
12. Gallagher CJ, Gregory WM, Jones AE, Stansfield AG, Richards MA, Dhaliwal HS *et al*. Follicular lymphoma: prognostic factors for response and survival. *J Clin Oncol* 1986; 4:1470–1480.
13. Hainsworth JD, Litchy S, Shaffer DW, Lackey VL, Grimaldi M, Greco FA. Maximizing therapeutic benefit of rituximab: maintenance therapy versus retreatment at progression in patients with indolent non-Hodgkin's lymphoma: a randomized phase II trial of the Minnie Pearl Cancer Research Network. *J Clin Oncol* 2005; in press.
14. Berinstein NL, Grillo-López AJ, White CA, Bence-Bruckler I, Maloney D, Czuczman M *et al*. Association of serum Rituximab (IDEC-C2B8) concentration and anti-tumor response in the treatment of recurrent low-grade or follicular non-Hodgkin's lymphoma. *Ann Oncol* 1998; 9:995–1001.
15. Gordon LN, Grow WB, Pusateri A, Douglas V, Mendenhall NP, Lynch JW. Phase II trial of individualized rituximab dosing for patients with CD20-positive lymphoproliferative disorders. *J Clin Oncol* 2005, in press.

16. Winkler U, Jensen M, Manzke O, Schulz H, Diehl V, Engert A. Cytokine-release syndrome in patients with B-cell chronic lymphocytic leukemia and high lymphocyte counts after treatment with an anti-CD20 monoclonal antibody (Rituximab, IDEC-C2B8). *Blood* 1999; 94:2217–2224.

17. Nguyen DT, Amess JA, Doughty H, Hendry L, Diamond LW. IDEC-C2B8 anti-CD20 (rituximab) immunotherapy in patients with low-grade non-Hodgkin's lymphoma and lymphoproliferative disorders: evaluation of response on 48 patients. *Eur J Haematol* 1999; 62:76–82.

18. Foran JM, Rohatiner AZ, Cunningham D, Popescu RA, Solal-Céligny P, Ghielmini M *et al*. European phase II study of rituximab (Chimeric anti-CD20 monoclonal antibody) for patients with newly diagnosed mantle-cell lymphoma and previously treated mantle-cell lymphoma, immunocytoma, and small B-cell lymphocytic lymphoma. *J Clin Oncol* 2000; 18:317–324.

19. Huhn D, von Schilling C, Wilhelm M, Ho AD, Hallek M, Kuse R *et al*. Rituximab therapy of patients with B-cell chronic lymphocytic leukemia. *Blood* 2001; 98:1326–1331.

20. Hainsworth JD, Litchy S, Barton JH, Houston GA, Hermann RC, Bradof JE *et al*. Single-agent rituximab as first-line and maintenance treatment for patients with chronic lymphocytic leukemia or small lymphocytic lymphoma: a phase II trial of the Minnie Pearl Cancer Research Network. *J Clin Oncol* 2003; 21:1746–1751.

21. Fisher RI, Gaynor ER, Dahlberg S, Oken MM, Grogan TM, Mize EM *et al*. Comparison of a standard regimen (CHOP) with three intensive chemotherapy regimens for advanced non-Hodgkin's lymphoma. *N Engl J Med* 1993; 328:1002–1006.

22. Gordon LI, Harrington D, Andersen J, Colgan J, Glick J, Neiman R *et al*. Comparison of a second-generation combination chemotherapeutic regimen (m-BACOD) with a standard regimen (CHOP) for advanced diffuse non-Hodgkin's lymphoma. *N Engl J Med* 1992; 327:1342–1349.

23. Vose JM, Link BK, Grossbard ML, Czuczman M, Grillo-López A, Gilman P *et al*. Phase II study of rituximab in combination with CHOP chemotherapy in patients with previously untreated, aggressive non-Hodgkin's lymphoma. *J Clin Oncol* 2001; 19:389–397.

24. Vose JM, Link BK, Grossbard ML, Czuczman M, Grillo-López AJ, Benyunes M *et al*. Long term follow-up of a phase II study of rituximab in combination with CHOP chemotherapy in patients with previously untreated aggressive non-Hodgkin's lymphoma (NHL). *Blood* 2002; 100(suppl 1):361a (abstract 1396).

25. Coiffier B, Lepage E, Briere J, Herbrecht R, Tilly H, Bouabdallah R *et al*. CHOP chemotherapy plus rituximab compared with CHOP alone in elderly patients with diffuse large B-cell lymphoma. *N Engl J Med* 2002; 346:235–242.

26. Feugier P, Van Hoof A, Sebban C *et al*. Long-term results of the R-CHOP study in the treatment of elderly patients with diffuse large B-cell lymphoma: a study by the Group d'Etude des Lymphome de l'Adulte. *J Clin Oncol* 2005; (Epub ahead of print).

27. Pfreundschuh MG, Trumper L, Ma D, Osterborg A, Pettingell R, Trneny M *et al*. Randomized intergroup trial of first line treatment for patients <=60 years with diffuse large B-cell non-Hodgkin's lymphoma (DLBCL) with a CHOP-like regimen with or without the anti-CD20 antibody rituximab – early stopping after the first interim analysis. *Proc Am Soc Clin Oncol* 2004; 22:558s (abstract 6500).

28. Sehn LH, Donaldson J, Chhanabhi M, Fitzgerald C, MacPherson N, O'Reilly SE *et al*. Introduction of combined CHOP-rituximab therapy dramatically improved outcome of diffuse large-B-cell lymphoma (DLBC) in British Columbia (BC). *Blood* 2003; 102(suppl 1):abstract 88.

29. Habermann TM, Weller E, Morrisson VA, Cassileth PA, Cohn J, Dakhil S *et al*. Rituximab-CHOP versus CHOP with or without maintenance rituximab in patients 60 years of age or older with diffuse large B-cell lymphoma (DLBCL): an update. *Blood* 2004; 104(suppl 1):abstract 127.

30. Howard OM, Gribben JG, Neuberg DS, Grossbard ML, Poor C, Janicek MJ *et al*. Rituximab and CHOP induction therapy for newly diagnosed mantle-cell lymphoma: molecular complete responses are not predictive of progression-free survival. *J Clin Oncol* 2002; 20:1288–1294.

31. Ghielmini M, Schmitz S-FH, Cogliatti S, Bertoni F, Waltzer U, Fey MF *et al*. Effect of single agent rituximab given at the standard schedule or as prolonged treatment in patients with mantle cell lymphoma. *J Clin Oncol* 2005; in press.

8

Interferon-alpha in lymphoid malignancies

J.-L. Harousseau, V. Dubruille

Interferon-alpha (IFN-α) has a diverse range of activities that can be used in the treatment of haematological malignancies.

IFN-α has immunomodulatory [1, 2] and anti-angiogenic properties [3] that may indirectly influence tumour growth. IFN-α directly affects cell growth by causing cell cycle arrest in G1 [4, 5] and can induce apoptosis [6]. IFN-α can also induce differentiation of a wide range of normal and malignant cells [7]. This pleiotropic cytokine has clinical activity in a variety of haematological malignancies including lymphoproliferative disorders. The availability of recombinant IFN-α2a and IFN-α2b has opened the way for clinical studies in different indications. In the 1980s there was great enthusiasm for IFN-α in the treatment of hairy cell leukaemia (HCL), multiple myeloma (MM) and follicular lymphoma (FL). However, the side-effects and the cost of this treatment have always been a concern and have prompted re-evaluation of its clinical benefit. Moreover, in all these diseases, newer agents have shown a high efficacy/toxicity ratio and are currently used in preference to IFN-α in a majority of cases. Therefore, it is of interest to summarise the current results and use of IFN-α in lymphoproliferative disorders.

IFN-α IN HAIRY CELL LEUKAEMIA

In 1984, Quesada and colleagues [8] published the results of partially purified IFN-α in the treatment of 7 patients with HCL. This publication initiated a new era in the treatment of this rare chronic B-cell lymphoproliferative disorder, which until that time could only be treated by splenectomy. A large multi-centre study on 195 patients confirmed that IFN-α has activity in HCL, with 82% overall response rate [9] but complete remissions were rare (7%); most responses were partial and were of relatively short duration if unmaintained. Although relapses occurred, patients could be re-treated with IFN-α and survival rates were greatly improved [10]. The estimated survival of patients treated with IFN-α was 85–90% at 5 years [9–11]. IFN-α was used at relatively low doses (3 million units 3 times a week) for HCL.

Maintenance therapy with IFN-α has been shown to delay relapses, is reasonably well tolerated by most patients and is not associated with late development of resistance [12]. Moreover, haematological response can improve with time on treatment. However, this strategy raises the issue of the long-term toxicity of IFN-α. Lower doses of IFN-α (≤1 million units; MU) have been shown to be less toxic but less effective [13].

Jean-Luc Harousseau, MD, Professor of Haematology, Hotel Dieu, University Hospital, Nantes, France.
Viviane Dubruille, PhD, Doctor of Haematology, Hotel Dieu, University Hospital, Nantes, France.

The introduction of purine analogues completely changed the management of HCL since 2-deoxycoformycin (Pentostatin) and 2-chloro-deoxy adenosine (2-CDA) (Cladribine) have been found to be more effective with longer duration of remissions following a short course of therapy.

A randomised study compared IFN-α (3 MU 3 times a week) vs. deoxycoformycin (4 mg/m^2 every 2 weeks) in 313 previously untreated patients [14]. Deoxycoformycin resulted in a significantly higher overall response rate (79 vs. 38%) and complete remission rate (76 vs. 11%) than IFN-α. As a consequence, relapse-free survival was dramatically longer with deoxycoformycin (p < 0.0001). However, with a median follow-up time of 57 months, there was no difference in overall survival but 104 of 159 patients treated with IFN-α were crossed over to receive deoxycoformycin at relapse vs. only 10 crossing over per 154 patients initially treated with deoxycoformycin. A large retrospective study on long-term outcome in 238 patients treated with deoxycoformycin (4 mg/m^2 every 2 weeks) confirmed that the complete remission rate was very high (79%), and that the relapse rate was low (15%) [15]. As a consequence, the 5-year survival was 88%.

The results for 2-CDA (0.1 mg/kg/day, 7-day continuous infusion) are comparable to those reported for deoxycoformycin. A large multi-centre open study of 979 previously treated or untreated patients showed an 87% response rate including 50% complete remissions [16]. With a median follow-up time of 52 months, the 4-year disease-free survival was 84% and the 4-year survival was 86%.

Long-term follow-up of 358 patients with HCL treated in a single centre (Scripps Clinic) with 2-CDA was evaluated [17]. The response rate was very high (98% including 91% complete remissions). Remissions were prolonged with a treatment failure rate of only 19% at 4 years (16% in patients with complete response). The overall survival was 96% at 4 years. These results were confirmed in a more recent evaluation on 207 patients with at least 7 years of follow-up for which the overall survival remained at 97% at 108 months [18].

While treatment with IFN-α needs to be continued for relatively long periods of time, treatment with purine analogues is short and predictable: 10–12 IV injections every 2 weeks with deoxycoformycin, 5–7 days IV infusion or S/C injections [19] with 2-CDA.

Since these drugs are immunosuppressive agents, the issue of short- and long-term toxicity was raised. However, in all large series, the incidence and severity of early opportunistic infections were unremarkable. In several retrospective studies, the incidence of second malignancies was slightly higher than the rate expected for the same age group [20–22]. This increased frequency may be mostly related to prolonged survival of patients immunocompromised because of their disease. All authors concluded that nucleoside analogues could be safely administered to patients with HCL. In one report, the incidence of the second neoplasms was unexpectedly high in patients with HCL treated with IFN-α [23] but this was not confirmed by other investigators and IFN-α therapy does not appear to exert any oncogenic effect in such patients [24, 25].

Considering the success of purine analogues, the role of IFN-α in the management of HCL appears to be limited. At the present time, IFN-α is reserved for the rare patients who fail purine analogue therapy.

IFN-α IN MULTIPLE MYELOMA

Twenty-five years after the first publication of purified natural IFN-α in MM [26] the role of IFN-α in the disease remains unclear [27]. Pilot studies reported remissions in refractory or relapsed MM with an overall response around 20% [28]. In newly diagnosed patients, again approximately 20% responses were observed [29–32], but the rate and the duration of response with IFN-α were inferior to those achieved with conventional chemotherapy. IFN-α was then evaluated as maintenance therapy for patients who respond to their initial treatment, or in combination with chemotherapy.

Table 8.1 IFN-α in maintenance after conventional chemotherapy in multiple myeloma. Results of published randomised trials with p values

	Number of patients	Progression-free survival	Survival
Pulsoni et al. [34]	101	0.001	NS
Salmon et al. [35]	211	NS	NS
Browman et al. [36]	181	0.0003	0.07
Westin et al. [37]	125	<0.0001	NS
Ludwig et al. [38]	100	0.02	NS
Peest et al. [39]	117	NS	NS
Drayson et al. [40]	283	0.09	NS
Blade et al. [41]	92	0.04	NS
Capnist et al. [42]	92	NS	NS

NS = Not significant.

IFN-α AS MAINTENANCE THERAPY AFTER CONVENTIONAL CHEMOTHERAPY

In 1990, an Italian multi-centre randomised study showed that patients responding to their initial chemotherapy had a significantly longer remission when they received maintenance therapy with IFN-α (3 MU/m^2 3 times a week) compared to patients without further treatment (median 26 vs. 14 months) [33]. Although this difference was highly significant, the benefit in terms of overall survival was not and further analysis confirmed that overall survival was not increased by maintenance with IFN-α [34]. Although no significant survival advantage was obtained, these results prompted a number of other prospective randomised trials and at least 9 randomised studies have been fully published [34–42]. Results are summarised in Table 8.1. Five out of these 9 trials showed a better progression-free survival in the IFN-α arm compared to the control arm, but in none of these studies the overall survival was significantly prolonged. However, the majority of these trials have probably been too small to show a significant improvement in survival.

Considering that this treatment might have a moderate, but still clinically meaningful, survival benefit, the Myeloma Trialists' Collaborative Group performed a meta-analysis of all randomised trials (either published or not) [43]. This study was based on the individual patient data supplied by the investigators. This overview of 1,543 patients showed a significant improvement of both response duration (p < 0.00001) and progression-free survival with IFN-α (p < 0.00001). The median time to progression was increased by about 6 months. Overall survival was also significantly improved by IFN-α (p = 0.04) with a median survival increased by 7 months.

IFN-α IN COMBINATION WITH CHEMOTHERAPY AS INDUCTION TREATMENT

The rationale for combining IFN-α with chemotherapy is the demonstration of an *in vitro* synergy with cytotoxic agents [44–46]. Again, at least 9 randomised trials have evaluated IFN-α in combination with various chemotherapy regimens (in more than 50 patients) [47–53]. The results are summarised in Table 8.2. In only one small study were the results in favour of the combination with IFN-α. The response rate was significantly superior in 2 studies and the progression-free survival in 2 studies. There was no significant overall survival benefit in 8 of the 9 trials.

Again a meta-analysis was performed on individual data of 2,469 patients [43]. Response rate was slightly, but significantly, better with IFN-α and progression-free survival was significantly longer (p = 0.0003) with a median time to progression increased by 6 months. However, there was no survival benefit.

Table 8.2 IFN-α in combination with chemotherapy in multiple myeloma. Results of studies with 50 patients or more with p values

	Number of patients	Chemotherapy regimen	Response rate	Progression-free survival	Overall survival
Montuoro et al. [47]	50	MP	0.05	<0.025	<0.025
Corrado et al. [48]	84	MP	NS	NS	NS
Osterborg et al. [49]	110	MP	<0.001	NS	NS
Cooper et al. [50]	272	MP	NS	NS	NS
Capnist et al. [42]	67	MP	NS	0.06	NS
Ludwig et al. [38]	256	VMCP	NS	0.05	NS
Oken et al. [51]	485	VBMCP	NS	0.07	NS
Casassus et al. [52]	282	VMCP/VBAP	NS	NS	NS
Joshua et al. [53]	113	CBAP	NS	0.005	NS

MP = melphalan-prednisone; VMCP = vincristine, melphalan, cyclophosphamide, prednisone; VBMCP = vincristine, BCNU, mephalan, cyclophosphamide, prednisone; VBAP = vincristine, BCNU, adriamycin, prednisone; CBAP = cyclophosphamide, BCNU, adriamycin, prednisone; NS = not significant.

CURRENT SITUATION

When adding trials with IFN-α in combination with chemotherapy to trials with mainten-ance IFN-α, the Myeloma Trialists' Collaborative Group showed a significant prolongation of progression-free survival (33 vs. 24% at 3 years, median 23 vs. 17 months) [43]. Overall survival was somewhat better with IFN-α (53 vs. 49% at 3 years, p = 0.01) but survival ben-efit was restricted to smaller trials. Another meta-analysis based only on published results showed similar results, with median improvements of 4.6 months in relapse-free and 3.7 months in overall survival [54]. Prolongation of remission without prolongation of survival was also observed in a large trial conducted by the Nordic Myeloma Study Group in which patients were randomly allocated to receive IFN-α through induction treatment, plateau phase and relapse [55]. This data raises the question of whether a 6-month prolongation of the remission with a marginal, if any, survival benefit justifies the cost and side-effects of this therapy. A quality-of-life study was integrated into the Nordic randomised trial [56]. During the first year of treatment, the occurrence of side-effects induced a moderate reduc-tion of the global quality-of-life score. Although response duration was prolonged by 6 months there was no quality-of-life benefit to compensate this early impairment.

In their meta-analysis, the Myeloma Trialists' Collaborative Group failed to show that the benefit of IFN-α differed between subgroups of patients. Good-risk patients or patients in complete remission after induction chemotherapy did not benefit more than the other patients [43].

After a period of great enthusiasm in the early 1990s, the use of IFN-α in the context of conventional chemotherapy in MM has dramatically decreased, mostly because many investigators were reluctant to use an expensive and potentially toxic drug in return for a relatively minor effect.

IFN-α IN THE CONTEXT OF AUTOLOGOUS STEM CELL TRANSPLANTATION

In younger patients (up to the age of 65), two randomised studies have shown that autolo-gous stem cell transplantation (ASCT) is superior to conventional chemotherapy and ASCT is now considered as the standard of care [57–58]. In a recently published Italian study, the use of 2 courses of intermediate-dose melphalan (100 mg/m^2) supported by ASCT was also shown to be superior to the classical melphalan-prednisone combination up to the age of 70 [59]. In all three studies, IFN-α was given as maintenance therapy and in the 1990s this approach was commonly used.

However, the clinical benefit of IFN-α after ASCT has never been demonstrated by a randomised trial. To date, only one study evaluating the impact of IFN-α compared to control patients in this setting has been published [60]. While both progression-free and overall survival were significantly longer at 4 years in the IFN-α maintenance arm, with a longer follow-up these differences ceased to be significant, because most patients ultimately relapsed and/or succumbed to their disease. However, this was a small study with only 85 randomised patients and the survival benefit of IFN-α might have been masked by the fact that half of the patients in the control arm received IFN-α after relapse.

Björkstrand and colleagues [61] have evaluated the impact of IFN-α maintenance in patients after ASCT in a retrospective European Registry analysis. In this study, 473 patients who received IFN-α maintenance treatment in complete or partial response after ASCT were compared with 419 similar patients who did not. Median overall and progression-free survival were significantly better in the IFN-α group (78 vs. 47 months, 29 vs. 20 months, respectively). The difference was more pronounced in patients who achieved only partial remission after ASCT.

However, a large randomised trial performed by a U.S. multi-centre intergroup did not show any benefit of maintenance with IFN-α after ASCT [62]. Although maintenance IFN-α (alone or in combination with corticosteroids) is still used by many investigators after ASCT, this will probably change in the near future. Thalidomide or its potentially more potent analogue (Revlimid®) is currently being tested for this indication and preliminary results with thalidomide are encouraging [63].

IFN-α IN NON-HODGKIN'S LYMPHOMA

Early clinical trials have shown that while IFN-α has no role in the treatment of patients with high-grade non-Hodgkin's lymphoma (NHL), it has clinical activity in low-grade NHL [64]. Given as a single agent, IFN-α induced 40–55% responses with approximately 10% complete remission in Phase II studies [64–65]. Phase III randomised trials were then designed to evaluate the impact of IFN-α in the overall management of low-grade NHL (mostly follicular type).

INITIAL TREATMENT IN FOLLICULAR NHL WITH A LOW TUMOUR BURDEN

A randomised study compared IFN-α with no initial treatment or with prednimustine in 193 patients with newly diagnosed FL with a low tumour burden [66]. Overall response to therapy was not reduced in the delayed treatment arm and initial treatment with IFN-α did not significantly increase survival. IFN-α is not indicated in this situation.

IFN-α AS MAINTENANCE THERAPY IN FOLLICULAR LYMPHOMAS

As in MM, IFN-α has been evaluated in low-grade NHL and mostly in FL as maintenance therapy in patients responding to their initial treatment.

Results of four large randomised trials appear to be controversial as shown in Table 8.3. In a recently published study, 384 patients in complete remission after 6 cycles of standard-dose chemotherapy with cyclophosphamide, epirubicin, vincristine, prednisone and bleomycin were randomly allocated to receive IFN-α three times a week for one year or no further treatment. Event-free and overall survival were significantly longer in the IFN-α arm [67]. The German Low-Grade Lymphoma Study Group reported a significant advantage in favour of IFN-α maintenance in terms of disease-free survival (median 37 vs. 20

Table 8.3   IFN-α as maintenance therapy in patients with follicular lymphoma responding to initial chemotherapy (p values)

	Number of patients	Induction chemotherapy	IFN-α	PFS	OS
Fisher et al. [70]	268	ProMACE/MOPP	2 MU/m² 3 × W	0.25	0.65
Hagenbeek et al. [69]	242	CVP	3 MU 3 × W	0.054	0.32
Aviles et al. [67]	384	CEOP-B	5 MU 3 × W	<0.01	0.001
Unterhalt et al. [68]	247	CVP or mitoxantrone/ prednisone	5 MU 3 × W	0.003	NA

PFS = Progression-free survival; OS = overall survival; ProMACE/MOPP = procarbazine, methotrexate, adriamycin, cyclophosphamide, etoposide/methotrexate, oncovin, procarbazine, prednisone; CVP = cyclophosphamide, vincristine, prednisone; CEOP-B = cyclophosphamide, epirubicin, vincristine, prednisone, bleomycin; MU = million units; 3 × W = 3 times weekly; NA = not available.

months in the control arm and 49 vs. 27% 4-year disease-free survival) [68]. In the European Organisation for Research and Treatment of Cancer (EORTC) study, 242 patients responding to a non-intensive induction chemotherapy with cyclophosphamide, vincristine and prednisone were also randomised between IFN-α maintenance and no further treatment. There was a trend in favour of IFN-α maintenance as regards time to progression, but no significant survival benefit [69]. In the Southwest Oncology Group (SWOG) study on 268 patients responding to the more intensive combination chemotherapy ProMACE/MOPP (procarbazine, methotrexate, adriamycin, cyclophosphamide, etoposide/ methotrexate, oncovin, procarbazine, prednisone), neither progression-free nor overall survival were significantly improved by IFN-α maintenance [70].

A recent randomised trial by the German Low-Grade Lymphoma Study Group compared ASCT and IFN-α maintenance in 260 patients in complete or partial remission after induction chemotherapy [71]. ASCT significantly improved progression-free survival compared with IFN-α (at 5 years 64.7 vs. 33.3%, p < 0.0001).

IFN-α IN COMBINATION WITH CHEMOTHERAPY IN FOLLICULAR LYMPHOMAS

In 1993, the Groupe d'Etudes des Lymphomes de l'Adulte published a randomised study comparing the combination of IFN-α plus a CHOP-like chemotherapy regimen (123 patients) vs. the same regimen without IFN-α (119 patients) [72]. Compared with the chemotherapy regimen alone, the combination of chemotherapy and IFN-α increased the response rate, and significantly improved the median time to treatment failure and the 3-year overall survival.

An updated analysis of this study confirmed, with a median follow-up of 6 years, that the combination of chemotherapy plus IFN-α still significantly improved median progression-free (2.9 vs. 1.5 years) and overall survival (not reached vs. 5.6 years) [73].

At the same time, the Eastern Cooperative Oncology Group (ECOG) published the same type of study in 249 patients with low- or intermediate-grade NHL treated with a CHOP-like regimen with or without IFN-α. There was a longer time to progression of borderline significance in favour of the IFN-α arm, but no survival benefit [74]. An updated analysis with a median follow-up of 12 years confirms that the combination significantly prolonged time to treatment failure (median 2.4 vs. 1.4 years) and induced a clinically but not statistically significant prolongation of overall survival (7.8 vs. 5.7 years) [75].

These two large studies support the addition of IFN-α to an anthracycline-based induction regimen in patients with low-grade NHL with a high tumour burden. Furthermore, a quality-of-life adjusted survival analysis applied to the French trial showed that the clinical benefits of IFN-α can significantly offset the associated grade 3 or worse toxic effects [76].

CURRENT SITUATION

Several randomised studies have evaluated the impact of IFN-α given both in combination with induction chemotherapy and as maintenance therapy [77–80]. It is more difficult to interpret these trials including a double randomisation. A recent meta-analysis of updated individual data in 1,922 patients from 10 Phase III randomised studies has evaluated the role of IFN-α in low-grade NHL (with and/or following chemotherapy) [81]. The addition of IFN-α to initial chemotherapy does not significantly influence the response rate. The differences in 5- and 10-year remission duration are 11 and 10%, respectively, in favour of IFN-α therapy. In the IFN-α arms, the 5- and 10-year survival rates are improved by 5.5 and 8%, respectively. However, there is a significant heterogeneity between the 10 studies. The survival advantage appeared to be restricted to the following conditions:

- relatively intensive initial chemotherapy
- dose ≥5 MU
- cumulative dose ≥36 MU per month
- with chemotherapy rather than as maintenance

All these results favour of the use of IFN-α in follicular NHL, at least in the conditions defined by the meta-analysis. However, the introduction of immunotherapy with monoclonal antibodies is probably going to change this scenario. Monotherapy with rituximab induces approximately 50% responses in relapsed low-grade NHL [82] and is capable of inducing complete and molecular remission in previously untreated patients [83, 84].

The combination of rituximab and chemotherapy appears to be superior to chemotherapy alone in terms of response rate, complete (and even molecular) remission rate and progression-free survival [85–87]. Extending treatment with multiple courses of rituximab prolongs time to treatment failure to 3–5 years [83, 88].

The role of IFN-α in combination with chemotherapy should therefore be re-evaluated in this new context. Preliminary results indicate that the combination of chemotherapy, IFN-α and rituximab appears be superior to chemotherapy plus IFN-α in terms of event-free survival and could compare favourably with rituximab-chemotherapy combinations [88, 89].

IFA-α IN OTHER LYMPHOPROLIFERATIVE DISORDERS

Most phase II clinical evaluations of IFN-α in patients with advanced chronic lymphocytic leukaemia have shown a low level of activity [90]. Although preliminary results in patients at early stages were encouraging [91], IFN-α has never been developed in this indication, mostly because of the superior activity of other agents (fludarabine, alemtuzumab and rituximab-containing regimes).

Some results have been observed in Waldenstrom's macroglobulinaemia [92–93], but again, they were not attractive enough to justify a clinical development in this indication where purine analogues, and more recently rituximab, have been shown to be very active.

A recently published randomised study has evaluated the impact of IFN-α maintenance in 88 patients with indolent non-follicular NHL responding to their initial chemotherapy [94]. No significant prolongation of progression-free survival was observed.

SUMMARY

IFN-α is effective in HCL but has largely been rapidly replaced by purine analogues. In MM, IFN-α given with chemotherapy or as maintenance therapy prolongs remission duration, but the survival benefit is marginal. It is still used after ASCT but will probably be replaced in the near future by thalidomide and its analogues.

In FL, IFN-α is useful specially when given in combination with relatively intensive chemotherapy for patients with a high tumour burden. However, the rapid development of strategies combining chemotherapy and immunotherapy with anti-CD20 antibodies will reduce its role or at least prompt re-evaluation of its impact.

REFERENCES

1. Borden EC, Ball LA. Interferons: biochemical, cell growth inhibitory and immunological effects. *Prog Hemat* 1981; 12:299–339.
2. Stark GR, Kerr IM, Williams BR *et al*. How cells respond to interferon. *Annu Rev Biochem* 1998; 67:227–264.
3. Dinney CP, Bielenberg DR, Perrotte P *et al*. Inhibition of basic fibroblast growth factor expression, angiogenesis and growth of human bladder carcinoma in mice by systemic interferon alpha administration. *Cancer Res* 1998; 58:808–814.
4. Arora T, Jelinek DF. Differential myeloma cell responsiveness to interferon-alpha correlates with differential induction of p19 (INK4 d) and cyclin D2 expression. *J Biol Chem* 1998; 273:11799–11805.
5. Sangfelt O, Erikson S, Castro J *et al*. Molecular mechanisms underlying interferon-alpha G0/G1 arrest: CKI mediated regulation of G1 cdk complexes and activation of pocket proteins. *Oncogene* 1999; 18:2798–2810.
6. Chen Q, Gong B, Mahmoud-Ahmed AS *et al*. Apo2L/Trial and Bcl-2 related proteins regulate type I interferon induced apoptosis in multiple myeloma. *Blood* 2001; 98:2183–2192.
7. Rossi G. Interferons and cell differentiation. In: Gresser I (ed) Interferon VI. Academic Press, London; 1985; pp 31–68.
8. Quesada JR, Reuben J, Manning JT *et al*. Alpha interferon for induction of remission in hairy-cell leukemia. *N Engl J Med* 1984; 310:15–18.
9. Golomb HM, Fefer A, Goide DW *et al*. Survival experience of 195 patients with hairy-cell leukemia treated in a multi-institutional study with interferon alpha. *Leuk Lymphoma* 1991; 4:99–102.
10. Ratain MJ, Golomb HM, Vardiman JW *et al*. Relapse after interferon alfa-2b therapy for hairy-cell leukemia: analysis of prognostic variables. *J Clin Oncol* 1998; 6:1714–1722.
11. Berman E, Heller G, Kempin S *et al*. Incidence of response and long-term follow-up in patients treated with recombinant interferon alfa-2a. *Blood* 1990; 75:839–847.
12. Smith JW, Longo DL, Urba WJ *et al*. Prolonged, continuous treatment of hairy-cell leukemia patients with recombinant interferon-alpha 2a. *Blood* 1991; 78:1664–1671.
13. Golomb HM, Ratain MJ, Fefer A *et al*. Low-dose interferon alpha-2b for the induction of remission of hairy cell leukaemia: a multi-institutional study of 49 patients. *Leuk Lymphoma* 1991; 5:335–340.
14. Grever M, Kopecky K, Foucar MK *et al*. Randomized comparison of pentostatin versus interferon alfa-2a in previously untreated patients with hairy-cell leukemia: an intergroup study. *J Clin Oncol* 1995; 13:947–982.
15. Maloisel F, Benboubker L, Gardembas M *et al*. Long-term outcome with pentostatin treatment in hairy-cell leukemia. A French retrospective study of 238 patients. *Leukemia* 2003; 17:45–51.
16. Cheson BD, Sorensen JM, Vena DA *et al*. Treatment of hairy-cell leukemia with 2-chlorodeoxyadenosine via the Group C protocol Mechanism of the National Cancer Institute: a report of 979 patients. *J Clin Oncol* 1998; 16:3007–3017.
17. Saven A, Burian C, Koziol JA *et al*. Long term follow-up of patients with hairy cell leukemia after cladribine treatment. *Blood* 1998; 92:1918–1926.
18. Goodman GR, Burian C, Koziol JA *et al*. Extended follow-up of patients with hairy cell leukemia after treatment with cladribine. *J Clin Oncol* 2003; 21:891–896.
19. Von Rohr A, Schmitz SF, Tichelli A *et al*. Treatment of hairy cell leukemia with cladribine by subcutaneous bolus injection: a phase II study. *Ann Oncol* 2002; 13:1641–1649.
20. Kurzrock R, Strom SS, Estey E *et al*. Second cancer risk in hairy cell leukemia: analysis of 350 patients. *J Clin Oncol* 1997; 15:1803–1810.
21. Au WY, Klasa RJ, Gallagher R *et al*. Second malignancies in patients with hairy cell leukemia in British Columbia: a 20-year experience. *Blood* 1998; 92:1160–1164.
22. Cheson BD, Vena DA, Barrett JJ. Second malignancies as a consequence of nucleoside analog therapy for chronic lymphoid leukemias. *J Clin Oncol* 1999; 17:2454–2460.

23. Kampmeier P, Spielberger R, Dickstein J *et al*. Increased incidence of second neoplasms in patients treated with interferon alpha 2b for hairy cell leukemia: a clinicopathologic assessment. *Blood* 1994; 83:2931–2938.
24. Troussard X, Henry-Amar M, Flandrin G. Second cancer risk after interferon therapy. *Blood* 1994; 84:3242–3243.
25. Federico M, Zinzani PL, Frassoldati *et al*. Risk of second cancers in patients with hairy cell leukemia: long-term follow-up. *J Clin Oncol* 2002; 20:638–666.
26. Mellstedt H, Aahre A, Björkholm M *et al*. Interferon therapy in myelomatosis. *Lancet* 1979; 1:245–247.
27. Bataille R, Harousseau JL. Multiple myeloma. *N Engl J Med* 1997; 336:1657–1664.
28. Cooper MR. Interferon in the management of multiple myeloma. *Semin Oncol* 1988; 15:21–25.
29. Ahre A, Bjorkholm M, Osterborg A *et al*. High doses of natural alpha-interferon (alpha-IFN) in the treatment of multiple myeloma: a pilot study from the Myeloma Group of Central Sweden. *Eur J Haematol* 1998; 41:123–130.
30. Quesada JR, Alexanian R, Hawkins M *et al*. Treatment of multiple myeloma with recombinant alpha-interferon. *Blood* 1996; 67:275–278.
31. Ahre A, Bjorkholm M, Mellstedt H *et al*. Human leukocyte interferon and intermittent high-dose melphalan-prednisone administration in the treatment of multiple myeloma: a randomised clinical trial from the Myeloma Group of Central Sweden. *Cancer Treat Rep* 1984; 68:1331–1338.
32. Ludwig H, Cortelezzi A, Scheithauer W *et al*. Recombinant interferon alpha-2c versus polychemotherapy (VMCP) for treatment of multiple myeloma: a prospective randomized trial. *Eur J Cancer Clin Oncol* 1986; 22:1111–1117.
33. Mandelli F, Avvisati G, Amadori S *et al*. Maintenance treatment with recombinant interferon alfa-2b in patients with multiple myeloma responding to conventional induction chemotherapy. *N Engl J Med* 1990; 322:1430–1434.
34. Pulsoni A, Avvisati G, Teresa-Petrucci M *et al*. The Italian experience on interferon as maintenance treatment in multiple myeloma: ten years after. *Blood* 1998; 92:2184–2186
35. Salmon SE, Crowley JJ, Grogan TM *et al*. Combination chemotherapy, glucorticoids and interferon alpha in the treatment of multiple myeloma: a Southwest Oncology Group study. *J Clin Oncol* 1994; 12:2405–2414.
36. Browman GP, Bergsagel D, Sicheri D *et al*. Randomized trial of interferon maintenance in multiple myeloma: a study of the National Cancer Institute of Canada Clinical Trials Group. *J Clin Oncol* 1995; 13:2354–2360.
37. Westin J, Rodjer S, Turesson P *et al*. Interferon alfa-2b versus no maintenance therapy during the plateau phase in multiple myeloma: a randomized study. *Br J Haematol* 1995; 89:561–568.
38. Ludwig H, Cohen AM, Polliack A *et al*. Interferon alpha for induction and maintenance in multiple myeloma: results of two multicenter randomized trials and summary of other studies. *Ann Oncol* 1995; 6:467–476.
39. Peest D, Deicher H, Coldewey R *et al*. A comparison of polychemotherapy and Melphalan/prednisone for primary remission induction and interferon alpha for maintenance treatment in multiple myeloma. A prospective trial of the German Myeloma Treatment Group. *Eur J Cancer* 1995; 31A:145–151.
40. Drayson NT, Chapman CE, Dunn JA *et al*. MRC trial of alpha2b-interferon maintenance therapy in first plateau phase of multiple myeloma. *Br J Haematol* 1998; 101:195–202.
41. Blade J, San Miguel J, Escudero ML *et al*. Maintenance treatment with interferon alpa-2b in multiple myeloma: a prospective randomized trial from Pethema. *Leukemia* 1998; 12:1144–1148.
42. Capnist G, Vespignani M, Spriano M *et al*. Impact of interferon at induction chemotherapy and maintenance treatment for multiple myeloma. Preliminary results of a multicenter study by the Italian non-Hodgkin's lymphoma Cooperative Study. *Acta Oncol* 1994; 33:527–529.
43. The Myeloma Trialist's Collaborative Group: Interferon as therapy for multiple myeloma: an individual patient data overview of 24 randomized trials and 4,012 patients. *Br J Haematol* 2001; 113:1020–1034.
44. Aapro MS, Alberts DS, Salmon SE. Interactions of human leucocyte interferon with vinca alkaloids and other chemotherapeutic agents against human tumors in clonogenic assay. *Cancer Chemother Pharmacol* 1983; 10:161–166.
45. Balkwill FR, Moodey EM. Positive interactions between interferon and cyclophosphamide or adriamycin in a human tumor model system. Cancer Res 1985; 44:906–908.
46. Welander CE, Morgan TM, Homesley HD *et al*. Combined recombinant human interferon alpha 2 and cytotoxic agents studied in the clonogenic assay. *Int J Cancer* 1985; 35:721–729.
47. Montuoro A, De Rosa L, De Balsio A *et al*. Alpha-2 interferon/melphalan/prednisone versus melphalan plus prednisone in previously untreated patients with multiple myeloma. *Br J Haematol* 1990; 76:365–368.

48. Corrado C, Flores A, Pavlosky S et al. Randomized trial of melphalan prednisone with or without recombinant alfa-2 interferon (ralphaZIFN) in multiple myeloma. *Proc Am Soc Clin Oncol* 1991; 10:304a.

49. Osterborg A, Bjorkholm M, Bjoneman M et al. Natural interferon alpha in combination with melphalan/prednisone versus melphalan/prednisone in the treatment of multiple myeloma stages II and III: a randomized study from the Myeloma Group of Central Sweden. *Blood* 1993; 81:1428–1434.

50. Cooper MR, Dear K, McIntyre OR et al. A randomized clinical trial comparing melphalan/prednisone with or without interferon alpha-2b in newly diagnosed patients with multiple myeloma: a Cancer and Leukemia Group B Study. *J Clin Oncol* 1993; 11:155–160.

51. Oken MM, Leong T, Kay NE et al. The effect of adding interferon or high-dose cyclophosphamide to VBMCP to treat multiple myeloma results of an ECOG phase III trial. *Blood* 1995; 86(suppl 1):441a.

52. Casassus P, Pegourie-Bandelier B, Sadouna A et al. Randomized comparison of interferon with VMCP/VBAP as the induction phase of untreated multiple myeloma: results of the KIF multicentric trial. *Blood* 1995; 86(suppl 1):441a.

53. Joshua DE, Penny R, Mathews JP et al. Australian Leukaemic Study Group Myeloma II: a randomized trial of intensive combination chemotherapy with or without interferon in patients with myeloma. *Br J Haematol* 1995; 6:467–476.

54. Fritz E, Ludwig H. Interferon α treatment in multiple myeloma: meta-analysis of 30 randomized trials among 3,948 patients. *Ann Oncol* 2000; 11:1427–1436.

55. The Nordic Myeloma Study Group. Interferon-alpha 2b added to melphalan-prednisone for initial and maintenance therapy in multiple myeloma: a randomized, controlled trial. *Ann Intern Med* 1996; 124:212–222.

56. Wisloff F, Hjorth M, Kaasa S et al. Effect of interferon on the health related quality of life of multiple myeloma patients: results of a Nordic randomized trial comparing melphalan-prednisone and melphalan-prednisone + alpha-interferon. *Br J Haematol* 1996; 94:324–332.

57. Attal M, Harousseau JL, Stoppa AM et al. A prospective, randomized trial of autologous bone marrow transplantation and chemotherapy in multiple myeloma. *N Engl J Med* 1996; 335:91–97.

58. Child JA, Morgan GJ, Davies FC et al. High-dose chemotherapy with hematopoietic stem-cell rescue for multiple myeloma. *N Engl J Med* 2003; 348:1875–1883.

59. Palumbo A, Bringhen S, Petrucci MT et al. Intermediate-dose melphalan improves survival of myeloma patients aged 50–70: results of a randomized controlled trial. Blood 2004; 104:3052–3057.

60. Cunningham D, Powles R, Malpas J et al. A randomised trial of maintenance interferon following high-dose chemotherapy in multiple myeloma: long-term follow-up results. *Br J Haematol* 1998; 102:495–502.

61. Bjorkstrand B, Svensson H, Goldschmidt H et al. Alpha-interferon maintenance treatment is associated with improved survival after high-dose treatment and autologous stem cell transplantation in patients with multiple myeloma: retrospective registry study from the European Group for *Blood* and Marrow Transplantation (EBMT). *Bone Marrow Transplant* 2001; 27:511–515.

62. Crowley J, Fonseca R, Greipp P et al. Comparable survival in newly diagnosed multiple myeloma (MM) after VAD induction with high dose therapy using melphalan 140 mg/m^2 + TBI 12 Gy (MEL + TBI) versus standard therapy with VBMCP and no benefit from interferon (IFN) maintenance: final clinical results of Intergroup Trial S9321 in the context of IFM 90 and MRC VII trials. *Blood* 2004; 104:156a–157a.

63. Attal M, Harousseau JL, Leyvraz S et al. Maintenance treatment with Thalidomide after autologous transplantation for myeloma: first analysis of a prospective randomized study of the Intergroupe Francophone du Myelome (IFM99–02). *Blood* 2004; 104:155a.

64. Gaynor ER, Fischer RI. Clinical trials of α-Interferon in the treatment of non-Hodgkin's lymphoma. *Semin Oncol* 1991; 18:12–17.

65. Foon KA, Roth MS, Bunn PAJ. Interferon therapy of non-Hodgkin's lymphoma. *Cancer* 1987; 59:601–604.

66. Brice P, Bastion Y, Lepage E et al. Comparison in low-tumor burden follicular lymphoma between an initial no treatment policy, prednimustine and interferon alpha: a randomized study from the Groupe d'Etude des Lymphomes Folliculaires Groupe d'Etude des Lymphomes de l'Adulte. *J Clin Oncol* 1997; 15:1110–1117.

67. Aviles A, Neri N, Huerta-Guzman J et al. Interferon alpha 2b as maintenance therapy improves outcome in follicular lymphoma. *Leuk Lymphoma* 2004; 45:2247–2251.

68. Unterhalt M, Hermann R, Koch P et al. Long term interferon alpha maintenance prolongs remission duration in advanced low grade lymphomas and is related to the efficacy of initial cytoreductive chemotherapy. *Blood* 1996; 88(supp 1):453a.

69. Hagenbeek A, Carde P, Meerwaldt JH *et al*. Maintenance of remission with human recombinant interferon alfa-2a in patients with stages III and IV low-grade malignant non-Hodgkin's lymphoma. European Organization for Research and Treatment of Cancer Lymphoma Cooperative Group. *J Clin Oncol* 1998; 16:41–47.

70. Fisher RI, Dana BW, Le Blanc M *et al*. Interferon alpha consolidation after intensive chemotherapy does not prolong the progression-free survival of patients with low-grade non-Hodgkin's lymphoma: results of the Southwest Oncology Group randomized phase III study 8809. *J Clin Oncol* 2000; 18:2010–2016.

71. Lenz G, Dreyling M, Schiegnitz E *et al*. Myeloablative radiochemotherapy followed by autologous stem cell transplantation in first remission prolongs progression-free survival in folicular lymphoma: results of a prospective randomized trial of the German low-grade lymphoma Study Group. *Blood* 2004; 104:2667–2674

72. Solal-Celigny P, Lepage E, Brousse N *et al*. Recombinant interferon alfa-2b combined with a regimen containing doxorubicin in patients with advanced follicular lymphoma. Groupe d'Etudes des Lymphomes de l'Adulte. *N Engl J Med* 1993; 329:1608–1614.

73. Solal-Celigny P, Lepage E, Brousse N *et al*. Doxorubicin-containing regimen with or without interferon alfa-2b for advanced follicular lymphomas: final analysis of survival and toxicity in the Groupe d'Etude des Lymphomes Folliculaires 86 Trial. *J Clin Oncol* 1998; 16:2332–2338.

74. Smalley RW, Anderson JW, Hawkins MJ *et al*. Interferon alfa combined with cytotoxic chemotherapy for patients with non-Hodgkin's lymphoma. *N Engl J Med* 1992; 327:1336–1341.

75. Smalley RW, Weller E, Hawkins MJ *et al*. Final analysis of the ECOG I-COPA trial (E6484) in patients with non-Hodgkin's lymphoma treated with interferon alfa (IFN alpha 2a) plus an anthracycline-based induction regimen. *Leukemia* 2001; 15:1118–1122.

76. Cole BF, Solal-Celigny P, Gelber RD *et al*. Quality-of-life adjusted survival analysis of interferon alfa-2b treatment for advanced follicular lymphoma: an aid to clinical decision making. *J Clin Oncol* 1998; 16:2339–2344.

77. Rohatiner A, Radford J, Deakin D *et al*. A randomised controlled trial to evaluate the role of interferon as initial and maintenance therapy in patients with follicular lymphoma. *Br J Cancer* 2001; 85:29–35.

78. Peterson BA, Petroni GR, Oken MM *et al*. Cyclophosphamide versus cyclophosphamide plus interferon alfa-2b in follicular low-grade lymphoma. *Proc Am Soc Clin Oncol* 1997; 16:14a.

79. Chisesi T, Gongiu M, Contu A *et al*. Randomized study of chlorambucil (CB) compared to interferon alfa-2b combined with CB in low-grade non-Hodgkin's lymphoma: an interim report of a randomized study. Non-Hodgkin's Lymphoma Cooperative Study. *Eur J Cancer* 1991; 24:531–533.

80. Arranz R, Garcia-Alfonso P, Sobrino P *et al*. Role of interferon alfa-2b in the induction and maintenance treatment of low grade non-Hodgkin's lymphoma: results form a prospective, multicenter trial with double randomization. *J Clin Oncol* 1998; 16:1538–1546.

81. Rohatiner AZS, Gregory WM, Peterson B *et al*. Meta-analysis to evaluate the role of interferon in follicular lymphoma. *J Clin Oncol* 2005; online.

82. McLaughlin P, Grillo-Lopez AJ, Link BK *et al*. Rituximab chimeric anti-CD20 monoclonal antibody therapy for relapsed indolent lymphoma. Half of patients respond to a four-dose treatment. *J Clin Oncol* 1998; 16:2825–2833.

83. Hainsworth JD, Burrism HA, Morrissey LH *et al*. Rituximab monoclonal antibody as initial therapy for patients with low-grade non-Hodgkin's lymphoma. *Blood* 2000; 95:3052–3056.

84. Colombat P, Salles G, Brousse N *et al*. Rituximab (anti-CD20 monoclonal antibody) as single first-line therapy for patients with follicular lymphoma with a low tumor burden: clinical and molecular evaluation. *Blood* 2001; 97:101–106.

85. Czucman MS, Weaver R, Alkuzweny B *et al*. Prolonged clinical and molecular remission in patient with low-grade follicular non-Hodgkin's lymphoma treated with rituximab plus CHOP chemotherapy: 9-year follow-up. *J Clin Oncol* 2004; 23:4659–4664.

86. Hiddeman W, Dreyling MH, Forstpointner R *et al*. Combined immuno-chemotherapy (R-CHOP) significantly improves time to treatment failure in first line therapy of follicular lymphoma: results of a prospective randomized trial of the German Low Grade lymphoma study group. *Blood* 2003; 102:104a.

87. Marcus R, Imrie K, Belch A *et al*. An international multicenter, randomized open-label, phase III trial comparing rituximab added to CVP chemotherapy to CVP chemotherapy alone in untreated stage III/IV follicular non-Hodgkin's lymphoma. *Blood* 2003; 102:28a.

88. Ghielmini M, Schmitz SF, Cogliatti SB *et al*. Prolonged treatment with rituximab in patients with follicular lymphoma significantly increases event-free survival and response duration with the standard weekly × 4 schedules. *Blood* 2004; 103:4416–4423.

89. Salles GA, Foussard C, Mounier N *et al*. Rituximab added to αIFN + CHVP improves the outcome of follicular lymphoma patients with a high tumor burden: first analysis of the GELA-GOELAMS FL-2000 randomized trial in 359 patients. *Blood* 2004; 104:49a.

90. Schiffer CA. Interferon studies in the treatment of patients with leukemia. *Semin Oncol* 1991; 18(suppl 1):1–6.

91. Rozman C, Montserrat E, Vinolas N *et al*. Recombinant alpha2-interferon in the treatment of B chronic lymphocytic leukaemia in early stages. *Blood* 1988; 71:1295–1298.

92. Rotoli B, De Renzo A, Frigeri F *et al*. A phase II trial on alpha-interferon effect in patients with monoclonal IgM gammopathy. *Leuk Lymphoma* 1994; 13:463–469.

93. Legouffe E, Rossi JF, Laporte JP *et al*. Treatment of Waldenstrom's macroglobulinemia with very low doses of alpha interferon. *Leuk Lymphoma* 1995; 19:337–342.

94. Baldini L, Brugiatelli M, Luminari S *et al*. Treatment of indolent B-cell non follicular lymphomas: final results of the LL01 randomized trial of the Gruppo Italiano per la Studio dei Lymphomi. *J Clin Oncol* 2003; 21:1459–1465.

9

Radioimmunotherapy safety: radiation protection, administration guidelines, isotope comparison, and quality of life issues

B. T. Brinker, L. I. Gordon

INTRODUCTION

The U.S. Food and Drug Administration (FDA) approved two radioimmunotherapeutic agents, Yttrium-90 (^{90}Y) ibritumomab tiuxetan (Zevalin; IDEC Pharmaceuticals Corporation, San Diego, CA) in 2002 and Iodine-131 (^{131}I) tositumomab (Bexxar; Corixa Corporation, South San Francisco, CA and GlaxoSmithKline, Philadelphia, PA) in 2003 for the treatment of relapsed or refractory low-grade, follicular, or transformed B-cell lymphoma. Yttrium-90 ibritumomab was approved in Europe in January 2004 (Zevalin; Schering AE, Berlin, Germany) and is at present the only radioimmunotherapy (RIT) available in Europe for this indication. Considered a scientific and clinical breakthrough, these radiolabelled monoclonal antibodies (MAbs) combined the targeted immune mechanisms of anti-CD20 immunotherapy with cytolytic ionising radiation to give patients durable remissions with minimal toxicity. Investigators reported response rates of 60–80% for patients with heavily pre-treated low-grade, follicular, and transformed lymphomas who were treated with ^{90}Y ibritumomab tiuxetan and ^{131}I tositumomab in phase I and II trials [1–8]. For responding patients, median disease-free survival was 6–14 months. With activity also observed in patients who were refractory to the anti-CD20 MAb, rituximab (Rituxan; Cellgene, Cambridge, MA), the clinical potential of these promising agents continues to expand [9, 10].

Though other radioimmunoconjugates have been developed, ^{90}Y ibritumomab tiuxetan and ^{131}I tositumomab remain the principle agents of RIT. Tositumomab is a murine, anti-CD20 antibody that targets the CD20 antigen on B lymphocytes. The antibody is directly chelated to ^{131}I to create the radiolabelled MAb, ^{131}I tositumomab. The formation of ^{90}Y ibritumomab tiuxetan requires the linker protein, tiuxetan, to chelate ^{90}Y to the murine, anti-CD20 immunoglobulin, ibritumomab.

There are no randomised studies to compare the efficacy of ^{131}I tositumomab and ^{90}Y ibritumomab tiuxetan, though an FDA-mandated trial is in progress. However, there are additional points to consider when selecting a radioimmunoconjugate for treatment. These agents have differences in terms of anti-tumour activity, radiation safety, treatment protocol, and toxicity that can impact clinical efficacy and patient's quality of life. The differences are due to the inherent qualities of ^{90}Y and ^{131}I. Understanding how the radioisotope emission

Brett Thomas Brinker, MD, Hematology/Oncology Fellow, Division of Hematology/Oncology, Northwestern University Feinberg School of Medicine, Chicago, Ilinois, USA.

Leo I. Gordon, MD, Abby & John Friend Professor of Cancer Research, Chief, Division of Hematology/Oncology, Northwestern University Feinberg School of Medicine, Division of Hematology/Oncology, Chicago Ilinois, USA.

Table 9.1 Comparison of physical and clinical characteristics of ^{90}Y and ^{131}I

Property	^{131}I	^{90}Y
Particle type	Beta, gamma	Beta
Particulate energy (MeV)[1]	Gamma 0.36, Beta 0.6	2.2
Path length (mm)	0.8	5.3
Half-life (days)	8.1	2.6
Stability	Stable radioimmunoconjugate with tositumomab	Requires tiuxetan-chelating agent to form stable radioimmunoconjugate
Immunoconjugate dissociation	De-halogenation possible due to longer half-life and if Mab bound to internalising antigens	<1% dissociation observed [14]
Imaging/Therapy	Imaging and therapy performed with ^{131}I Mab	No gamma rays for imaging. Requires ^{111}In for imaging
Dosimetry	Required. Based on clearance of tracer dose of ^{131}I	Not required. Dosing determined by patient weight and platelet count
Elective admission for therapy	Possibly gamma rays increase radiation-exposure risk to patient contacts. Out-patient therapy if patient suitable and release guidelines are followed.	No. Outpatient therapy is routine. Release guidelines are necessary.
Cost	Low	High

[1]Million electron volts.

profile affects the radiolabelled MAb may provide guidance when selecting the best agent for each patient. This chapter will compare the advantages and disadvantages of ^{90}Y and ^{131}I and their respective radioimmunoconjugates. Factors that will be discussed include the properties of each radionuclide and radiation safety for patient, healthcare worker, and patient family, as well as therapy administration, treatment toxicities, and the impact that these factors have on a patient's quality of life.

RADIOISOTOPE PROPERTIES

Radioisotopes vary in the type of radioactive emission, energy, path length, and half-life as well as biodistribution and stability. While a clearly superior radioisotope has not been identified, certain properties make radionuclides more attractive for immunoconjugation. Early RIT trials were conducted with ^{131}I for several reasons: it was inexpensive, investigators were familiar with its use in the treatment of thyroid disease, the radiolabelling techniques available were well defined, and both imaging (gamma emission) and therapeutic (beta emission) benefits were achievable with the same isotope. While other radionuclides have been used to construct radioimmunoconjugates in addition to ^{131}I including ^{125}I, ^{186}Re, ^{67}Cu, and others, ^{90}Y gained popularity among investigators because it was a high-energy, pure beta-emitting isotope that did not emit potentially harmful gamma particles. Table 9.1 compares several properties of ^{131}I and ^{90}Y that are discussed in detail below.

PARTICLE EMISSIONS

Radionuclides emit one or more of three types of radioactive particles called alpha, beta, or gamma photons with low, intermediate, and high tissue penetration, respectively (Figure 9.1). Alpha emissions have a high linear energy transfer with a particularly short range. Beta emissions have a longer range of emissions and gamma particles have the longest path length of

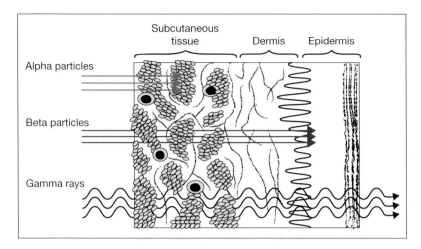

Figure 9.1 Comparative tissue penetration of particulate and electromagnetic radiation/reproduced with permission [30].

the three photon types. For RIT, emission path length is clinically relevant because alpha and beta emissions are not able to pass through the epidermis of patients treated with these isotopes, and the risk of radiation exposure to the environment is essentially non-existent. Gamma waves, on the other hand, are longer and are able to pass through the epidermis of treated patients. This property has clinical utility because the gamma emissions can be detected for imaging and can be used to document appropriate tumour uptake of gamma-emitting radioimmunoconjugates. Gamma waves can be problematic, however, because there are significant radiation safety concerns with these long-range emissions. When utilised in high doses, patients treated with isotopes that emit gamma waves have required isolation to prevent radiation exposure to family members, other patients, and heathcare workers.

^{131}I emits both gamma and beta particles, which makes both imaging and treatment with ^{131}I tositumomab possible. Patients treated with ^{131}I tositumomab, however, have also required strict in-patient isolation due to the environmental exposure risk. ^{90}Y emits only beta particles. While there is no gamma decay and subsequent radiation risk that necessitates in-patient administration of ^{90}Y ibritumomab tiuxetan, the use of additional gamma-emitting isotopes such as Indium-111 (^{111}In) is necessary for imaging purposes. Until recently, one major advantage of ^{90}Y ibritumomab tiuxetan was that patients could be treated on an out-patient basis while patients receiving ^{131}I tositumomab required one week of hospitalisation. The Nuclear Regulatory Commission (NRC) has published new guidelines, however, that permit most patients treated with ^{131}I tositumomab to receive therapy as out-patients [11].

ENERGY, PATH LENGTH, AND HALF-LIFE

^{131}I beta photons are emitted with a maximum energy of 0.61 MeV (million electron volts) and half-life of 8.1 days. Ninety percent of the particle emissions are released within a path length of 0.8 mm that is cytotoxic over several cell diameters. By contrast, ^{90}Y beta particles have a maximum energy of 2.2 MeV with a shorter half-life of 2.6 days. Whether it is more efficacious for a radionuclide to have higher energy with shorter half-life or lower energy with longer half-life is debatable. The shorter half-life of ^{90}Y correlates more closely with the half-life of its carrier antibody which may, however, reduce the risk of dissociation and non-specific radiation to healthy tissue. ^{90}Y beta photons are emitted over a path length of 5.3 mm. This is approximately seven times the length of ^{131}I photons and translates to a cytotoxic radius of 100–200 cell diameters [12]. This is a potential advantage for ^{90}Y-radiolabelled MAbs because the greater percentage of energy distributed over a longer path length allows for increased cytotoxicity for both targeted and neighbouring tumour cells through a 'bystander' effect. Clinically, ^{90}Y may be better suited to treating large or poorly vascu-larised tumours where antibody penetration is poor or to treat tumours that have weak or heterogeneous CD20 expression on tumour cells. In one phase III trial of patients with low-grade non-Hodgkin's lymphoma (NHL) treated with RIT, multi-variate analysis demon-strated that improved response rates were associated with treatment of bulky disease (tumour size ≥5 cm) with ^{90}Y ibritumomab tiuxetan [13]. Enhanced response rates were also observed when patients with nonbulky disease (tumour size <500 g) received ^{131}I tositu-momab [4]. Accordingly, ^{90}Y treatment may not be optimal for patients with smaller, less bulky disease as the longer particle path length of ^{90}Y emissions may expose a greater pro-portion of normal tissue to radiation compared with tumour cells.

STABILITY OF RADIOIMMUNOCONJUGATES

In general, ^{131}I forms stable radioimmunoconjugates and by comparison to ^{90}Y ibritumomab tiuxetan, the process of linking ^{131}I to its carrier anti-CD20 antibody, tositumomab, is straight-forward. The radiochemistry of ^{90}Y ibritumomab tiuxetan is complex and requires the chelat-ing protein, tiuxetan, to link ^{90}Y to ibritumomab. The radiolabelled MAb is stable, however, and the dissociation of ^{90}Y from ibritumomab *in vitro* is less than 1% per day [14, 15]. Of some concern, however, is the propensity for ^{131}I to dissociate through de-halogenation from its car-rier MAb. This process can be problematic as iodine and ^{131}I are released into the bloodstream and free radionuclide can result in non-specific radiation exposure to normal tissue. While a considerable amount of free ^{131}I is excreted in the urine, the radionuclide can also localise to the thyroid and cause end-organ damage, such as hypothyroidism. The particularly long half-life of ^{131}I may increase the risk of de-halogenation to some degree. However, the great-est risk of de-halogenation occurs when ^{131}I MAbs are targeted to antigens that internalise upon antibody binding. Because bound CD20 does not internalise, de-halogenation is less problematic for ^{131}I tositumomab. In addition, the risk of thyroid toxicity has been signifi-cantly reduced with the practice of administering supersaturated potassium iodine (SSKI) or Lugol's solution to block iodine uptake in the thyroid at the time of ^{131}I exposure [1].

DOSIMETRY

There are essentially two techniques that have been used to determine the dose of radio-immunoconjugate to administer to patients that will maximise tumour reduction and minimise toxicity to normal organs [16]. Utilising both gamma emissions for imaging and therapeutic beta emissions with the same radionuclide, ^{131}I tositumomab administration requires stan-dard dosimetry [3, 17]. Due to variability in ^{131}I urinary excretion between patients and pos-sible de-halogenation, this technique is well suited for ^{131}I ibritumomab as calculations arrive at a patient-specific dose to achieve the best ratio between therapeutic benefit and toxicity. For dosimetry calculations, the dose of radiolabelled MAb is based on dose-limiting toxicity to a specific organ: red marrow or the total body in the case of non-myeloablative RIT and secondary organs (lung, liver, kidneys) for myeloablative therapy. Patients receive an attenu-ated dose of radiolabelled tracer prior to a higher, therapeutic dose. Based on this pre-therapy dose, imaging can demonstrate the proper biodistribution of the radioimmunoconjugate and calculations can predict clearance of the radiolabelled MAb. Assuming a proportional rela-tionship of radiation exposure to critical organs between tracer and therapeutic dosing levels, a safe therapeutic dose can be determined. For ^{131}I tositumomab, therapeutic doses in the range of 50–160 mCi are administered to achieve a maximum tolerated dose of 65–75 cGy for patients with platelet counts greater than 150,000/μl.

A second method determines the dose of radioimmunoconjugate based on a fixed amount of radionuclide activity adjusted for body weight or body surface area. In this setting, if a standardised dose of radiolabelled MAb demonstrates a predictable rate of clearance with acceptable toxicity for a defined patient population, pre-therapy dosimetry calculations can be discontinued. Dosimetry studies in early clinical trials of ^{90}Y ibritumomab tiuxetan were conducted to predict the biodistribution, absorbed radiation to tumour end organs, and to correlate absorbed radiation with end-organ toxicity. Because ^{90}Y does not emit gamma photons, dosimetry requires a tracer dose of gamma-emitting ^{111}In for imaging. In a phase I/II trial of 56 patients with relapsed and refractory NHL receiving treatment with ^{90}Y ibritumomab tiuxetan, dosimetry calculations were used to predict absorbed radiation dose to tumour, marrow, and solid organs. After administration of a tracer dose of ^{111}In chelated to ibritumomab, serial blood sampling, quantitative gamma camera imaging, and MIRDOSE3 software (Radiation Internal Dose Information Center, Oak Ridge Institute for Science and Education, Oak Ridge, TN) were used to demonstrate that radiation exposure did not exceed pre-specified limits of 20 Gy to solid organs and 3 Gy to red marrow, and that all patients were able to receive a therapeutic dose of ^{90}Y ibritumomab tiuxetan. Furthermore, transient haematotoxicity correlated with pre-treatment haematological function and not the estimated radiation dose to red marrow [18]. Dosimetry studies were also conducted in a ^{90}Y ibritumomab tiuxetan phase III trial and demonstrated that haematotoxicity did not correlate with standard dosimetric parameters [19]. These findings are consistent with ^{90}Y data that demonstrated little dissociation of the ^{90}Y ibritumomab tiuxetan immunoconjugate and minimal inter-patient variability of radionuclide urinary clearance [14, 15, 20]. On the basis of these studies, non-myeloablative ^{90}Y ibritumomab tiuxetan is now administered to patients with low-grade B-cell lymphoma at a standard dose of 0.4 mCi/kg for platelet counts greater than 150,000/ml or at a reduced dose of 0.3 mCi/kg for platelet counts of 100,000–149,000/ml.

RADIATION PROTECTION

Because ^{90}Y isotopes do not emit tissue-penetrating gamma photons, there is little risk of radiation exposure to healthcare workers, patients' family members, and others who come in contact with patients treated with ^{90}Y ibritumomab tiuxetan. Patients receive ^{90}Y ibritumomab tiuxetan on an out-patient basis and can be released immediately after treatment with few restrictions [15]. General release guidelines are available and provide an opportunity to discuss a few precautionary points with patients (Table 9.2).

Out-patient treatment with ^{90}Y ibritumomab tiuxetan is in accordance with guidelines published by the NRC [21]. According to the NRC, the out-patient administration of radiotherapy limits the radiation exposure of patient contacts to 500 mrem. For ^{90}Y ibritumomab tiuxetan, in-patient treatment would require an initial dose of at least 38,500 mCi to exceed the out-patient limit. Because treatment doses are in the range of 20–30 mCi and are approximately 1,000-fold less than the NRC limit, the out-patient administration of ^{90}Y ibritumomab is safe and acceptable. A study of family members of patients treated with ^{90}Y ibritumomab tiuxetan also determined that the radiation exposure to patient contacts was low. In the trial, 13 family members with close patient contact were asked to wear dosimeters for 7 days after patients received ^{90}Y ibritumomab tiuxetan. The median radiation exposure was 3.5 mrem and was within the range of normal background radiation [22].

Radiation precautions that restrict patient contact such as shielding, minimising time of exposure, and maximising distance from the radioactive source are not necessary for healthcare personnel who work with ^{90}Y ibritumomab tiuxetan. However, providers should exercise universal precautions when preparing, transporting, or administering ^{90}Y ibritumomab tiuxetan. Direct contact with body fluids should be avoided and gloves should be worn. Normal amounts of blood from menstruation, cuts, or haemorrhoids do not contain a significant

Table 9.2   Patient release instructions after treatment with ^{90}Y ibritumomab tiuxetan [31]

For 3 days after treatment:
- Clean up spilled urine and dispose of body-fluid-contaminated material so that others will not inadvertently handle it (i.e., flush down the toilet or place in a plastic bag in household trash)
- Wash hands thoroughly after using the toilet for one week after treatment
- Use condoms for sexual relations

enough amount of radioactivity to be an exposure risk [15]. The ^{90}Y radioimmunoconjugate can be transported safely in plastic or acrylic vial shields. Transportation in lead containers is not recommended due to bremsstrahlung radiation — increased radioactive emissions that are a result of the interaction between emitted particles from radionuclides and heavy metals.

Before the NRC published the revised criteria in 1997, the requirement for out-patient administration of radioactive materials was based on the total dose activity administered to patients. This placed patients receiving ^{131}I immunoconjugates at a tremendous disadvantage because all patients required in-patient admission for several days after treatment. When the NRC changed the guidelines to its current definition based on radiation absorbed by maximally exposed patient contacts, the out-patient administration of ^{131}I tositumomab became possible.

Several studies have documented that the radiation absorbed by close patient contacts is below the NRC limit of 500 mrem. In one study, 26 family members of 22 patients receiving ^{131}I tositumomab wore dosimeters for 2–17 days after RIT treatment. All radiation doses received by caregivers were within the NRC out-patient limit (range 17–409 mrem), and the authors concluded that administration of ^{131}I tositumomab can be performed confidently on an out-patient basis [23]. In a larger study of 139 patients treated with ^{131}I tositumomab, the mean estimated dose to the maximally exposed individuals was 306 mrem (range 195–496 mrem) and all patient contacts were under the NRC limit [24].

In summary, it is now possible to treat patients receiving ^{131}I tositumomab as out-patients. Release instructions have been developed in accordance with the NRC guidelines and are essential to ensure that the radiation exposure to maximally exposed patient contacts is under the 500 mrem limit established by the NRC (Table 9.3). The release instructions are more extensive than the ^{90}Y ibritumomab guidelines but with ample time for review and questions, patients can adhere to the temporary restrictions.

QUALITY OF LIFE

There are several aspects of therapy with radiolabelled immunoconjugates that impact the quality of life of patients. Points to consider include the method of RIT administration, cost, and short- and long-term toxicities. Both ^{131}I tositumomab and ^{90}Y ibritumomab tiuxetan require approximately one week for delivery of therapy. Unlabelled anti-CD20 antibodies (unlabelled tositumomab prior to ^{131}I tositumomab and rituximab prior to ^{90}Y ibritumomab tiuxetan) are administered prior to the tracer and therapeutic doses of the radioimmuno-conjugates to bind non-tumour antigen and enhance biodistribution of the radiolabelled immunoconjugates. Because ^{131}I tositumomab produces gamma and beta emissions, a single 5 mCi tracer dose is given for imaging and dosimetry, respectively. Serial whole body counts are taken over several days after the tracer dose to ensure tumour targeting and to determine the final therapeutic dose. ^{90}Y ibritumomab requires ^{111}In-labelled ibritumomab for imaging to document proper biodistribution. Because the dose of ^{90}Y ibritumomab is determined by patient weight and platelet count and not dosimetry calculations, administration may be easier for clinicians. This last point may be an advantage for ^{90}Y ibritumomab, as the ease of weight-based dosing has the potential for delivery by medical oncologists who are approved

Table 9.3 Patient release instructions after treatment with ^{131}I tositumomab [32]

For 4–7 days after treatment:
- Sleep in a separate bed (≥6 feet apart)
- Keep ≥6 feet from children and pregnant women
- Do not take long trips
- Limit time spent in public places
- Use a separate bathroom
- Sit while urinating
- Wash hands frequently
- Drink plenty of liquids
- Use separate eating utensils
- Wash laundry separately, avoid using disposable items
- Avoid sexual contact

to work with radioactive materials. In the case of ^{131}I tositumomab, the expertise of trained nuclear medicine physicians is necessary for dosimetric calculations.

Previously, the need for hospitalisation for recipients of ^{131}I tositumomab placed patients at a tremendous disadvantage compared with patients treated with ^{90}Y immunoconjugates. The temporary isolation from family members and limited time allowed with healthcare personal could contribute to a sense of isolation, anxiety, and poor patient education. However, the new NRC guidelines have allowed more patients to receive out-patient ^{131}I therapy. Though the release guidelines with ^{131}I tositumomab are more limiting than with ^{90}Y tositumomab tiuxetan, the difference should not have a tremendous impact on patient quality of life.

To date, a cost analysis comparison has not been reported between the two RIT agents. In general terms, ^{131}I is a much less expensive radionuclide than [90]Y. Because ^{90}Y ibritumomab requires the use of ^{111}In for imaging, therapy with this radioimmunoconjugate may be more expensive and this may affect clinical decision making for certain patients. However, use of ^{131}I tositumomab may require hospitalisation that could add to the cost of therapy.

Safety data for ^{90}Y ibritumomab tiuxetan and ^{131}I tositumomab demonstrate that both agents are safe and well tolerated by patients with adequate marrow reserves who are treated for low-grade or transformed NHL. The dose-limiting toxicity for each radioimmunoconjugate is reversible, delayed myelosuppression. An analysis of 349 patients treated with ^{90}Y tositumomab tiuxetan in five phase I/II U.S. studies demonstrated that haematotoxicity was transient with nadir counts occurring at 7–9 weeks after therapy and recovery 1–4 weeks thereafter [25]. Grade 4 neutropaenia, thrombocytopaenia, and anaemia were reported in 30, 10, and 4% of patients, respectively. Grade 3 or 4 bleeding events occurred in 2% of patients, and 7% of patients were hospitalised with infections (3% with neutropaenia). Similarly, in a review of 677 patients treated with ^{131}I tositumomab, grade 4 neutropaenia, thrombocytopaenia, and anaemia occurred in 16, 3, and 2% of patients, respectively [26]. Grade 3 or 4 haematological nadirs usually appeared 4–6 weeks after treatment and recovered to grade 2 toxicity by 8–9 weeks. Grade 3 or 4 bleeding events occurred in 1% of treated patients and serious infections were observed in 5% of patients.

The non-haematological toxicities were also similar between the two radioimmunoconjugates for patients treated for relapsed or refractory low-grade and transformed NHL. For patients treated with ^{90}Y ibritumomab tiuxetan, grade 1 and 2 non-haematological events were reported in 279 of 349 patients (80%) in the integrated analysis of phase I/II trials during the 13-week treatment period [25]. The most frequent symptoms were asthenia (35%), nausea (25%), and chills (21%). Grade 3 and 4 toxicities occurred in 39 patients (11%) and included asthenia in 6 patients (2%) and abdominal pain in 4 patients (1%). Infections were reported in 29% of patients. In a larger multicentre, phase II trial of ^{131}I tositumomab, transient toxicity thought secondary to therapy was observed in 44 of 47 patients (96%). The most common toxicities were fatigue (32%), nausea (30%), fever (26%), and vomiting (15%). Infections were reported in only 13% of patients. Though clinically silent, an elevated TSH was observed in 2–8% of patients despite pre-treatment with SSKI in early phase II trials of ^{131}I tositumomab [2–4].

The incidence of human anti-mouse antibodies (HAMA) or anti-chimeric antibodies (HACA) to the carrier MAbs appears somewhat higher in patients treated with ^{131}I tositumomab. Of 211 patients treated with ^{90}Y ibritumomab who were evaluated for HAMA/HACA, 3 patients (1%) developed HAMA and one patient (<1%) developed HACA for a total incidence of 1.4% [25]. HAMA was observed in 0–17% of patients treated with ^{131}I tositumomab in phase I/II trials [2–4]. In a multi-centre expanded access study report of 359 patients with advanced B-cell NHL, the incidence of HAMA was 8% [27]. The higher incidence of HAMA may be due to administration of unlabelled tositumomab for ^{131}I tositumomab therapy, whereas the chimeric antibody rituximab is used with ^{90}Y ibritumomab tiuxetan. In all reported cases of HAMA or HACA, however, patients did not experience adverse sequelae.

The long-term risk of treatment-related myelodysplastic syndrome (tMDS) and acute myelogenous leukaemia (tAML) also appear similar between ^{90}Y ibritumomab tiuxetan and ^{131}I tositumomab. In either case, the risk of tMDS or tAML appears to correlate with the amount of chemotherapy received prior to RIT. Only 10 of 770 (1.3%) patients treated with ^{90}Y ibritumomab tiuxetan since 1993 have developed secondary AML or MDS [28]. A review of 1,071 patients treated with ^{131}I tositumomab in seven trials demonstrated that 13 of 995 patients (1.3%) who received chemotherapy prior to RIT had confirmed pathologic evidence of tMDS/tAML [29]. For 76 previously-untreated patients with follicular lymphoma who received ^{131}I tositumomab as initial therapy, Kaminski and colleagues reported 0% incidence of tMDS/tAML after a median follow-up of 5.1 years [33].

SUMMARY

Clinicians now have two highly effective agents to treat patients with refractory or relapsed low-grade or transformed NHL. However, the decision to choose one radiolabelled Mab over the other is not yet clear. Because clinical trials that compare the two agents are not yet available, an understanding of the nature of the radionuclides used to construct the radioimmunoconjugates may provide direction. Apparent differences that may impact clinical decision-making include patient tumour burden, ease of administration, radiation safety, and the need for hospitalisation to administer therapy. However, there does not appear to be a clinically significant difference in treatment toxicity between the two agents. Prospective trials that directly compare the two agents are necessary to distinguish efficacy, safety, and the impact on patients quality of life.

REFERENCES

1. Kaminski MS *et al*. Iodine-131-anti-B1 radioimmunotherapy for B-cell lymphoma. *J Clin Oncol* 1996; 14:1974–1981.
2. Kaminski MS *et al*. Radioimmunotherapy with iodine ^{131}I tositumomab for relapsed or refractory B-cell non-Hodgkin lymphoma: updated results and long-term follow-up of the University of Michigan experience. *Blood* 2000; 96:1259–1266.
3. Vose JM *et al*. Multicenter phase II study of iodine-131 tositumomab for chemotherapy-relapsed/refractory low-grade and transformed low-grade B-cell non-Hodgkin's lymphomas. *J Clin Oncol* 2000; 18:1316–1323.
4. Kaminski MS *et al*. Pivotal study of iodine I 131 tositumomab for chemotherapy-refractory low-grade or transformed low-grade B-cell non-Hodgkin's lymphomas. *J Clin Oncol* 2001; 19:3918–3928.

5. Davies AJ *et al*. Tositumomab and iodine I 131 tositumomab for recurrent indolent and transformed B-cell non-Hodgkin's lymphoma. *J Clin Oncol* 2004; 22:1469–1479.

6. Witzig TE *et al*. Phase I/II trial of IDEC-Y2B8 radioimmunotherapy for treatment of relapsed or refractory CD20(+) B-cell non-Hodgkin's lymphoma. *J Clin Oncol* 1999; 17:3793–3803.

7. Gordon LI *et al*. Durable responses after ibritumomab tiuxetan radioimmunotherapy for CD20+ B-cell lymphoma: long-term follow-up of a phase 1/2 study. *Blood* 2004; 103:4429–4431.

8. Wiseman GA *et al*. Ibritumomab tiuxetan radioimmunotherapy for patients with relapsed or refractory non-Hodgkin lymphoma and mild thrombocytopenia: a phase II multicenter trial. *Blood* 2002; 99:4336–4342.

9. Witzig TE *et al*. Treatment with ibritumomab tiuxetan radioimmunotherapy in patients with rituximab-refractory follicular non-Hodgkin's lymphoma. *J Clin Oncol* 2002; 20:3262–3269.

10. Horning SJ, Lucas JB, Younes A *et al*. Iodine-131 tositumomab for non-Hodgkin's lymphoma (NHL) in patiens who progressed after treatment with rituximab: results of a multi-center phase II study. *Blood* 2000; 96:508a.

11. Nuclear Regulatory Commission. Regulatory Guide 8.39: release of patients administered radioactive materials.

12. Kuzel TM, Rosen ST. Radioimmunotherapy of Lymphomas and Leukemias. In: Henkin RE, Boles MA, Dillehay GL *et al*. (eds). *Nuclear Medicine* Mosby, St Louis, MO, 1996, 549–601.

13. Witzig TE *et al*. Randomized controlled trial of yttrium-90-labeled ibritumomab tiuxetan radioimmunotherapy versus rituximab immunotherapy for patients with relapsed or refractory low-grade, follicular, or transformed B-cell non-Hodgkin's lymphoma. *J Clin Oncol* 2002; 20:2453–2463.

14. Chinn PC *et al*. Preclinical evaluation of 90Y-labeled anti-CD20 monoclonal antibody for treatment of non-Hodgkin's lymphoma. *Int J Oncol* 1999; 15:1017–1025.

15. Wagner HN, Jr *et al*. Administration guidelines for radioimmunotherapy of non-Hodgkin's lymphoma with (90)Y-labeled anti-CD20 monoclonal antibody. *J Nucl Med* 2002; 43:267–272.

16. DeNardo GL *et al*. Role of radiation dosimetry in radioimmunotherapy planning and treatment dosing. *Crit Rev Oncol Hematol* 2001; 39:203–218.

17. Kaminski MS *et al*. Radioimmunotherapy of B-cell lymphoma with [131I]anti-B1 (anti-CD20) antibody. *N Engl J Med* 1993; 329:459–465.

18. Wiseman GA *et al*. Phase I/II 90Y-Zevalin (yttrium-90 ibritumomab tiuxetan, IDEC-Y2B8) radioimmunotherapy dosimetry results in relapsed or refractory non-Hodgkin's lymphoma. *Eur J Nucl Med* 2000; 27:766–777.

19. Wiseman GA *et al*. Biodistribution and dosimetry results from a phase III prospectively randomized controlled trial of Zevalin radioimmunotherapy for low-grade, follicular, or transformed B-cell non-Hodgkin's lymphoma. *Crit Rev Oncol Hematol* 2001; 39:181–194.

20. Wiseman GA *et al*. Radiation dosimetry results and safety correlations from 90Y-ibritumomab tiuxetan radioimmunotherapy for relapsed or refractory non-Hodgkin's lymphoma: combined data from 4 clinical trials. *J Nucl Med* 2003; 44:465–474.

21. Criteria for the release of individuals administered radioactive materials—NRC. Final rule. *Fed Regist* 1997; 62:4120–4133.

22. Wiseman GA, Leigh B, Witzig T, *et al*. Radiation exposure is very low to the family members of patients treated with yttrium-90 Zevalin and to CD-20 monoclonal antibody therapy for lymphoma. *Eur J Nucl Med* 2001; 28:1198.

23. Rutar FJ *et al*. Outpatient treatment with (131)I-anti-B1 antibody: radiation exposure to family members. *J Nucl Med* 2001; 42:907–915.

24. Siegel JA *et al*. A practical methodology for patient release after tositumomab and (131)I-tositumomab therapy. *J Nucl Med* 2002; 43:354–363.

25. Witzig TE *et al*. Safety of yttrium-90 ibritumomab tiuxetan radioimmunotherapy for relapsed low-grade, follicular, or transformed non-Hodgkin's lymphoma. *J Clin Oncol* 2003; 21:1263–1270.

26. Kaminski M, Gregory S, Fehrenbacher L, Magnuson D, Cheever M, Frenette G et al. Acute and delayed hematologic toxicities associated with Bexxar therapy are modest: overall experience in patients with low-grade and transformed low-grade NHL. *Blood* 2001; 98:339a.

27. Schenkein D, Leonard J, Harwood S *et al*. Interim safety results of Bexxar in a large multicenter expanded access study. *Proc Am Soc Clin Oncol*, 2001; 20:285a.

28. Czuczman M, WT, Gaston I *et al*. Zevalin radioimmunotherapy is not associated with an increased incidence of secondary myelodysplastic syndrome (MDS) or acute myelogenous leukemia (AML). *Blood* 2002; 100:357a–358a.

29. Bennett JM *et al*. Assessment of treatment-related myelodysplastic syndromes and acute myeloid leukemia in patients with non-Hodgkin's lymphoma treated with Tositumomab and Iodine I 131 Tositumomab (BEXXAR®). *Blood* 2005 in press.
30. Woolton R, Radiation Protection of Patients. Cambridge University Press, Cambridge, England, 1993.
31. Zevalin (ibritumomab tiuxetan) prescribing information. IDEC Pharmaceuticals Corporation, San Diego, CA, 2002.
32. Bexxar (tositumomab and iodine-131 tositumomab) prescribing information. Corixa Corporation, Seattle, WA, 2003.
33. Kaminski MS, Tuck M, Estes J *et al*. [131]I- tositumomab therapy as initial treatment for follicular lymphoma. *N Engl J MEd* 2005; 352:441–449.

10

Radioimmunotherapy with Yttrium-90-labelled ibritumomab tiuxetan (Zevalin™) for B-cell non-Hodgkin's lymphoma

T. E. Witzig

INTRODUCTION

Immunotherapy with monoclonal antibodies has become an integral part of the treatment of B-cell non-Hodgkin's lymphomas (NHL). Rituximab, an unlabelled monoclonal antibody to the CD20 antigen, was the first monoclonal antibody to be approved by the FDA for the treatment of cancer. This approval, in 1997, was based in part on the results of a pivotal clinical trial that treated 166 patients, with relapsed B-cell NHL, with rituximab 375 mg/m^2 weekly $\times$ 4. The overall response rate (ORR) was 48% with 6% complete remission (CR) and a 13-month time-to-progression (TTP) [1]. Rituximab is now widely used as a single agent for relapsed patients and combined with chemotherapy as initial treatment [2–4]. High response rates have also been demonstrated in previously untreated patients with low-grade NHL [5–10]. Immunotherapy has clearly been a major advance in the treatment of NHL; however, patients with advanced stage low-grade NHL are still considered 'treatable but not usually curable'. New treatments are needed that build upon the success of rituximab immunotherapy.

RADIOIMMUNOTHERAPY

Radioimmunotherapy (RIT) is a relatively new treatment for NHL that involves the linking of a high-energy, short-path length radionuclide to an antibody to form a radioimmunoconjugate (RIC). The goal of RIT is to use the targeting feature of a monoclonal antibody to focus radiation on the target cell population while sparing nearby normal tissues. The RIC kills tumour cells by the direct effects of the antibody, such as antibody-dependent cellular cytotoxicity, as well as the effects of ionising low-dose-rate radiation [11]. The radionuclide can potentially be attached to any antibody. The choice of antibody depends on the antigenic profile of the tumour cell to be targeted. Ideal targets are those antigens that are expressed on tumour cells but not normal cells, so as to avoid toxicity to normal organs. Cell surface antigens that are not internalised or shed from the cell surface are preferred. Administration of the RIC is preceded by a dose of cold antibody in order to deplete normal blood B cells and block non-specific binding sites resulting in improved tumour to normal organ biodistribution. There are many different radionuclides that have been linked to antibodies for the treatment of cancer [12, 13]. Yttrium-90 (^{90}Y) and iodine-131 (^{131}I) are currently in common use and are commercially available (Table 10.1).

Thomas E. Witzig, MD, Professor of Medicine, Division of Internal Medicine and Hematology, Mayo Clinic, Rochester, Minnesota, USA.

Table 10.1 Characteristics of radionuclides currently used in radioimmunotherapy

Parameter	$^{131}Iodine$	$^{90}Yttrium$
Gamma emission	Yes	No
Beta emission	Yes	Yes
Beta emission path length	0.8 mm	5 mm
Theoretical half-life	8 days	2.4 days
Free radioisotope	Thyroid/Stomach	Bone
Administration	Out-patient in most states	Out-patient
Pre-treatment cold antibody required?	Yes	Yes
Useful for imaging and dosimetry?	Yes	No (^{111}In required as a surrogate)

The application of RIT to treat B-cell NHL was a logical choice because NHL is typically sensitive to radiation delivered by conventional external sources. Unfortunately, the widespread nature of these tumours makes it difficult to encompass all tumour sites into a radiation field without compromising marrow function. Initial studies of RIT in lymphoma used polyclonal antibodies [14]; however, most RIC today are murine monoclonal antibodies [15, 16]. Recent studies of RIT targeting a variety of tumour antigens on NHL cells have indeed demonstrated tumour regressions with very few side-effects in normal organs other than myelosuppression [17–33].

There are two Food and Drug Administration (FDA)-approved RIC for B-cell NHL – ibritumomab tiuxetan (Zevalin™, Biogen Idec, San Diego, CA and Cambridge, MA) and tositumomab (Bexxar™, Corixa and GlaxoSmithKline, Seattle, WA) [16, 34, 35]. Both RIC target the CD20 antigen. CD20 is a good target for RIT because CD20 expression is restricted to normal B cells, almost all B-cell NHLs are CD20+, CD20 is not internalised into the cell nor expressed on other normal tissues (including stem cells), and depletion of normal B cells by these antibodies has not led to significant short- or long-term side-effects.

IBRITUMOMAB TIUXETAN (ZEVALIN™)

Ibritumomab is a murine anti-CD20 antibody from which the human chimeric antibody rituximab (Rituxan and MabThera; IDEC Pharmaceuticals Corp, San Diego, CA and Genentech, Inc, South San Francisco, CA) was engineered. Ibritumomab was attached to tiuxetan, an MX-DTPA linker-chelator to form Zevalin™ (Biogen Idec). Tiuxetan forms a covalent, urea-type bond with ibritumomab and chelates the radionuclide *via* 5 carboxyl groups. Zevalin is then reacted with either Indium-111 (^{111}In) for tumour imaging and dosimetry or with ^{90}Y for therapeutic RIT. ^{90}Y emits pure beta radioactivity with a path length of approximately 5 mm. Zevalin must be handled and injected by personnel certified by the Nuclear Regulatory Commission. Thus, administration of RIT is a team effort between the haematologist/oncologist who is caring for the patient and the Nuclear Medicine Physician or Radiation Oncologist who will administer the Zevalin.

Because there is no gamma emission from ^{90}Y, useful tumour and normal organ images require ^{111}In-Zevalin to produce high-quality images of the tumour and normal organs for dosimetry and biodistribution studies (Figure 10.1) Previous studies have demonstrated that the gamma radiation from the ^{111}In-Zevalin can be used for imaging and dosimetry and that these results accurately predict ^{90}Y-Zevalin biodistribution [36]. In the USA, the FDA requires that patients receive ^{111}In-Zevalin followed by two scans (a third scan is optional) to

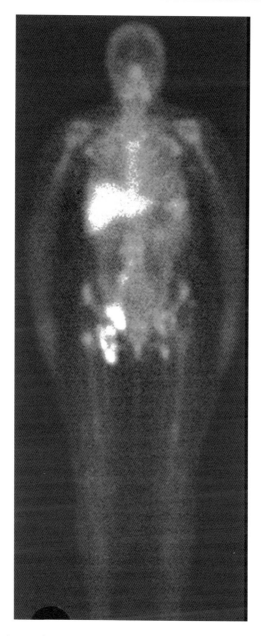

Figure 10.1 ^{111}In-Zevalin images demonstrate excellent tumour targeting in the right inguinal region as well as uptake in the liver. The liver uptake is typically about 500 cGy [60].

ensure that there is no abnormal biodistribution. Formal dosimetry is not required in the non-transplant setting because the dose of ^{90}Y-Zevalin is based on weight (maximum 32 mCi for those patients over 80 kg) and platelet count (0.3 mCi/kg for patients with platelet count ≥100,000 and 0.4 mCi/kg for those with platelet counts ≥150,000). In Europe and other countries imaging may not be required. Biodistribution studies have demonstrated that the initial image on the day of ^{111}In-Zevalin shows activity in the blood pool with images on subsequent days showing no blood pool activity and progressive uptake in tumour sites. There is virtually no renal uptake and only 7% of the Zevalin is excreted through the kidneys in 7 days. There is typically activity noted in the liver even in situations without known lymphomatous involvement of the liver. When calculations have been performed, the liver typically receives about 500 cGy of radiation [37–42]. To date, there has been no hepatoxicity from Zevalin.

Rituximab 250 mg/m^2 is administered before each dose of Zevalin, using standard infusion pre-medications (acetaminophen and diphenhydramine) and infusion schedules. Zevalin is provided as a solution containing 3.2 mg of the immunoconjugate in 2 ml of saline solution. Although the Zevalin antibody is murine, human anti-mouse antibody (HAMA) development is very rare [24] with Zevalin, probably because only 1.3 ml of the solution is typically required. The Zevalin is administered as an out-patient over 10 min and infusion-related reactions are rare; specialised isolation rooms are not required because the beta radiation from ^{90}Y is effectively shielded with plastic or acrylic [41, 43]. Patients may be released immediately after treatment in accordance with current Nuclear Regulatory Commission guidelines [43]. Patients and family members are recommended to avoid direct exposure to the patient's body fluids such as blood, urine, and stool. The dose of radiation to family members of the patient is similar to background radiation [44]. Men are recommended to wear condoms during sexual intercourse for one week after Zevalin [43].

CLINICAL RESULTS OF ZEVALIN RADIOIMMUNOTHERAPY FOR RELAPSED NHL

Clinical trials to assess toxicity and efficacy of Zevalin were initially limited to patients with relapsed disease (Table 10.2). In most studies, the patients were to have measurable disease, bone marrow with <25% involvement with NHL, absolute neutrophil count (ANC) ≥1,500, platelet count ≥100,000, normal renal and liver function, and <25% of the bone marrow previously treated with external beam radiotherapy. Patients were excluded from these trials if they had CNS lymphoma, HIV infection, or HIV-related NHL, chronic lymphocytic leukaemia (CLL), pleural or peritoneal fluid that was positive for lymphoma, known myelodysplasia, or history of a prior allogeneic or autologous stem cell transplant. Table 10.3 summarises the tumour responses observed in the trials; each trial is discussed in detail below.

PHASE I STUDIES OF ZEVALIN

There were two phase I trials of Zevalin. The first study enrolled 14 patients with relapsed low or intermediate CD20+ B-cell NHL [20]. In this trial, cold ibritumomab was given before single doses of Zevalin and stem cells were cryopreserved in case of prolonged myelosuppression. The patients were imaged twice with ^{111}In-Zevalin – the first imaging was performed without unlabelled ibritumomab; the second was performed following unlabelled ibritumomab. A comparison of the two sets of ^{111}In-Zevalin images demonstrated that pre-dosing with cold ibritumomab improved biodistribution of the Zevalin. Patients were then treated with ^{90}Y-Zevalin in cohorts of 3–4 with doses ranging from 13.5 to 50 mCi. Only 2 patients (both had received 50 mCi of ^{90}Y-Zevalin) required re-infusion of stem cells. The maximum tolerated dose (MTD) without the use of stem cells was 50 mCi and doses ≤40 mCi were not myeloablative [20]. The ORR was 79% (11/14) with 36% CR, and 43% partial remission (PR).

The second phase I trial used rituximab 250 mg/m^2 as the unlabelled antibody before Zevalin, because it was felt that rituximab was less likely to cause a HAMA human anti-chimeric antibody (HACA) than murine ibritumomab [25, 45]. An additional goal of the second phase I trial was to determine the MTD of ^{90}Y-Zevalin that could be given to patients without the use of stem cells or prophylactic growth factors and to treat additional patients

Table 10.2 Summary of the clinical trials of ibritumomab tiuxetan (Zevalin)

Trial #	N	Goal	Reference
IDEC 106-02	14	■ Used cold ibritumomab prior to ⁹⁰Y-Zevalin ■ Determine MTD of ⁹⁰Y-Zevalin	[20]
IDEC 106-03	51	■ Determine dose of rituximab prior to ¹¹¹In-Zevalin ■ Determine MTD of ⁹⁰Y-Zevalin	[25, 39]
IDEC 106-04	143	■ Randomised trial of rituximab vs. ⁹⁰Y-Zevalin to determine if efficacy of ⁹⁰Y-Zevalin is superior	[23, 44]
IDEC 106-05	30	■ Efficacy and toxicity of 0.3 mCi/kg ⁹⁰Y-Zevalin for patients with platelet count of 100–149 K × 10^6/l	[22]
IDEC 106-06	54	■ Efficacy and toxicity of 0.4 mCi/kg ⁹⁰Y-Zevalin for patients refractory to rituximab	[42]
Safety analysis	349	■ Evaluate the side-effects experienced by patients treated with Zevalin on clinical trials	[24, 59]

^{90}Y = Yttrium-90; ^{111}In = indium-111; MTD = maximum tolerated dose.

Table 10.3 Response rates to Zevalin radioimmunotherapy in trials without stem cell support

Trial	n	ORR	CR	DR
Phase I [20]	14	79	36	–
Phase I/II [25]	51	67	26	11.7+
Randomised [23]	73	80	30	14.2 (0.9–28.9)
Rituximab refractory [42]	54	74	15	6.4 (0.5–≥24.9)
Phase II for patients with thrombocytopaenia [22]	30	83	43	11.7 (3.6–≥23.4)

ORR = Overall response rate; CR = complete remission; DR = duration of response.

at the MTD in a phase II study. There was no provision for re-treatment [25]. Fifty-one patients were enrolled and the study concluded that 250 mg/m^2 was the optimal dose of rituximab to be used before ^{111}In-Zevalin imaging and ^{90}Y-Zevalin therapy [25]. Dosimetry predicted that all patients were eligible for ^{90}Y-Zevalin [46]. The doses of ^{90}Y-Zevalin used in the phase I/II trial were 0.2–0.4 mCi/kg; 5 patients received 0.2, 15 received 0.3, and 30 patients received 0.4 mCi/kg. The dose was capped at 32 mCi for patients over 80 kg. All patients who received 0.4 mCi/kg were able to recover bone marrow function without prophylactic growth factors or stem cells. The dose was not increased to >0.4 mCi/kg because substantial myelosuppression was already being obtained with 0.4 mCi/kg and stem cells had not been collected pre-Zevalin. The efficacy portion of the phase I/II trial demonstrated a 67% ORR in all patients with 26% CR. In patients with low-grade NHL, the ORR was even higher at 82% with 26% CR [25]. The median TTP for responders was 15.4 months; the duration of response (DR) was 11.7+ months. Long-term follow-up indicated that 24% of the responding patients had a TTP >3 years and some were over 5 years out without needing further treatment [45].

ZEVALIN TREATMENT IN PATIENTS WITH MILD THROMBOCYTOPAENIA

Many patients with relapsed NHL have mild thrombocytopaenia from an enlarged spleen or from previous treatment. The phase I study suggested that 0.4 mCi/kg may be too myelo-suppressive for these patients. Thus, a separate trial using a reduced-dose ^{90}Y-Zevalin (0.3 mCi/kg) for patients with platelet counts between $100,000–149,000 \times 10^6/l$ was designed. Thirty patients were treated in this study and the ORR was 83% with 43% CR/unconfirmed complete response (CRu). The TTP was 9.4 months in all patients and 12.6 months in responders [22]. The median DR was 11.7 months ($3.6–\geq23.4$). Haematological toxicity was the primary toxicity with a median nadir ANC of $600 \times 10^6/l$ (grade IV in 33% of patients). The median nadir platelet count was $26,500 \times 10^6/l$ (grade IV in 13% of patients).

RANDOMISED TRIAL OF ZEVALIN VS. RITUXIMAB

After the phase I/II trials suggested a high ORR with Zevalin, it was important to test Zevalin in a randomised study. At the time this study was initiated, rituximab was just becoming FDA approved (1997) and it was not difficult to find rituximab-naïve patients. Patients were randomised to receive either 0.4 mCi/kg (maximum of 32 mCi) of ^{90}Y-Zevalin or rituximab 375 mg/kg weekly $\times$ 4 [23]. 143 patients were randomised in this trial – 73 received Zevalin and 70 rituximab. The analysis of all 143 patients found an ORR (International Workshop NHL criteria [47]) of 80% with ^{90}Y-Zevalin compared to 56% for rituximab (p = 0.002). The CR rate of 30% in the ^{90}Y-Zevalin arm was also higher than the 16% found with rituximab (p = 0.04). The median DR was 14.2 months (0.9–28.9). The Kaplan–Meier (K–M) estimated median TTP was 11.2+ months (range, 0.8–31.5+ months) for the ^{90}Y-Zevalin group compared with 10.1+ months (range, 0.7–26.1 months) for the rituximab group (p = 0.173). However, the estimated time to next therapy (TTNT) for patients with non-transformed histology indicates a significantly longer TTNT for Zevalin patients (17.8+ months; range, 2.1–21.7+) than for rituximab patients (11.2 months; range, 1.3–19.0+; p = 0.040).

STUDIES OF ZEVALIN IN RITUXAN-REFRACTORY PATIENTS

In 2005, many patients receive rituximab as part of induction therapy; therefore, it was important to learn what the ORR to Zevalin was in the rituximab-refractory patient population. Fifty-four patients were observed in a study that treated patients who had failed to respond with a PR or CR to rituximab or had a response that lasted <6 months with a standard dose of 0.4 mCi/kg of ^{90}Y-Zevalin and were followed without further therapy [48]. The median age was 54 years (range, 34–73), 95% of patients had follicular NHL, 32% had bone marrow involvement, and 74% had bulky disease (≥5 cm). This patient group was heavily pre-treated with a median of four prior therapies. The dosimetry determined by ^{111}In-Zevalin was acceptable in all 27 cases in which it was performed. The median nadir ANC was $700 \times 10^6/l$ and in 35% of patients it was grade IV. The median nadir platelet count was $33,000 \times 10^6/l$ and was grade IV in 9%. The ORR using International Workshop criteria [47] was 74% with 15% CR. The median TTP estimated by the K-M method is 6.8 months (range, 1.1–25.9+) with 30% of data censored. Median TTP in the 40 responders is 8.7 months (range, 1.7–25.9+), with 28% of data censored. The median DR estimated by K–M is 6.4 months (range, 0.5–24.9+).

STUDIES OF ZEVALIN IN RELAPSED MANTLE CELL LYMPHOMA

Limited numbers of patients with relapsed mantle cell NHL have been treated with Zevalin. Although the malignant cells in mantle cell lymphoma (MCL) strongly express CD20, the disease often heavily infiltrates the marrow making these patients ineligible for

RIT studies. Oki and colleagues [49] reported on 15 patients with relapsed MCL that received treatment with Zevalin. There were 5 objective responses (33%) with all responses being CR/CRu. The median TTP was 4.9 months for all patients and the median DR was 5.7 months. Thus it appears that in relapsed MCL patients, the ORR to single-agent Zevalin is lower than observed for low-grade NHL or large cell NHL. Current trials are using Zevalin after R-CHOP (rituximab, cyclophosphamide, doxorubicin, vincristine, prednisone) induction for patients with previously untreated MCL. This approach uses the RIT at a time of minimal residual disease. It will be several years before it will be known whether this strategy can improve the otherwise relentless relapses that typically occur in the MCL patient group.

ZEVALIN IN RELAPSED DIFFUSE LARGE CELL LYMPHOMA

Patients with relapsed large cell lymphoma who are in good health, less than 75 years of age, and with chemosensitive disease are usually treated with high-dose therapy with stem cell rescue. However, elderly patients, or those who are not candidates for transplant do not have good therapeutic options and can be considered candidates for trials of RIT. In the phase I trial of Zevalin [25] there were 14 patients with relapsed large cell NHL and 43% responded. A recent trial in Europe treated 104 patients with relapsed or refractory diffuse large cell NHL with a single dose of Zevalin 0.4 mCi/kg (maximum of 32 mCi). They found an ORR of 44% for the entire group with 55% of rituximab-naïve patients responding compared to 19% of patients with prior treatment with rituximab-containing regimens. Further follow-up of the patients and full publication of the results are needed before conclusions on the use of Zevalin RIT in this setting can be made [50]. Current trials in the Eastern Cooperative Oncology Group for diffuse large cell NHL are focusing on using Zevalin as adjuvant therapy after completion of R-CHOP induction. The aim is to increase the rate of CR and TTP.

LONG-TERM RESPONDERS

Gordon and co-workers [51] recently reported long-term follow-up on patients that enrolled on the randomised study that compared Zevalin with rituximab [23]. Although this study was designed to enroll rituximab-naïve patients and was not powered for TTP, the authors continued to follow the groups for progression. At a median follow-up of 44 months, there was a trend towards longer median TTP (15 vs. 10.2 months; p = 0.07), DR (16.7 vs. 11.2 months; p = 0.44) and TTNT (21.1 vs. 13.8 months; p = 0.27) in follicular NHL patients treated with Zevalin compared with the rituximab control arm. In patients achieving a CR/CRu, the median TTP was 24.7 months for patients treated with Zevalin compared with 13.2 months for rituximab-treated patients (p = 0.41), and ongoing responses of >5 years have been observed.

RE-TREATMENT WITH RADIOIMMUNOTHERAPY

There has been limited experience of re-treatment of patients with RIT. Wahl and colleagues [52] re-treated 13 patients with Bexxar and 62% (8/13) responded with 31% (4/13) CR. No grade IV toxicity was noted and only one patient developed a HAMA. Wiseman and co-workers [53] reported preliminary results on a phase I trial where all patients were treated with two sequential doses of Zevalin. The first dose was 0.4 millicurie (mCi)/kg and the phase I dose levels for the second dose delivered 3–6 months after the first dose are 0.2, 0.3, and 0.4 mCi/kg. This trial is ongoing and is currently using growth factor support to reduce haematological toxicity. This trial is also integrating position emission tomography (PET) scanning before each dose to learn the relationship of PET positivity and response to Zevalin (Figure 10.2).

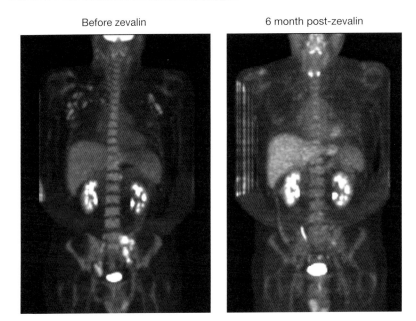

Figure 10.2   Left: Position emission tomography (PET) scan pre-Zevalin demonstrating uptake in bilateral axillary nodes, right neck nodes, and bilateral pelvic nodes. Right: Repeat PET scan 6 months after a single dose of Zevalin 0.4 mCi/kg. Uptake in previously involved nodes has cleared consistent with a complete remission.

HIGH-DOSE RADIOIMMUNOTHERAPY WITH STEM CELL SUPPORT

It is clear that the primary dose-limiting toxicity of RIT for NHL is myelosuppression and normal organ toxicity to organs other than marrow has not been a problem. It is possible that much higher doses of RIT could be given if stem cells were harvested and re-infused after RIT. Indeed, this approach has been pioneered by Press and colleagues using Bexxar [54, 55]. Phase I trials of Zevalin plus chemotherapy and autologous stem cell transplant are ongoing to learn the safety and efficacy of Zevalin in the transplant setting [56–59]. In these trials ^{111}In-Zevalin imaging and dosimetry are necessary to calculate the dose of ^{90}Y-Zevalin to be administered to deliver the phase I centigray (cGy) dose to the critical organ. Winter and colleagues are conducting a trial of high-dose Zevalin with standard BEAM (BCNU, etoposide, ara-C, melphalan) chemotherapy and stem cell support in patients with relapsed NHL [56, 59]. This phase I study started with 100 cGy to the critical organ (liver, lung, or kidney) and the investigators have recently reported results up through to the 900-cGy cohort [56, 59]. To date, there has been no dose-limiting toxicity and patients continue to be accrued to the study.

Nademanee and co-workers [57, 58] recently reported updated results on 31 patients treated with Zevalin, high-dose etoposide and cyclophosphamide, and stem cell transplant. In this trial the dose of Zevalin was calculated to provide a maximum radiation dose of 1,000 cGy to normal organs. The median dose of Zevalin was 70.8 mCi (range, 36.6–105). At a median of 21 months, the 2-year estimated overall survival (OS) and disease-free survival (DFS) is 93% (95% CI, 86–96%), and 80% (95% CI, 64–96%), respectively. These two ongoing studies have yet to define the maximal tolerated dose of Zevalin that can be delivered with stem cells. It is encouraging that the number of mCi of Zevalin that was administered in this setting is clearly much higher than the maximum dose of 32 mCi that is approved for use in patients without stem cell support. Whether this will translate into meaningful improvement in OS post-transplant will require randomised trials after the MTD of Zevalin in this setting has been determined.

PREVIOUSLY UNTREATED PATIENTS

RIT is approved for use in previously treated patients. Because Zevalin has been well tolerated in patients with relapsed NHL, it is attractive to test its use earlier in the course of disease. Kaminski and colleagues [60] reported on 76 patients with Stage III or IV follicular NHL that received Bexxar as initial therapy: 95% of the patients had a response and 75% had a CR. After a median follow-up of 5.1 years, the actuarial 5-year progression-free survival (PFS) for all patients was 59% with a median PFS of 6.1 years. It is not clear whether this regimen is curative because approximately 4.4% of patients are still relapsing each year after 3 years. This is an exciting result but cannot yet be considered as the standard of care. It is likely that randomised trials will be necessary [61].

Sweetenham and co-workers [62] are performing a similar study with Zevalin using standard doses of Zevalin to previously untreated patients with stages III or IV follicular NHL. This study differs from the Kaminski study in that patients will be administered rituximab maintenance every 6 months for 2 years. Early results on 8 patients that were evaluable for response showed an ORR of 100% with 62% CR (5/8) and 38% PR (3/8) [62]. This study will obviously require more patients and longer follow-up to learn the precise role of Zevalin and rituximab maintenance as treatment for patients with newly diagnosed follicular NHL.

Another approach is to utilize RIT as adjuvant therapy after induction chemoimmunotherapy. This approach has been piloted and found to be safe [63, 64]. A large randomised trial in Europe is being conducted where patients receive induction chemotherapy and then randomisation to observation or a single dose of Zevalin RIT. The results of this trial have the potential to change clinical practice.

SUBSEQUENT THERAPY AFTER RADIOIMMUNOTHERAPY

Since the CR rate with Zevalin is about 30% and approximately 20–25% of patients have long-term DFS, it is apparent that most patients treated with Zevalin will subsequently require additional therapy. Ansell and colleagues [65, 66] examined the subsequent therapy administered to 58 patients who had relapsed after receiving Zevalin 0.4 mCi/kg. The median number of subsequent treatments received was 2 (range, 1–7). Eight patients had stem cells collected from the peripheral blood after Zevalin and one of these required a marrow harvest in addition to the blood collection. All 8 engrafted. The other patients received a variety of chemotherapy regimens as detailed in the report [65, 66]. In summary, in this selected group of patients who had met all of the criteria for inclusion into a Zevalin trial, subsequent chemotherapy was feasible and tolerable. Stem cells were able to be collected and successful transplants performed. Although this data is encouraging, it should not be interpreted that stem cells will always be able to be collected on all patients after Zevalin. In patients that have received extensive chemotherapy or external beam radiation therapy, stem cells can be difficult to collect, even in the absence of RIT [67]. If the patient is considered to be a strong candidate for autologous transplant, then stem cells should be collected before RIT.

SAFETY OF RADIOIMMUNOTHERAPY

The safety of Zevalin RIT has been reported in each trial and also in aggregate [24, 68]. Infusion-related toxicities were typically Grade 1 or 2 and were associated with the rituximab infusion; there were no further infusion-related reactions when the [111]In- or ^{90}Y-Zevalin was

Table 10.4   Haematological toxicity experienced with anti-CD20 radioimmunoconjugates

Study	Neutrophils		Platelets		Haemoglobin	
	Nadir × 10⁶/l	% grade 4 (<500 × 10⁶/l)†	Nadir × 10⁶/l	% grade 4 (<10,000 × 10⁶/l)††	Nadir (g/dl)	% grade 4 (<6.5 g/dl)
Phase I [25]	1,100	27	49,500	10	–	–
Randomised [23]	900	32	42,000	6	10.8	1
Phase II for patients with thrombocytopaenia [22]	600	33	26,500	13	10.1	3
Rituximab-refractory [42]	700	35	33,000	9	9.9	4

†Grade 4 neutropaenia is <500 × 10⁶/l.
†† Grade 4 thrombocytopaenia is <10,000 × 10⁶/l.

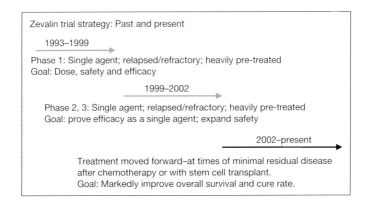

Figure 10.3   Overview of goals for Zevalin radioimmunotherapy trials.

administered at the conclusion of the rituximab. No significant normal organ toxicity was noted. The main toxicity noted was myelosuppression with the nadir haemoglobin, white blood cell (WBC), and platelet counts typically occurring at 7–9 weeks and lasting approximately 1–4 weeks depending on the method of calculation (Table 10.4). Following the 0.4 mCi/kg dose, Grade 4 neutropaenia, thrombocytopaenia and anaemia occurred in 30, 10, and 3% of patients, respectively, and following the 0.3 mCi/kg dose in 35, 14, and 8%. Bone marrow involvement with lymphoma at study entry was present in 146 patients (42%). Patients with any degree of bone marrow involvement had a significantly greater incidence of Grade 4 neutropaenia ($p = 0.001$), thrombocytopaenia ($p = 0.013$), and anaemia ($p = 0.040$) than patients with no bone marrow involvement. The incidence of Grade 4 haematological toxicity increased with increasing levels of bone marrow involvement at baseline. Seven percent of patients were hospitalised with infection (3% with neutropaenia) and 2% had Grade 3 or 4 bleeding events. Myelodysplasia or acute myelogenous leukaemia was reported in 5 patients (1%) 8–34 months after treatment and all of these patients had been previously treated with alkylating agents. The HAMA rate in the studies with Zevalin has been very low (<1%) [24].

SUMMARY

The results of the phase I, phase II, and randomised trials discussed above document that the single doses of Zevalin are safe and efficacious in patients with relapsed B-cell NHL. RIT produces a response rate of approximately 80%, and 25–30% of patients obtain a CR. The primary toxicity is myelosuppression and this is dose limiting if stem cell support is not used. Overall patient acceptance of Zevalin is high with an excellent quality of life.

All the patients in the above trials have had relapsed disease. Current trials are now moving the Zevalin treatment earlier up the disease course after chemotherapy or with stem cell support (Figure 10.3). These trials aim to build on the known effectiveness of radiotherapy in NHL, the targeting ability of Zevalin, and the results of single-agent studies that demonstrate that Zevalin works best on low-bulk disease. The aim of these trials is to increase the CR rate and TTP so that patients with low-grade NHL will become curable.

ACKNOWLEDGEMENTS

Supported in part by CA87912 and CA97274.

REFERENCES

1. McLaughlin P, Grillo-Lopez AJ, Link BK, Levy R, Czuczman MS, Williams ME *et al*. Rituximab chimeric anti-CD20 monoclonal antibody therapy for relapsed indolent lymphoma: half of patients respond to a four-dose treatment program. *J Clin Oncol* 1998; 16:2825–2833.
2. Czuczman MS, Grillo-Lopez AJ, White CA, Saleh M, Gordon L, LoBuglio AF *et al*. Treatment of patients with low-grade B-cell lymphoma with the combination of chimeric anti-CD20 monoclonal antibody and CHOP chemotherapy. *J Clin Oncol* 1999; 17:268–276.
3. Vose JM, Link BK, Grossbard ML, Czuczman M, Grillo-Lopez A, Gilman P *et al*.Phase II study of rituximab in combination with CHOP chemotherapy in patients with previously untreated, aggressive non-Hodgkin's lymphoma. *J Clin Oncol* 2001; 19:389–397.
4. Coiffier B, Lepage E, Briere J, Herbrecht R, Tilly H, Bouabdallah R *et al*. CHOP chemotherapy plus rituximab compared with CHOP alone in elderly patients with diffuse large-B-cell lymphoma. *N Engl J Med* 2002; 346:235–242.
5. Witzig TE, Vukov AM, Habermann TM, Geyer S, Kurtin PJ, Friedenberg WR *et al*. Rituximab therapy for patients with newly diagnosed, advanced-stage, follicular grade I non-Hodgkin's lymphoma: a phase II trial in the North Central Cancer Treatment Group. *J Clin Oncol* 2005; 18:18.
6. Ghielmini M, Schmitz SF, Cogliatti SB, Pichert G, Hummerjohann J, Waltzer U *et al*. Prolonged treatment with rituximab in patients with follicular lymphoma significantly increases event-free survival and response duration compared with the standard weekly × 4 schedule. *Blood* 2004; 103:4416–4423.
7. Hainsworth JD, Burris HA, Morrissey LH, Litchy S, Scullin DC, Bearden JD *et al*. Rituximab monoclonal antibody as initial systemic therapy for patients with low-grade non-Hodgkin lymphoma. *Blood* 2000; 95:3052–3056.
8. Hainsworth JD, Litchy S, Barton JH, Houston GA, Hermann RC, Bradof JE *et al*. Single-agent rituximab as first-line and maintenance treatment for patients with chronic lymphocytic leukemia or small lymphocytic lymphoma: a phase II trial of the Minnie Pearl Cancer Research Network. *J Clin Oncol* 2003; 21:1746–1751.
9. Hainsworth JD, Litchy S, Burris HA, 3rd, Scullin DC, Jr, Corso SW, Yardley DA *et al*. Rituximab as first-line and maintenance therapy for patients with indolent non-Hodgkin's lymphoma. *J Clin Oncol* 2002; 20:4261–4267.
10. Colombat P, Salles G, Brousse N, Eftekhari P, Soubeyran P, Delwail V *et al*. Rituximab (anti-CD20 monoclonal antibody) as single first-line therapy for patients with follicular lymphoma with a low tumor burden: clinical and molecular evaluation. *Blood* 2001; 97:101–106.

11. Hernandez MC, Knox SJ. Radiobiology of radioimmunotherapy with 90Y ibritumomab tiuxetan (Zevalin). *Semin Oncol* 2003; 30:6–10.
12. Fritzberg A, Meares C. Metallic radionuclides for radioimmunotherapy. In: PAF, Abrams AR (ed.) Radioimmunotherapy of Cancer. Marcel Dekker Inc, New York; 2000, pp 57–79
13. DeNardo GL, Kennel SJ, Siegel JA, Denardo SJ. Radiometals as payloads for radioimmunotherapy for lymphoma. *Clin Lymphoma* 2004; 5:S5–S10.
14. Vriesendorp HM, Herpst JM, Germack MA, Klein JL, Leichner PK, Loudenslager DM *et al.* Phase I-II studies of yttrium-labeled antiferritin treatment for end-stage Hodgkin's disease, including Radiation Therapy Oncology Group 87–01 [published erratum appears in *J Clin Oncol* 1991; 9:1516]. *J Clin Oncol* 1991; 9:918–928.
15. Cheson BD. Radioimmunotherapy of non-Hodgkin lymphomas. *Blood* 2003; 101:391–398.
16. Friedberg JW. Radioimmunotherapy for non-Hodgkin's lymphoma. *Clin Cancer Res* 2004; 10:7789–7791.
17. Liu SY, Eary JF, Petersdorf SH, Martin PJ, Maloney DG, Appelbaum FR *et al.* Follow-up of relapsed B-cell lymphoma patients treated with iodine-131-labeled anti-CD20 antibody and autologous stem-cell rescue. *J Clin Oncol* 1998; 16:3270–3278.
18. Kaminski MS, Zasadny KR, Francis IR, Milik AW, Ross CW, Moon SD *et al.* Radioimmunotherapy of B-cell lymphoma with [131I]anti-B1 (anti-CD20) antibody. *N Eng J Med* 1993; 329:459–465.
19. Kaminski MS, Zasadny KR, Francis IR, Fenner MC, Ross CW, Milik AW *et al.* Iodine-131-anti-B1 radioimmunotherapy for B-cell lymphoma. *J Clin Oncol* 1996; 14:1974–1981.
20. Knox SJ, Goris ML, Trisler K, Negrin R, Davis T, Liles TM *et al.* Yttrium-90-labeled anti-CD20 monoclonal antibody therapy of recurrent B-cell lymphoma. *Clin Cancer Res* 1996; 2:457–470.
21. Press OW, Eary JF, Appelbaum FR, Martin PJ, Nelp WB, Glenn S *et al.* Phase II trial of 131I-B1 (anti-CD20) antibody therapy with autologous stem cell transplantation for relapsed B cell lymphomas. Lancet 1995; 346:336–340.
22. Wiseman GA, Gordon LI, Multani PS, Witzig TE, Spies S, Bartlett NL *et al.* Ibritumomab tiuxetan radioimmunotherapy for patients with relapsed or refractory non-Hodgkin lymphoma and mild thrombocytopenia: a phase II multicenter trial. *Blood* 2002; 99:4336–4342.
23. Witzig TE, Gordon LI, Cabanillas F, Czuczman M, Emmanouilides C, Joyce R *et al.* Randomized controlled trial of 90Y-labeled ibritumomab tiuxetan radioimmunotherapy versus rituximab immunotherapy for patients with relapsed or refractory low-grade, follicular, or transformed B-cell non-Hodgkin's lymphoma. *J Clin Oncol* 2002; 20:2453–2463.
24. Witzig TE, White CA, Gordon LI, Wiseman GA, Emmanouilides C, Murray JL *et al.* Safety of Yttrium-90 ibritumomab tiuxetan radioimmunotherapy for relapsed low-grade, follicular, or transformed non-Hodgkin's lymphoma. *J Clin Oncol* 2003; 21:1263–1270.
25. Witzig TE, White CA, Wiseman GA, Gordon LI, Emmanouilides C, Raubitschek A *et al.* Phase I/II trial of IDEC-Y2B8 radioimmunotherapy for treatment of relapsed or refractory CD20(+) B-cell non-Hodgkin's lymphoma. *J Clin Oncol* 1999; 17:3793–3803.
26. DeNardo SJ, DeNardo GL, Kukis DL, Shen S, Kroger LA, DeNardo DA *et al.* 67Cu-2IT-BAT-Lym-1 pharmacokinetics, radiation dosimetry, toxicity and tumor regression in patients with lymphoma. *J Nucl Med* 1999; 40:302–310.
27. Kaminski M, Estes J, Zasadny K, Francis I, Ross C, Tuck M *et al.* Radioimmunotherapy with iodine 131I tositumomab for relapsed or refractory B-cell non-Hodgkin lymphoma: updated results and long-term follow-up of the University of Michigan experience. *Blood* 2000; 96:1259–1266.
28. Press O, Eary J, Gooley T, Gopal A, Liu S, Rajendran J *et al.* A phase I/II trial of iodine-131-tositumomab (anti-CD20), etoposide, cyclophosphamide, and autologous stem cell transplantation for relapsed B-cell lymphomas. *Blood* 2000; 96:2934–2942.
29. Kaminski MS, Zelenetz AD, Press OW, Saleh M, Leonard J, Fehrenbacher L *et al.* Pivotal study of iodine I 131 tositumomab for chemotherapy-refractory low-grade or transformed low-grade B-cell non-Hodgkin's lymphomas. *J Clin Oncol* 2001; 19: 3918–3928.
30. Vose JM, Colcher D, Gobar L, Bierman PJ, Augustine S, Tempero M *et al.* Phase I/II trial of multiple dose 131Iodine-MAb LL2 (CD22) in patients with recurrent non-Hodgkin's lymphoma. *Leuk Lymphoma*, 2000; 38:91–101.
31. Vose JM, Wahl RL, Saleh M, Rohatiner AZ, Knox SJ, Radford JA *et al.* Multicenter phase II study of iodine-131 tositumomab for chemotherapy-relapsed/refractory low-grade and transformed low-grade B-cell non-Hodgkin's lymphomas. *J Clin Oncol* 2000; 18:1316–1323.

32. Juweid ME, Stadtmauer E, Hajjar G, Sharkey RM, Suleiman S, Luger S et al. Pharmacokinetics, dosimetry, initial therapeutic results with 131I- and (111)In-/90Y-labeled humanized LL2 anti-CD22 monoclonal antibody in patients with relapsed, refractory non-Hodgkin's lymphoma. Clin Cancer Res 1999; 5:3292S–3303S.

33. Waldmann TA, White JD, Carrasquillo JA, Reynolds JC, Paik CH, Gansow OA et al. Radioimmunotherapy of interleukin-2R alpha-expressing adult T-cell leukemia with Yttrium-90-labeled anti-Tac [see comments]. Blood 1995; 86:4063–4075.

34. Dillman RO. Radiolabeled Anti-CD20 Monoclonal Antibodies for the Treatment of B-Cell Lymphoma. J Clin Oncol 2002; 20:3545–3557.

35. Witzig TE. Radioimmunotherapy for B-cell non-Hodgkin's lymphoma. In: Hoffman R, Benz EJ, Jr, Shattil SJ, Furie B, Cohen HJ, Silberstein LE, McGlave P (eds.), Hematology: Basic Principles and Practice Elsevier, Churchill, Livingstone, Philadelphia, 2005, pp 1045–1055.

36. Chinn PC, Leonard JE, Rosenberg J, Hanna N, Anderson DR. Preclinical evaluation of 90Y-labeled anti-CD20 monoclonal antibody for treatment of non-Hodgkin's lymphoma. In J Oncol 1999; 15:1017–1025.

37. Wiseman GA, Leigh B, Erwin WD et al. Radiation Dosimetry Results From a Phase II Trial of Ibritumomab Tiuxetan (Zevalin) Radioimmunotherapy for Patients With Non-Hodgkin's Lymphoma and Mild Thrombocytopenia. Cancer Biother Radiopharm 2003; 18:165–178.

38. Wiseman GA, Kornmehl E, Leigh B et al. Radiation dosimetry results and safety correlations from 90Y-ibritumomab tiuxetan radioimmunotherapy for relapsed or refractory non-Hodgkin's lymphoma: combined data from 4 clinical trials. J Nucl Med 2003; 44:465–474.

39. Wiseman GA, White C, Erwin W et al. Zevalin biodistribution and dosimetry estimated normal organ absorbed radiation doses are not affected by prior therapy with rituximab. Blood 1999; 94 (Suppl):92a.

40. Wiseman GA, Leigh B, Erwin WD et al. Radiation dosimetry results for Zevalin radioimmunotherapy of rituximab-refractory non-Hodgkin lymphoma. Cancer 2002; 94:1349–1357.

41. Wiseman GA, Leigh BR, Dunn WL, Stabin MG, White CA. Additional radiation absorbed dose estimates for Zevalin radioimmunotherapy. Cancer Biother Radiopharm 2003; 18:253–258.

42. Wiseman GA, White CA, Sparks RB et al. Biodistribution and dosimetry results from a phase III prospectively randomized controlled trial of Zevalin radioimmunotherapy for low-grade, follicular, or transformed B-cell non-Hodgkin's lymphoma. Crit Rev Oncol Hematol 2001; 39:181–194.

43. Wagner HN, Jr, Wiseman GA, Marcus CS, Nabi HA, Nagle CE, Fink-Bennett DM et al. Administration guidelines for radioimmunotherapy of non-Hodgkin's lymphoma with (90)Y-labeled anti-CD20 monoclonal antibody. J Nucl Med 2002; 43:267–272.

44. Wiseman G, Leigh B, Witzig T, Gansen DN, White C. Radiation exposure is very low to the family members of patients treated with yttrium-90 Zevalin™ anti-CD20 monoclonal antibody therapy for lymphoma. European J Nucl Med 2001; 28:1198.

45. Gordon LI, Molina A, Witzig T, Emmanouilides C, Raubtischek A, Darif M et al. Durable responses after ibritumomab tiuxetan radioimmunotherapy for CD20+ B-cell lymphoma: long-term follow-up of a phase 1/2 study. Blood 2004; 103:4429–4431.

46. Wiseman G, White C, Stabin M, Witzig T, Spies S, Silverman D et al. Phase I/II 90Y-Zevalin (yttrium-90 ibritumomab tiuxetan, IDEC-Y2B8) radioimmunotherapy dosimetry results in relapsed or refractory non-Hodgkin's lymphoma. Eur J Nucl Med 2000; 27:766–777.

47. Cheson B, Horning S, Coiffier B, Shipp M, Fisher R, Connors J et al. Report of an international workshop to standardize response criteria for non-Hodgkin's lymphoma. J Clin Oncol 1999; 17:1244–1253.

48. Witzig TE, Flinn IW, Gordon LI, Emmanouilides C, Czuczman MS, Saleh MN et al. Treatment with ibritumomab tiuxetan radioimmunotherapy in patients with rituximab-refractory follicular non-Hodgkin's lymphoma. J Clin Oncol 2002; 20:3262–3269.

49. Oki Y, Pro B, Delpassand E, Ballaster V, McLaughlin P, Romaguera J et al. Phase II Study of Yttrium 90 (90Y) ibritumomab tiuxetan (Zevalin®) for treatment of patients with relapsed and refractory mantle cell lymphoma (MCL). Blood 2004; 104:Abstract 2632.

50. Morschhauser F, Huglo D, Martinelli G et al. Yttrium-90 Ibritumomab Tiuxetan (Zevalin) for Patients with Relapsed/Refractory Diffuse Large B-Cell Lymphoma Not Appropriate for Autologous Stem Cell Transplantation: Results of an Open-Label Phase II Trial. Blood 2004; 110:Abstract 130.

51. Gordon LI, Witzig T, Molina A, Czuczman M, Emmanouilides C, Joyce R et al. Yttrium 90-labeled ibritumomab tiuxetan radioimmunotherapy produces high response rates and durable remissions in patients with previously treated B-cell lymphoma. Clin Lymphoma 2004; 5:98–101.

52. Wahl RL, Tidmarsh G, Kroll S. Successful retreatment of non-Hodgkin's lymphoma with iodine-131 anti-B1 antibody. *Proc Am Soc Clin Oncol* 1998; 17:40a (abstract 156).

53. Wiseman G, Colgan J, Inwards D, Micallef IN, Porrata LF, Gansen DN *et al.* Yttrium-90 Zevalin phase I sequential dose radioimmunotherapy trial of patients with relapsed low grade and follicular B-cell non-Hodgkin's lymphoma (NHL): preliminary results. *Blood* 2002; 100:358a (abstract 1387).

54. Press OW, Eary JF, Appelbaum FR, Martin PJ, Badger CC, Nelp WB *et al.* Radiolabeled-antibody therapy of B-cell lymphoma with autologous bone marrow support [see comments]. *N Engl J Med* 1993; 329:1219–1224.

55. Gopal AK, Gooley TA, Maloney DG, Petersdorf SH, Eary JF, Rajendran JG *et al.* High-dose radioimmunotherapy versus conventional high-dose therapy and autologous hematopoietic stem cell transplantation for relapsed follicular non-Hodgkin lymphoma: a multivariable cohort analysis. *Blood* 2003; 102:2351–2357.

56. Winter JN, Inwards D, Erwin W, Wiseman G, Rademaker A, Patton DR *et al.* Zevalin dose-escalation followed by high-dose BEAM and autologous peripheral blood progenitor cell (PBPC) Transplant in non-Hodgkin's lymphoma: early outcome results. *Blood* 2002; 100:411a (abstract 1597).

57. Nademanee A, Forman SJ, Molina A, Kogut N, Fung HC, Yamauchi D *et al.* High-dose radioimmunotherapy with yttrium 90 (90Y) ibritumomab tiuxetan with high-dose etoposide (VP-16) and cyclophosphamide (CY) followed by autologous hematopoietic cell transplant (AHCT) for poor-risk or relapsed B-cell non-Hodgkin's lymphoma (NHL): update of a phase I/II trial. *J Clin Oncol* 2004; 22:559.

58. Nademanee AP, Molina A, Forman SJ, Kogut N, Yamauchi D, Liu A *et al.* A phase I/II trial of high-dose radioimmunotherapy (RIT) with Zevalin in combination with high-dose etoposide (VP-16) and cyclophosphamide (CY) followed by autologous stem cell transplant (ASCT) in patients with poor-risk or relapsed B-cell non-Hodgkin's lymphoma (NHL). *Blood* 2002; 100:182a (abstract 679).

59. Winter JN. Combining yttrium 90-labeled ibritumomab tiuxetan with high-dose chemotherapy and stem cell support in patients with relapsed non-Hodgkin's lymphoma. *Clin Lymphoma* 2004; 5:S22–S26.

60. Kaminski MS, Tuck M, Estes J, Kolstad A, Ross CW, Zasadny K *et al.* 131I-Tositumomab therapy as initial treatment for follicular lymphoma. *N Engl J Med* 2005; 352:441–449.

61. Connors JM. Radioimmunotherapy – hot new treatment for lymphoma. *N Engl J Med* 2005; 352:496–498.

62. Sweetenham JW, Dicke K, Arcaroli J, Kogel K, Rana TR, Rice LL. Efficacy and safety of Yttrium 90 (90Y) ibritumomab tiuxetan (Zevalin®) therapy with rituximab maintenance in patients with untreated low-grade follicular lymphoma. *Blood* 2004; 104:Abstract 2633.

63. Shipley DL, Spigel DR, Carrell DL, Dannaher C, Greco FA, Hainsworth JD. Phase II trial of rituximab and short duration chemotherapy followed by 90Y-ibritumomab tiuxetan as first-line treatment for patients with follicular lymphoma: A Minnie Pearl Cancer Research Network phase II trial. *J Clin Oncol* 2004; (Meeting Abstracts), 22:562–b.

64. Radford JA, Ketterer N, Sebban C *et al.* Ibritumomab Tiuxetan (Zevalin) Therapy Is Feasible and Safe for the Treatment of Patients with Advanced B-Cell Follicular NHL in First Remission: Interim Analysis for Safety of a Multicenter, Phase III Clinical Trial. *Blood* 2003; 102:408a.

65. Ansell SM, Ristow KM, Habermann TM, Wiseman GA, Witzig TE. Subsequent chemotherapy regimens are well tolerated after radioimmunotherapy with Yttrium-90 ibritumomab tiuxetan for non-Hodgkin's lymphoma. *J Clin Oncol* 2002; 20:3885–3890.

66. Ansell SM, Schilder RJ, Pieslor PC, Gordon LI, Emmanouilides C, Vo K *et al.* Antilymphoma treatments given subsequent to Yttrium 90 ibritumomab tiuxetan are feasible in patients with progressive non-Hodgkin's lymphoma: a review of the literature. *Clin Lymphoma* 2004; 5:202–204.

67. Micallef IN, Apostolidis J, Rohatiner AZ, Wiggins C, Crawley CR, Foran JM *et al.* Factors which predict unsuccessful mobilisation of peripheral blood progenitor cells following G-CSF alone in patients with non-Hodgkin's lymphoma. *Hematol J* 2000; 1:367–373.

68. Borghaei H, Wallace SG, Schilder RJ. Factors associated with toxicity and response to yttrium 90-labeled ibritumomab tiuxetan in patients with indolent non-Hodgkin's lymphoma. *Clin Lymphoma* 2004; 5:S16–S21.

11

Radioimmunotherapy combinations with other therapies for non-Hodgkin's lymphoma

C. Emmanouilides

INTRODUCTION

The introduction of targeted therapeutic approaches has revolutionised the field of cancer treatment over the last decade. In particular, the use of monoclonal antibodies has met with considerable success, firstly in the treatment of lymphoma and subsequently in other cancer types. Although engagement and direct interaction with selected surface proteins appear to be of therapeutic value, antibodies also constitute an excellent targeting system, marking selected cells for interaction with innate immune effector mechanisms, or by conjugation with moieties of therapeutic value. In contrast to the mixed results of the use of monoclonal antibodies as a means to deliver toxins, radioimmunotherapy (RIT) has been proven to be effective enough for the U.S. Food and Drug Administration to approve the first ever radioimmunoconjugate (RIC) for the treatment of a malignancy in February of 2002, when ^{90}Y-ibritumomab tiuxetan (Zevalin, ^{90}Y-IT) was licensed for the treatment of lymphoma. Nearly a year later, an earlier radioimmunotherapy product, ^{131}I-tositumomab (Bexxar, ^{131}I-T) was also approved for rituximab-refractory indolent or transformed lymphoma. Both agents are considered comparable in terms of efficacy or toxicity. Thus, CD20-based RIT for non-Hodgkin's lymphoma (NHL) follows the path first paved by the successful application of rituximab, an anti-CD20 monoclonal antibody widely used against B-cell malignancies. RIT has already been tested in a variety of tumour types, but its success in lymphoma is conferred by the relative radiosensitivity of the disease, and possibly by the therapeutic value of the direct engagement of CD20 by an antibody. RIT offers several advantages compared with external beam irradiation, because normal tissues overlying the tumour mass are prevented from significant radiation exposure; also, since the RIC is given intravenously, it provides systemic radiation treatment to known as well as unsuspected tumour cells. Obviously, the commercially available products are more advanced in clinical applications, although experimental agents for the treatment of lymphoma are under development as well.

The launching of RIT is presumed to be the first step in the development of a therapeutic modality that complements current treatments of NHL and will evolve into a robust and well-defined strategy for the management of this disease. However, the optimal incorporation of RIT into the therapeutic algorithm of NHL remains to be proven. Monotherapy studies with RICs in indolent or follicular NHL have defined a relatively consistent

Christos Emmanouilides, Associate Professor, UCLA, Interbalkan European Medical Center-Oncology, Pylaia, Thessaloniki.

response rate of 60–80%, with a duration of reponse (DR) of approximately one year [1–3]. Significant activity has been documented for patients with aggressive histologies such as diffuse large B-cell NHL and mantle cell lymphoma [4–6]. The activity of RIC is in general superior to what is observed with the naked anti-CD20 antibody rituximab, as shown in comparison studies or compared with historical controls. This is not surprising, given the fact that anti-CD20-based RIT combines the advantage of CD20 engagement with tumour irradiation. Given the successful incorporation of rituximab with standard chemotherapeutic treatments, it is only natural to try to define ways of combining RIT with standard therapy, be it chemotherapy or immunotherapy, expecting an additive, if not synergistic, effect. However, in sharp contrast with the use of rituximab, RIT-induced myelosuppression is an overlapping toxicity with chemotherapy-induced cytopaenia. For the most part, concurrent use with standard chemotherapy cycles is clearly impossible given the kinetics of the myelosuppression from RIT, with the characteristic nadir at week 6–8 and slow recovery of the counts that may last several weeks, unless innovative schedules are tried. On the other hand, applications of RIT as consolidation after remission induction, treating macroscopic or minimal residual disease, could theoretically offer a considerable prolongation of disease-free survival. Additionally, in situations eliminating myelosuppression from being the dose-limiting toxicity, i.e. in the context of autologous or allogeneic haematopoietic progenitor cell transplant, RIT can be a useful alternative or adjunct anti-lymphoma ablating method, either at standard or escalated doses. Since the administration of naked anti-CD20 antibody is an integral part of the delivery method of RIT, concurrent use with rituximab may offer little, if any, value. On the other hand, if a rituximab maintenance approach is elected for a given patient, it may be more reasonable to try to consolidate a remission of better quality, which is usually induced by RIT, rather than rituximab monotherapy; hence, combinations of RIT followed by rituximab consolidation may be very helpful in inducing and maintaining remissions in indolent lymphoma and such regimens are currently being explored.

THEORETICAL CONSIDERATIONS FOR COMBINATION STRATEGIES

Standard and well-defined criteria of conventional screening for RIT exclude patients with excessive bone marrow involvement by disease. Special attention should be paid to the myelotoxicity of RIT which, unlike chemotherapy, induces a rather late decrease of counts with nadir at weeks 6–8 followed by a gradual recovery over the ensuing weeks. Clearly, during the period of 2–3 months following administration of RIT, myelotoxic chemotherapy cannot be safely administered, as it may interfere with the recovery of marrow function. However, it is reasonable to assume a synergistic action of chemotherapy and RIT-based tumour radiation, so that it may be of interest to combine RIT with concurrent chemotherapy. For instance, RIT could be administered with the last cycle of a prescribed chemotherapy schedule in order to avoid cycle delay, but such a trial has not been conducted to date. Combination with chemotherapy may be easier to test in the context of stem cell rescue. In the latter case, dose escalation is possible, which has obvious therapeutic advantage. Myelosuppression ceases to be the dose-limiting toxicity, again raising the question of a maximum tolerated dose in this context. Pertinent to combination with chemotherapy is the fact that the radiation is delivered by the RIC over a period of several days, depending on the half-life of the isotope used so that, in essence, concurrent treatment is delivered even if the RIC is administered several days prior to chemotherapy. Aside from several studies that have been performed or are underway exploring the use of RIT as monotherapy or part of a megatherapy regimen requiring stem cell rescue, it is of note that there is one study underway that has been designed to deliver standard ^{90}Y-IT with the first cycle of CVP (cyclophosphamide, vincristine, prednisone) chemotherapy, whereas the subsequent CVP cycles are given 12 weeks later, at haematological recovery.

RIT may serve as a practical and convenient consolidation treatment after induction chemotherapy. Such a use offers several advantages. Firstly, full recovery of blood counts is assured at the time of RIT treatment. Secondly, the cytoreduction achieved by chemotherapy usually results in amelioration of bone marrow disease, so that the likelihood of considerable bone marrow involvement exceeding 25% is extremely low. This of course translates into reduced severity and duration of cytopaenia, which correlates with the extent of bone marrow involvement. The observed lack of increased risk of myelodysplasia or acute leukaemia with RIT permits its inclusion in a front-line regimen [7]. The rate of development of antibodies against the RIC (human anti-mouse antibodies, HAMA) may be less than that in the unmanipulated immune system, which may be particularly relevant in the case of ^{131}I-T. Furthermore, the impact of RIT in measurable residual disease could be quantified, i.e. one could know how many partial responses could be converted to complete ones. However, this should be viewed with caution, since ongoing shrinkage of involved nodes may occasionally occur for several months after conventional treatment as well, so that the true impact could only be assessed in the context of a randomised study which, fortunately, is underway. Prolongation of disease-free survival (DFS) is expected. Alternatively, because of the documented activity of RIT for indolent NHL, one could envision its use as a chemotherapy-sparing agent, so that patients receive fewer cycles of chemotherapy followed by RIT.

Several of the ongoing chemotherapy followed by RIT studies utilise rituximab as part of the induction regimen. The use of rituximab could be argued against, for fear that it will engage the CD20 epitopes of the lymphoma cells so that the RIC does not reach its target; however, the interaction of the antibody with its target should be viewed as a dynamic process of equilibrium with constant detachment of molecules and replacement by others. It should not be forgotten that the RIC is always stoichiometrically a much smaller quantity compared to the amount of naked anti-CD20 antibody given with it. In addition, RIT is known to be active even in the presence of measurable rituximab levels, as shown in the study of Zevalin in rituximab-refractory patients, supporting the use of RIT even in the presence of rituximab [2].

It appears, therefore, that the concept of antibody-based consolidation therapy has gained acceptance, given the results obtained with rituximab, and lends attractiveness to such a use for RIT as well. However, there are certain theoretical caveats for indiscrete consolidation treatment with RIT. By design, the ratio of beneficial radiation vs. radiation deposited to surrounding tissue depends on the size of the lymphomatous mass and the length of the path of radiation delivered. Since radiation is delivered within a sphere whose centre is the radioactive material, if one assumes micrometastatic single cell disease, most of the radiation of the lymphoma-attached radioconjugate will be delivered to the surrounding tissue, and as such, there will be a waste of radioactivity. On the other hand, the intensity of the radiation is stronger in the centre of such a sphere, so that the hypothesised single lymphomatous cell covered with RIC could still be exposed to sufficient radiation for clinical benefit, even without the crossfire effect, more so as it may already be damaged from the preceding chemotherapy.

At this point, the benefit of RIT for minimal, immeasurable disease is unknown. If, however, the response to preceding chemotherapy was not complete, then RIT may be an ideal agent to treat the remaining involved nodes, from the point of view of radiation physics, because of the crossfire effect. This hypothesis is supported by the clinical studies discussed below. In such cases, another question would be whether the relative resistance to chemotherapy preventing a complete response (CR) also predisposes to radioresistance. Based on the evidence of significant activity of RIT in patients with chemoresistant disease [1, 2], it appears that RIT still provides a benefit. Another concern of the consolidation use is whether a bone marrow in the process of recovering and regenerating from the effects of recent myelotoxic chemotherapy can safely sustain the effect of RIT, and if there is a minimum safe period separating the preceding chemotherapy from the subsequent RIT. Completed studies seem to indicate that an interval period of 5 weeks is sufficient for safe administration of RIT without unexpected toxicity, particularly myelosuppression.

It can be reasonably expected that the addition of RIT after a standard chemotherapy regimen will prolong the duration of the remission and time to progression. Whether the pre-emptive treatment of the residual disease with RIT may be more beneficial in terms of overall survival compared with reserving its use for the inevitable progression of the indolent lymphoma will remain an important question to be answered in the future.

Recently, studies documenting activity of RIT in lymphoma types other than indolent lymphoma have led to the development of consolidation studies in such histologies as well. Given the observed improvement of DFS when standard chemotherapy is combined with antibody-based treatment, one cannot exclude a significant benefit in such patients.

RADIOIMMUNOTHERAPY CONSOLIDATION (Table 11.1)

INDOLENT NHL

The largest experience of using consolidation RIT has been by the Southwest Oncology Group (SWOG), a large phase II study of 90 patients with untreated follicular lymphoma [8]. After an initial full course of CHOP (cyclophosphamide, adriamycin, vincristine, prednisone) chemotherapy, responding patients received ^{131}I-T as consolidation. The mean time between the end of chemotherapy and treatment with RIT was 35 days. RIT was well tolerated without excessive myelotoxicity, and 57% of the patients achieving less than a CR improved their remission with RIT. The overall response rate was 90% including 67% CRs, and the 2-year progression-free survival (PFS) was estimated at 81%. This sequential regimen (CHOP- ^{131}I-T) was now tested in a randomised fashion against CHOP-rituximab. The same RIC was tested after an abbreviated 3-cycle course of fludarabine [9], again as first-line treatment. The sequence induced a CR in 83% of the 35 evaluable patients. Grade 4 neutropaenia or thrombocytopaenia was noted in 34% and 29%, respectively.

Several studies are underway in the USA involving ^{90}Y-IT consolidation after chemotherapy. In the Sarah Cannon Cancer Center, a short 3-cycle regimen of CHOP-rituximab or CVP-rituximab was followed by ^{90}Y-IT, which was thus used as a chemotherapy-sparing agent [10]. ^{90}Y-IT was given 5–7 weeks after the last chemotherapy cycle. Among the 22 reported responding patients who completed the whole protocol, there were 13 partial responders to chemotherapy, 10 of which converted to CR after ^{90}Y-IT, for an overall CR rate of 86%. Limited grade 4 neutropaenia or thrombocytopaenia was seen (18 and 0%, respectively). Studies at Rush Presbyterian Cancer Center and MD Anderson Cancer Center are underway exploring the use of ^{90}Y-IT after fludarabine-mitoxantrone and fludarabine-mitoxantrone-dexamethasone-rituximab, respectively. A study of full course CHOP-rituximab consolidated by Zevalin followed by rituximab is being evaluated at the University of Pittsburg.

The above observations have led to a large proposed multi-centred randomised phase III study based in Europe and the United States, testing the role of ^{90}Y-IT as consolidation therapy. Patients with stage III and IV follicular NHL receive a first-line induction regimen chosen by the site investigators. Four hundred and fifteen responders have been randomised to either receive ^{90}Y-IT consolidation or observation, with the primary end point being the DFS. It is expected that this study, as well as the SWOG randomised study, will help to more precisely define the value of adding RIT consolidation to standard treatment. It is clearly very important to define the probable prolongation of the DFS as well as possible long-term toxicities. However, the advantage of this practice as opposed to the application of RIT at first relapse, both in terms of time to subsequent relapse and possibly survival, will probably require subsequent trials.

Table 11.1 Consolidation studies with ^{90}Y-Ibritumomab Tiuxetan (Zevalin)

Study	Status	Results
a) Follicular or indolent NHL		
Phase II		
Rituximab-CHOP or CVP × 3 cycles followed by ^{90}Y-IT [10]	Completed	CR: 86%
Fludarabine-mitoxantrone × 6 followed by ^{90}Y-IT	Ongoing	
Fludarabine-mitoxantrone-dexamethasone-rituximab followed by ^{90}Y-IT	Ongoing	
CHOP-rituximab × 6 followed by ^{90}Y-IT	Ongoing	
Phase III		
Any chemotherapy followed by randomisation to ^{90}Y-IT, or observation	Ongoing	
b) Aggressive NHL		
Phase II		
CHOP-rituximab (full course) followed by ^{90}Y-IT	Ongoing	
Phase III		
CHOP-rituximab followed by randomization to ^{90}Y-IT or observation	Planned	
Early stage		
CHOP × 6 followed by involved-field radiotherapy followed by ^{90}Y-IT	Ongoing	
CHOP-rituximab × 4 followed by ^{90}Y-IT	Ongoing	
c) Mantle cell NHL (Phase II)		
CHOP-rituximab × 4 followed by ^{90}Y-IT	Ongoing	
HyperCVAD-R followed by ^{90}Y-IT	Ongoing	

AGGRESSIVE NHL

The documentation of the considerable activity of ^{90}Y-IT in patients with relapsed or refractory diffuse large B-cell lymphoma as well as the hope for further improvement of the overall survival in such a group of patients has led to the initiation of consolidation studies which are in progress. In a Memorial Sloan-Kettering phase II study, patients receive ^{90}Y-IT consolidation after a CHOP-rituximab course, as first-line treatment. A similar design has been adopted for first-line treatment of mantle cell lymphoma by the Eastern Cooperative Oncology Group (ECOG). For the latter disease, at the MD Anderson Cancer Center, ^{90}Y-IT is given as consolidation after standard HyperCVAD/rituximab regimen. In relapsed aggressive NHL unsuitable for high-dose chemotherapy, the use of ^{90}Y-IT following salvage ifosfamide-carboplatin-etoposide-rituximab (R-ICE) is being explored.

It is intriguing to consider RIT as a possible substitute for external beam irradiation in limited disease. Two ongoing phase II studies are exploring its consolidative use in conjunction with external beam radiation after an abbreviated course of either CHOP (SWOG), or CHOP-rituximab (ECOG), in patients with early stage aggressive lymphoma. It may also be interesting to consider the use of RIT with external beam irradiation in refractory cases. Based on personal anecdotal experience, involved nodes can be treated with both ^{90}Y-IT and external irradiation without apparent additive toxicity.

STEM CELL TRANSPLANT (Table 11.2)

Studies at the University of Washington have documented the feasibility of escalating the doses of RIT in order to maximise anti-tumour efficacy and, using the infusion of autologous stem cells, avoid ensuring myeloablation. Several years ago, Press and colleagues [11] reported on the administration of ^{131}I-B1 anti-CD20 antibody (tositumomab) at myeloablative, dosimetry-based doses of 345–785 mCi in 22 patients with relapsed follicular lymphoma, inducing a CR in 16 of 21 of the patients and a 62% PFS at 2 years. In a subsequent analysis of this cohort expanded to 29 patients, a 42% 5-year PFS was reported; reversible acute cardiopulmonary toxicity was noted in 2 patients as dose-limiting toxicity, whereas 60%

Table 11.2 Transplant studies with ^{90}Y-IT (Zevalin)

Study	Other chemotherapy	Maximum ^{90}Y-IT dose
Autologous		
Phase I–II with escalating absorbed doses to critical organs [17]	BEAM	1,100 cGy (0.75 mCi/kg)
Phase II with 1,000 cGy to the liver [18]	VP-16/Cy	med 71 mCi, max 105 mCi, dose escalation continuing
Phase II standard ^{90}Y-IT	BEAM	Standard dose (0.4 mCi per kg)
Phase I with escalating absorbed doses to organ [19]	Monotherapy	24 cGy to liver (121.7 mCi), dose escalation continuing
Allogeneic		
Phase II non-ablative	Flu/Cy	Standard dose (0.4 mCi per kg)

developed elevated thyroid stimulating hormone (TSH) [12]. Although these results compared favourably with historical controls [13], the inconvenience of the administration of high doses of ^{131}I seems to have prevented the widespread use of such a treatment. In addition to the above study, which involved single-agent-escalated RIT, studies combining ^{131}I-T with with 60 mg/kg of etoposide and 100 mg/kg of cyclophosphamide showed that the maximum tolerated dose would be such that 22–25 Gy was delivered to critical organs, inducing a 68% PFS [14]. A similar approach was used in a small cohort of patients with relapsed mantle cell lymphoma and frequent long remissions [15]. A different group at the University of Nebraska recently reported a phase I study of up to standard doses of ^{131}I-T followed by high-dose BEAM (BCNU, etoposide, ara-C, mephalan), showing feasibility and promising DFS [16].

Several ongoing studies are also exploring the use of ^{90}Y-IT in the context of autologous stem cell transplant. At Northwestern University, a careful dose escalation of ^{90}Y-IT beginning with a dose below the conventional one has been performed in conjunction with the BEAM regimen, proving the feasibility of the combination in multiply relapsed B-cell lymphoma [17]. Cohorts of patients received as much ^{90}Y-IT as was possible prior to BEAM so that critical organs received pre-defined escalating doses of radiation. Dosimetry was performed using ^{111}In-IT. The doses of ^{90}Y-IT differed widely per cohort (0.5–0.75 mCi/kg for the 1,100 cGy cohort). There was no unexpected toxicity, though a case of transient veno-occlusive disease was noted. All patients engrafted and had a 50% 3-year DFS.

A somewhat different approach has been taken by researchers at City of Hope. In an escalated ^{90}Y-IT study, increased dose of ^{90}Y-IT was administered so that the liver received 1,000 cGy of radiation, again using ^{111}In-IT imaging [18]. A week later, patients received high-dose etoposide and cyclophosphamide, followed by the infusion of autologous stem cells on the 14th day after ^{90}Y-IT. The median dose of ^{90}Y-IT was 71 mCi (2.6 GBq), more than twice the standard (range 37–105 mCi). Thus, ^{90}Y-IT served as a substitute for historically-used total body irradiation. Over 40 patients have been treated so far and an excellent DFS of 80% at 2 years was noted in this selected group of patients with diverse histologies. In a parallel study at the same institution, standard ^{90}Y-IT was given, again 14 days prior to the infusion of autologous stem cells following BEAM chemotherapy, in over 20 patients, showing the feasibility of combining standard dose RIC as well. In another smaller phase I study of escalated myeloablative ^{90}Y-IT following cyclophosphamide-rituximab mobilisation, doses delivering up to 24 Gy to the liver with administration of up to 121.7 mCi were given and were generally well tolerated [19].

At MD Anderson, a study using ^{90}Y-IT prior to a reduced-dose regimen with a fludarabine-cyclophosphamide combination followed by allogeneic stem cell transplant is underway. Although it is too early to comment on results, this study follows the very exciting data obtained using rituximab with the same regimen and may prove to be useful for indolent refractory B-cell malignancies.

It should be pointed out that in all of these studies, there has been no adverse effect on stem cell engraftment and the recovery from high-dose-therapy-induced aplasia. In most studies, the time to neutrophil engraftment was 10 days as expected. All designs allow a minimum of 14 days between the administration of RIT and the infusion of stem cells, which seems to be a safe period. The use of RIT did not seem to increase other organ toxicity, although the studies need to mature before definitive conclusions can be made.

SUMMARY

The emergence of RIT has opened up exciting new prospects for the treatment of lymphoma. Encouraging phase II studies are suggestive of favourable results when RIT complements the cytoreduction achieved by chemotherapy, either in the form of sequential consolidation therapy, or in the context of escalated doses with haematopoetic cell rescue. If the principle of achieving maximum anti-tumour effect from combining different modes of attack is truly beneficial, then RIC may prove to be the ideal product, since they combine immunologic targeting and systemic radiation, two already active modalities, and can thus complement chemotherapy to provide a more effective therapeutic strategy. In particular, the lack of significant radiation hazard associated with the use of a beta-emitter in the case of ^{90}Y-IT facilitates a widespread application of such combinations. Fortunately, ongoing (phase II) and randomised studies are underway and the results, which are expected in the near future, will help to better define its therapeutic role. The time may not be too far away when RIT becomes an essential part of any stem cell transplant for B-cell malignancies or part of a standard first-line treatment regimen.

REFERENCES

1. Witzig TE, Gordon LI, Cabanillas F, Czuczman MS, Emmanouilides C, Joyce R et al. Randomized controlled trial of yttrium-90-labeled ibritumomab tiuxetan radioimmunotherapy versus rituximab immunotherapy for patients with relapsed or refractory low-grade, follicular, or transformed B-cell non-Hodgkin's lymphoma. J Clin Oncol 2002; 20:2453–2463.
2. Witzig TE, Flinn IW, Gordon LI, Emmanouilides C, Czuczman MS, Saleh MN et al. Treatment with ibritumomab tiuxetan radioimmunotherapy in patients with rituximab-refractory follicular non-Hodgkin's lymphoma. J Clin Oncol 2002; 20:3262–3269.
3. Emmanouilides C. Radioimmunotherapy in non-Hodgkin lymphoma. Semin Oncol 2003; 30:531–544.
4. Witzig TE, White CA, Wiseman GA, Gordon LI, Emmanouilides C et al. Phase I/II trial of IDEC-Y2B8 radioimmunotherapy for treatment of relapsed or refractory CD20+ B-cell non-Hodgkin's lymphoma. J Clin Oncol 1999; 17:3793–3803.
5. Morschauser F, Huglo D, Martinelli G, Paganelli G, Zinzani PL, Hadjiyiannakis D et al. Yttrium-90 ibritumomab tiuextan (Zevalin) for patients with relapsed/refractory diffues large B-cell lymphoma not appropriate for autologous stem cell transplantation: results of an open-label phase II trial. Blood 2004; 104:Abstract 130.
6. Oki Y, Pro B, Delpassand E, Ballaster V, McLaughlin P, Romaguera J et al. A phase II study of yttrium-90 ibritumomab tiuxetan (Zevalin) for treatment of patients with refractory mantle cell lymphoma (MCL). Blood 2004; 104:Abstract 2632.
7. Emmanouilides C, Czuczman MS, Revell S. Low incidence of treatment-related myelodysplastic syndrome and acute myelogenous leukemia in patients with non-Hodgkin's lymphoma treated with ibritumomab tiuxetan. J Clin Oncol (Proc Am Soc Clin Oncol) 2004; 22:6696a.
8. Press OW, Unger JM, Braziel RM et al. A phase II trial of CHOP chemotherapy followed by tositumomab for previously untreated follicular non-Hodgkin lymphoma: Southwest Oncology Protocol S9911. Blood 2003; 102:1602–1612.
9. Leonard JP, Coleman M, Kostakoglu L et al. Durable remissions from fludarabine followed by the iodine I-131 tositumomab Bexxar therapeutic regimen for patients with previously untreated follicular NHL. J Clin Oncol (Proc Am Soc Clin Oncol) 2004; 22:6518a.

10. Shipley DL, Spigel DR, Carrell DL *et al.* Phase II trial of rituximab and short duration chemotherapy followed by ^{90}Y-ibritumomab tiuxetan as first line treatment for patients with follicular lymphoma. *J Clin Oncol (Proc Am Soc Clin Oncol)* 2004; 22:6519a.

11. Press OW, Eary JF, Appelbaum FR *et al.* Phase II trial of 131I-B1 (anti-CD20) antibody therapy with autologous stem cell transplantation for relapsed B cell lymphomas. *Lancet* 1995; 346:336–340.

12. Liu SY, Eary JF, Petersdorf SH *et al.* Follow up of relapsed B-cell lymphoma patients treated with iodine-131-labeled anti-CD20 antibody and autologous stem cell rescue. *J Clin Oncol* 1998; 16:3270–3278.

13. Gopal AK, Gooley TA, Maloney DG *et al.* High-dose radioimmunotherapy versus conventional high dose therapy and autologous stem cell transplantation for relapsed follicular non-Hodgkin lymphoma: a multivariate cohort analysis. *Blood* 2003; 102:2351–2357.

14. Press OW, Eary JF, Gooley T *et al.* A phase I/II trial of iodine-131-tositumomab, etoposide, cyclophosphamide, and autologous stem cell transplantation for relapsed B-cell lymphomas. *Blood* 2000; 96:2934–2942.

15. Gopal AK, Rajendran JG, Petersdorf SH *et al.* High dose chemo-radioimmunotherapy with autologous stem cell support for relapsed mantle cell lymphoma. *Blood* 2002; 99:3158–3162.

16. Vose JM, Bierman PJ, Enke C *et al.* Phase I trial of iodine-131-tositumomab with high dose chemotherapy and autologous stem cell transplantation for relapsed non-Hodgkin's lymphoma. *J Clin Oncol* 2005; 23:461–467.

17. Winter JN, Inwards DJ, Spies S *et al.* ^{90}Y Ibritumomab Tiuxetan doses higher than 0.4 mCi/kg may be safely combined with high dose BEAM and autotransplant. *Blood* 2004; 104:1162a.

18. Nademanee A, Forman SJ, Molina A *et al.* High dose radioimmunotherapy with yttrium 90 ibritumomab tiuxetan with high dose etoposide and cyclophosphamide followed by autologous hematopoetic stem cell transplant for poor risk or relapsed B-cell NHL. Updae of a phase I/II trial. *J Clin Oncol (Proc Am Soc Clin Oncol)* 2004; 22:6504a.

19. Flinn IW, Hahl BS, Frey E *et al.* Dose finding trial of yttrium 90 ibritumomab tiuxetan with autologous stem cell transplantation in patients with relapsed or refractory B-cell lymphoma. *Blood* 2004; 104:897a.

12

^{131}I-Tositumomab therapy for the treatment of low-grade non-Hodgkin's lymphoma

A. J. Jakubowiak, M. S. Kaminski

INTRODUCTION

Tositumomab is a monoclonal antibody that selectively binds to CD20 antigen on the surface of normal and malignant B cells. Tositumomab can be labelled with iodine-131 (^{131}I) to yield ^{131}I-labelled tositumomab [1]. The combination of unlabelled and I 131-labelled tositumomab is registered as tositumomab and ^{131}I-tositumomab or Bexxar therapeutic regimen. ^{131}I-tositumomab belongs to a novel class of therapy for non-Hodgkin's lymphomas (NHLs) known as radioimmunotherapy (RIT). The activity of ^{131}I-tositumomab depends on several mechanisms of action, including ionising radiation from ^{131}I and on antibody-mediated mechanisms, such as antibody-dependent cellular cytotoxicity (ADCC), complement-dependent cytotoxicity (CDC) and induction of apoptosis. In June 2003, ^{131}I-tositumomab was approved by the U.S. Food and Drug Administration (FDA) for the treatment of patients with CD20-positive, follicular, NHL, with and without transformation, whose disease is refractory to rituximab and has relapsed following chemotherapy. On January 3, 2005, the FDA approved an expanded indication for ^{131}I-tositumomab. ^{131}I-tositumomab is now indicated for the treatment of patients with CD20 antigen-expressing relapsed or refractory, low-grade, follicular, or transformed NHL including patients with rituximab-refractory NHL.

RATIONALE

Unlabelled monoclonal antibodies have shown promising efficacy in the treatment of NHL. However, unlabelled antibodies, when used alone, rarely produce complete responses, presumably due to variable and incomplete penetration of antibodies into lymphoma cells. One of the ways of improving the efficacy of unlabelled antibodies is to use them as carriers of radiation. It is well established that lymphomas are exquisitely sensitive to ionising radiation and that relapses rarely occur in irradiated sites of disease. Radiolabelled antibodies can retain immune-mediated and other mechanisms of action against lymphoma cells and at the same time can overcome some of the inherent limitations of unlabelled antibodies. Because ionising particles emitted from the radioisotope can travel through a number of cell diameters, many tumour cells within a tumour can be killed by a single radiolabelled antibody bound to a tumour cell. In addition, crossfire of ionising particles is created from multiple

Andrzej J. Jakubowiak, MD, PhD, Assistant Professor of Internal Medicine, University of Michigan Medical Center, Ann Arbor, Michigan, USA.

Mark S. Kaminski, MD, Professor of Internal Medicine, University of Michigan Medical Center, Ann Arbor, Michigan, USA.

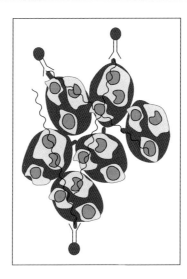

Figure 12.1   Crossfire effect in radioimmunotherapy[1].

radiolabelled antibodies bound to cells within a tumour, further intensifying the radiation dose to tumour cells (Figure 12.1). This effect is particularly important in bulkier tumours in which vascular access for antibodies to reach cells deep within a tumour may be limited. Furthermore, tumour cells either lacking the target antigen or expressing a small amount of antigen can be killed by crossfiring particles. Moreover, radiation from radiolabelled antibodies could be effective against tumour cells that have developed resistance to either immune or direct antibody cell killing. Therefore, radiolabelled antibodies can make use of multiple mechanisms of attack on tumour cells. Because systemic treatment with radiolabelled antibodies results in targeting of radiation to tumour sites *via* the specificity of the antibody, RIT, in contrast to conventional whole body irradiation, delivers more radiation to tumour sites than to normal tissues. Finally, in contrast to conventional external beam radiation therapy, in which radiation is delivered in a short pulse once a day, the radiation from RIT is delivered continuously at a lower dose rate. This difference may result in differing biological effects of radiation on exposed tumour cells.

Selection of an appropriate target for radiolabelled antibodies is critical for the success of this modality. Several potential targets have been considered; however, the CD20 antigen, which is expressed on the majority of B-cell lymphomas, was early recognised as a superior target of RIT of lymphoma. Importantly, CD20 is expressed only on normal and malignant B lymphocytes but not on lymphoid stem cells, allowing for reconstitution of B lymphocytes after elimination of CD20 cells by RIT. In addition, CD20 is considered to be a stable target for RIT because it is neither shed nor internalised to any significant degree upon antibody binding, allowing for extended continuous exposure to radiation after the antibody reaches its target.

COMPOSITION OF ^{131}I-TOSITUMOMAB

Tositumomab is the monoclonal antibody component of ^{131}I-tositumomab, while ^{131}I is the radionuclide used to label this antibody. Tositumomab, originally named anti-B1, is a

---

[1]Beta particles emitted by a radiolabelled antibody bound to multiple target antigens cross-travel through multiple cells, including cells to which antibody did not bind (Courtesy of Andrew Zelenetz, MD).

murine IgG2a antibody that is specific for the CD20 antigen (formerly known as the B1 antigen). CD20 is known to play a role in cell proliferation and differentiation and can act as a calcium channel. Importantly, it is expressed by approximately 90% of B-cell lymphomas. Tositumomab has the characteristics of a very efficient therapeutic antibody. Firstly, it is highly specific for B-cell lymphoma as a target. Furthermore, the murine Ig2a has a short plasma half-life. Preclinical studies provided evidence that tositumomab is effective in mediating CDC and ADCC as well as inducing apoptosis and cell-cycle arrest [2], providing additional mechanisms by which the lymphoma cell may be destroyed. In addition, tositumomab is capable of causing B-cell tumour regression *in vivo* in an animal model [2].

The ¹³¹I radioisotope that is coupled to tositumomab by a simple covalent reaction emits 0.6 Mev beta particles with a pathlength of 0.8 mm. Therefore, it can potentially deliver ionising radiation over approximately 60 lymphoma cell diameters, providing means for crossfire effects within a tumour as described above. ¹³¹I also emits low L.E.T. (linear energy transfer) gamma rays, which have longer pathlength that can be detected externally with a gamma camera or Geiger counter. Gamma rays from ¹³¹I have low energy and are not believed to contribute significantly to anti-tumour effects. While gamma rays do impose certain modest radiation precautions to limit the exposure of individuals in the vicinity, they are useful in monitoring the biodistribution and the rate of clearance of the radiolabelled antibody. This property of ¹³¹I is important since biodistribution and clearance rates can be significantly influenced by tumour burden, splenic size and the amount of bone marrow involvement and has been applied in the ¹³¹I-tositumomab regimen to provide an individualised dose for each patient, potentially avoiding over- and under-dosing if only a set dose were to be used (see below). Although the physical half-life of ¹³¹I is 8 days, biological clearance is rapid and is primarily through the kidneys and gut, allowing for treatment in an outpatient setting in the United States.

¹³¹I-TOSITUMOMAB THERAPEUTIC REGIMEN

The ¹³¹I-tositumomab therapeutic regimen consists of a dosimetric and therapeutic step (Figure 12.2). Each step involves administration of both unlabelled (cold) and radiolabelled (hot) antibody. Due to variability in the clearance rate of ¹³¹I-tositumomab between patients, individualised dosing is required. The dosimetric phase of the regimen involves delivery of a trace-labelled dose (5 millicuries; mCi) of ¹³¹I-tositumomab. This step is used to determine the therapeutic dose that minimises organ toxicity and maximises therapeutic benefit.

The dosing regimen and maximally tolerated dose were established in a Phase I/II single-centre study conducted at the University of Michigan [3]. A total of 59 patients with chemotherapy relapsed/refractory low-grade, transformed low-grade or *de novo* inter-mediate-grade lymphoma were enrolled. Inclusion criteria included limited bone marrow involvement with lymphoma (less than 25% of the haematopoietic marrow space), platelet counts of at least 100,000/mm³ and an absolute neutrophil count of at least 1,500/mm³, ade-quate renal function and an ability to comply with radiation safety instructions. These requirements were retained for all subsequent studies and continue to be followed in the clinical use of ¹³¹I-tositumomab.

In the dosimetric step, a one-hour intravenous infusion of 450 mg unlabelled tositumomab is followed by a 20-min infusion of 35 mg of trace dose (5 mCi) of ¹³¹I-tositumomab. The rationale for administering unlabelled antibody was confirmed in early animal and human biodistribution studies [4]. These showed that the tumour uptake of radiolabelled antibody is higher if unlabelled antibody is administered prior to the radioactive unlabelled dose than if given without the unlabelled pre-dose, presumably due to blocking of non-specific FC recep-tors and non-malignant B cells which may bind the CD20 antibody. The initial dose of unla-belled antibody is well tolerated, usually without (or with mild) infusion reactions. Fever,

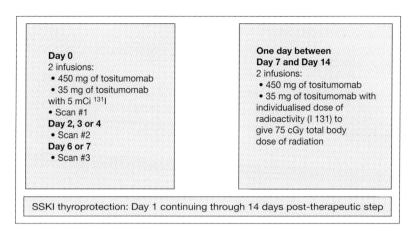

Figure 12.2   The ^{131}I-tositumomab therapeutic regimen[1].

rigors, mucosal oedema and hypotension may occur and may require that the infusion rate be slowed. More severe reactions, including anaphylaxis, have been observed, but only rarely. The trace-labelled ^{131}I-tositumomab is then administered within a couple of hours following the end of the cold tositumomab infusion.

During the dosimetric step of the ^{131}I-tositumomab regimen, gamma camera scans are obtained at baseline and at two other occasions over the ensuing week to evaluate the biodistribution of radiolabelled antibody and to determine the rate of clearance. This allows individualised dosing of radiolabelled antibody for each patient to deliver a desired total body dose (TBD). Factors affecting clearance of radiolabelled antibody and the patient-specific dose include a patient's weight, binding of antibody to normal B cells, degree of tumour burden, spleen size and degree of bone marrow involvement. Although variability in patient size can easily be corrected for using a standardised millicuries/body size radiation dose, other variables could be significant and more difficult to predict. The clearance rate of ^{131}I-tositumomab has varied as much as 5-fold in clinical trials [5] and the millicurie amount of ^{131}I-tositumomab required to administer a set TBD (75 cGy) of radiation varied from 56.8 to 153 mCi [3]. The more rapidly the antibody is cleared, the lower the delivered radiation TBD. It has been calculated that if patients had received a fixed 1.1-mCi/kg dosage of ^{131}I-tositumomab, 51% of the patients would have been under- or overdosed by at least 10%. Moreover, 10% of patients would have received ≤25% of the maximally tolerated TBD (75 cGy) and 6% would have been overdosed by ≥ 25% [6].

The rate of clearance of radiolabelled antibody is derived from the semilog plot of the percentage of radioactivity remaining at each of the dosimetric scans (Figure 12.3). The residence time of ^{131}I-tositumomab in hours corresponds to the value on the X-axis at which a best-fit line intersects the horizontal 37% activity line. The patient-specific dose of radiolabelled tositumomab (in mCi) required to deliver the desired therapeutic dose of total-body radiation is then calculated using the following equation:

Therapeutic dose (mCi) = [Activity hours (mCi hr)/residence time (hr)] × [desired TBD (cGy)/75 cGy]

Activity hours are derived from a table based on a calculation of the number of millicuries needed to result in a 75-cGy exposure of the total body for a given weight of a patient.

---

[1] The dosimetric step is used to calculate a therapeutic dose of ^{131}I-tositumomab individualised for each patient. SSKI = Saturated solution of potassium iodide.

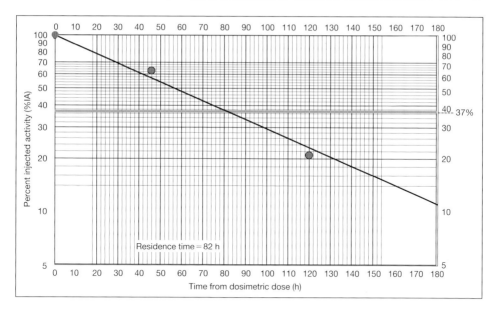

Figure 12.3   Graphic estimate of total body resistance time.

One to two weeks after the dosimetric dose infusion, the therapeutic step is administered. It again consists of infusion of 450 mg of unlabelled tositumomab followed by a 35 mg
of tositumomab labelled with patient-specific activity (in mCi) of ^{131}I. In order to protect the
thyroid gland from absorption of free ^{131}I which could be released from radiolabelled antibody, non-radioactive iodide such as a saturated solution of potassium iodide (SSKI) is
given orally, beginning the day before the dosimetric dose and ending 2 weeks after the
therapeutic dose.

For most patients, a maximally tolerated TBD is 75 cGy. The TBD is decreased to
65 cGy for patients with a platelet count of 100,000–149,000 platelets/mm³, and to
45–55 cGy for patients with a history of prior haematopoietic stem cell transplant. In contrast to chemotherapy regimens which usually required multiple cycles of therapy, the
^{131}I-tositumomab therapeutic regimen is completed at this juncture with no repeated cycles.

EFFICACY DATA IN RELAPSED/REFRACTORY LOW-GRADE OR TRANSFORMED LOW-GRADE LYMPHOMA

While a Phase I/II study was critical to establish the schedule and dosing of the
^{131}I-tositumomab therapeutic regimen, it also provided efficacy data. In this study carried
out at the University of Michigan, patients with relapsed or refractory low-grade or follicular lymphoma showed a high response rate (64% overall (OR), 38% complete (CR))
and long durations of remissions [3]. Particularly, patients with complete remission
achieved remissions lasting a median of 29.1 months and 7 patients have had remission of
7–11 years duration in the most recent update of the data. Patients with intermediate- or
high-grade lymphomas faired less well (41% OR, 0% CR). Based on this information, subsequent multi-centre trials focused on low-grade or follicular lymphoma and were conducted in patients with chemotherapy relapsed or refractory low-grade or transformed
low-grade lymphoma.

Efficacy data from multi-centre Phase II studies are summarised in Table 12.1. The RIT-
II-001 trial included 47 patients and was designed to validate the dosing methodology

Table 12.1 Summary of ^{131}I-tositumomab studies in rituximab-naïve patients

Study description/name	Overall response (%)	Median TTP (months) (range)	Complete response (%)	Median TTP (months) (range)
Chemotherapy refractory (RIT-I I-004)	47	13.2 (3.2–48.7)	20	48.7 (10.5–48.7)
Chemotherapy-relapsed or refractory (RIT-II-002*)	59	NR (3.2–58.9+)	36	NR (6.3–58.9+)
Chemotherapy-relapsed or refractory LG NHL (RIT-II-001)	49	14.4 (3.0+–62.1+)	26	60.1 (11.6–62.1+)
Chemotherapy-relapsed or refractory (RIT-I-000‡)	64	15.2 (3.7–95.8+)	38	29.1 (3.7–95.8+)

*Excludes patients who only received unlabelled Tositumomab(Arm B); NR = Not reached; ‡Excludes 17 patients with intermediate- and high-grade lymphoma.
LG NHL = Low-grade non-Hodgkin's lymphoma.; TTP = Time to progression.

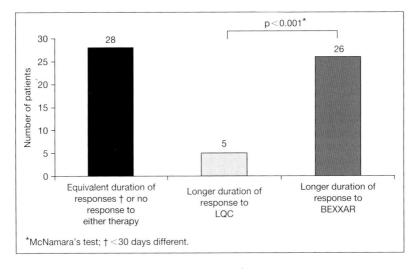

Figure 12.4 ^{131}I-tositumomab in chemotherapy-refractory NHL[1].

developed at Michigan [7]. Response rates and duration appeared to be comparable with those obtained in the original Phase I/II trial. The RIT-II-002 trial randomised 78 patients to receive either the tositumomab and ^{131}I-tositumomab regimen or the unlabelled tositumomab to determine the value added by the radionuclide component [8]. Patients treated on the radiolabelled antibody arm compared to those treated on the unlabelled antibody arm showed a higher OR (55 vs. 19%) and CR (33 vs. 8%). The RIT-II-004 study

---

[1]Paired comparison of duration of response to ^{131}I-tositumomab (n = 60) compared to the last chemotherapy regimen received prior to entering the RIT-II-004 trial. LQC = Last qualifying chemotherapy.

Table 12.2 Response rates to ^{131}I-tositumomab in chemotherapy-refractory NHL[1]

	Last qualifying chemotherapy (n = 60)	BEXXAR (n = 60)	p value*	p value†
Response	7/60(12%)	28/60(47%)	<0.001	NA
Median (95% CI) duration of response for responders (months)	4.1 (3.0–5.4)	11.7 (6.9–47.2)	<0.001	<0.001
Complete response	1/60(2%)	12/60(20%)	0.002	NA
Median (95% CI) duration of response for responders (months)	4.8 (NA)	47.2 (NA)	0.003	0.001

*P values for response rates based on McNamara's test vs. 0.50; †p values for duration based on generalised McNamara's test. Paired Prentice-Wilcoxon test for censored data for comparisons of duration. NA = Not applicable; CI = confidence interval.
[1]Data from RIT-II-004

enrolled 60 patients with chemotherapy-refractory disease (no response or response lasting less than 6 months to the last chemotherapy received). Using patients as their own control, the duration of response to the ^{131}I-tositumomab therapeutic regimen was compared to that of the last chemotherapy regimen the patient received [9]. In a paired analysis, the number of patients who achieved a longer duration of response to ^{131}I-tositumomab was about five times higher than the number of patients who had a longer duration to their last chemotherapy (p < 0.001) (Figure 12.4). In addition, patients treated with ^{131}I-tositumomab had a an OR of 47% and CR rate of 20% (compared with 12 and 2%, respectively, for the last chemotherapy) (Table 12.2). In summary, all four initial studies, including Phase I/II trial, showed high response rates and duration of responses in patients with relapsed or refractory low-grade or follicular lymphoma, including transformed follicular lymphoma previously treated with chemotherapy. Most remarkably, patients who achieved complete responses often experienced particularly long durations of responses lasting for years. Data from these studies established ^{131}I-tositumomab as an effective salvage regimen.

Patients enrolled in all early ^{131}I-tositumomab studies had either relapsed or were refractory to prior chemotherapy, but none of these patients had been previously treated with anti-CD20 therapy, notably rituximab. During the conduct of the above studies, rituximab was approved by the FDA for the treatment of patients with relapsed/refractory low-grade or follicular lymphoma. It thus became a new standard of care for such patients. It was therefore necessary to evaluate ^{131}I-tositumomab in rituximab-refractory patients to gain FDA approval. A multi-centre study was then conducted in 40 patients who had relapsed or were refractory to rituximab and who had also had prior chemotherapy [10]. Thirty-five of these patients were rituximab-refractory. Interestingly, response rates and response durations appeared quite similar to those in patients never exposed to rituximab. The OR and CR were 65 and 38%, respectively, and with a median follow-up of 39 months, the median duration of all responses was 24.5 months and the median for complete responses was not reached (Table 12.3). These data provided support for the first FDA-approved indication for ^{131}I-tositumomab, namely its use in rituximab-refractory patients.

In January 2005, the FDA approved an expanded indication for ^{131}I-tositumomab. The expanded indication now allows for the treatment of patients with CD20 antigen expressing relapsed or refractory, low-grade, follicular, or transformed NHL, including patients with

Table 12.3 Response to ^{131}I-tositumomab in patients relapsed after rituximab (n = 40)[1]

	Response Rate (%)	Median PFS (Months)
Overall response	65 (68)*	24.5**
Complete response[†]	38 (32)*	NR
Median duration of follow-up	39 months	

[1]35/40 patients were refractory to rituximab.
*Panel assessed.
**For confirmed responders; 10.4 months for all patients.
[†]Complete response rate = Pathological and clinical complete responses.
[‡]NR = Not reached, estimated 3-year progression-free survival (PFS) 73%.

rituximab-refractory NHL. Thus, the stipulation that patients had to be refractory to rituximab was dropped. The basis for this change was an integrated review of data on 250 patients from trials that included rituximab-naïve patients. The results of this analysis indicated that ^{131}I-tositumomab could result in remissions lasting over one year and extending to 10 years in 32% of these patients. For this durable response population, 44% had not progressed (range 2.5+–9.5+ years) with a median response duration of 45.8 months. The median duration of complete response had not been reached. Such durations of response are rarely encountered in heavily pre-treated patients with other therapies.

RETREATMENT WITH ^{131}I-TOSITUMOMAB AND OTHER TREATMENTS AFTER ^{131}I-TOSITUMOMAB

With the expanding use of RIT, it was important to determine how well patients could tolerate subsequent therapy and whether re-treatment with ^{131}I-tositumomab could be an option. Dosik and colleagues [11] have shown that a variety of chemotherapeutic regimens can be tolerated in patients who were refractory or relapsed after ^{131}I-tositumomab. Median time from ^{131}I-tositumomab therapy to progression in patients included in this study was 183 days. Pre-treatment blood counts were comparable to counts pre-^{131}I-tositumomab therapy except for slightly lower platelet counts. Of 60% of patients who received myelosuppressive chemotherapy after relapse (median 1 regimen, range 1–3), 16 (42%) were treated with anthracyclines, 13 (34%) with platinum and 9 (24%) with fludarabine. In addition, 9 patients (24%) went on to receive either autologous or allogeneic transplantation. Disease improvement was noted in most of these patients, while 15 died after further chemotherapy, predominantly from refractory lymphoma. Others have also observed that it is possible to successfully harvest haematopoietic stem cells after ^{131}I-tositumomab [12] but it is difficult to determine a true denominator of eligible patients.

With regard to re-treatment, a multi-centre study was conducted to determine the efficacy and safety of re-treatment with ^{131}I-tositumomab in 32 patients who had previously responded to ^{131}I-tositumomab and who had relapsed [13]. Fifty-six percent of the patients achieved a response for a median of 15.2 months. Twenty-five percent (8/32) achieved a CR lasting a median of 35 months with 5 of these patients continuing in CR from 1.8+ to 5.7+ years. Notably, while the median duration of response with re-treatment was not statistically different from that of the initial treatment, about half of re-responders had longer durations of response than they had with the first treatment. Reassuringly, the haematological toxicity of the second treatment with ^{131}I-tositumomab was comparable with that of the first.

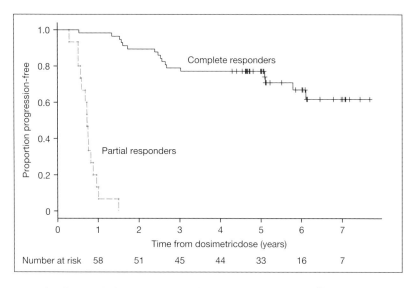

Figure 12.5   Progression-free survival in patients with follicular lymphoma given ^{131}I-tositumomab as front-line therapy[1].

EARLIER TREATMENT, INCLUDING FRONT-LINE TREATMENT

Given the promising results seen in heavily pre-treated patients, the outcome of this treatment when employed earlier in the management of low-grade lymphoma has been investigated. Davies and co-workers [14], have recently shown that ^{131}I-tositumomab is very active when it is used as a treatment for either a first or second recurrence after chemotherapy. In this group of patients, the OR was 76% and CR was 49%, suggesting a higher response rate than in the more heavily pre-treated patients in other ^{131}I-tositumomab trials. With a median follow-up of 3 years, the median duration of response was 1.3 years for all responders and was not reached for complete responders.

Moving the treatment up even earlier, a study was conducted at the University of Michigan in 76 previously untreated patients with advanced-stage follicular lymphoma [15]. The OR and CR were 95 and 75%, respectively. The 5-year progression-free survival was 59% for all patients and 77% for those who achieved a complete response (Figure 12.5). The median progression-free survival for all patients was 6.1 years at a median follow-up period of 5.1 years. These data obtained with a one-week treatment course are comparable with the best results published for front-line treatment of follicular lymphoma, including arduous regimens taking months to complete. Further randomised clinical studies investigating front-line RIT compared to extended chemotherapy treatments are warranted.

[131]I-tositumomab has also been given in sequence after a course of initial cytoreductive chemotherapy such as CHOP (cyclophosphamide, doxorubicin, vincristine and prednisolone), fludarabine and CVP (cyclophosphamide, vincristine and prednisolone) in the front-line setting [16–18]. The results from these trials are promising. All of these studies show very high ORs and CRs, including a significant rate of conversion from partial to CR with the addition of ^{131}I-tositumomab after the chemotherapy phase of treatment. Randomised trials are underway to examine the role of ^{131}I-tositumomab in the front-line setting. An inter-group

---

[1]Fifty-seven of the total of 76 patients (75%) had a complete response and 15 (20%) partial response.

Table 12.4 Haematologic toxicity (n = 230)

	Platelets	ANC	Haemoglobin
Grade 3/4*	53%	63%	29%
Median duration of grade 3/4	32 days	31 days	23 days
Grade 4†	21%	25%	5%
Median duration of grade 4	28 days	16 days	10 days
Median nadir	43,000/mm^3	690 cells/mm^3	10 gm/dl
Median time to nadir	34 days	43 days	47 days

*Grade 3/4 defined as platelets <50,000/mm^3, absolute neutrophil count (ANC) <1,000 cells/mm^3, haemoglobin <8.0 g/dl
†Grade 4 defined as platelets <25,000 mm^3, ANC<500 cells/mm^3, haemoglobin <6.5 g/dl

Southwest Oncology Group and Cancer and Leukemia Group B study is comparing a rituximab and CHOP combination with CHOP followed by ^{131}I-tositumomab consolidation.

The data from front-line studies and first and second relapse studies strongly suggest that RIT should be considered earlier in the course of treatment of this disease rather than waiting for the disease to become refractory to other treatments.

SAFETY

Combined data from early re-treatment trials and from newer studies provides compelling evidence that ^{131}I-tositumomab Treatment Regimen is safe and well tolerated. Acute adverse events were assessed in the 230 patients from the four initial studies. An additional analysis for long-term and serious adverse events included 765 patients from an expanded access program. Most of the acute non-haematological toxicities were similar to those seen with antibody infusions and were almost always grade 1 or 2. Only 7% of infusions required interruption or adjustment in rate because of side-effects. Haematological toxicity is summarised in Table 12.4. While most of patients developed ≥grade 3 haematological toxicities, only 8% of patients experienced a serious infection requiring hospitalisation, and haemorrhagic events were very rare. Only 27% of patients required one or more types of haematological support such as growth factors or transfusions. It is important to note that the time to haematological nadirs is significantly delayed when compared with standard chemotherapy and occurs 4–7 weeks after therapeutic dose of ^{131}I-tositumomab.

Because tositumomab is a mouse antibody, there was a concern that significant numbers of patients would develop human anti-mouse antibodies (HAMA). However, HAMA became detectable in only 10% of patients who had been previously treated with chemotherapy. In contrast, 63% of patients who received ^{131}I-tositumomab as their initial treatment eventually developed HAMA, probably reflecting a more immunocompetent state in these patients.

Another anticipated toxicity was the development of hypothyroidism, related to possible exposure of the thyroid gland to free ^{131}I released from ^{131}I-tositumomab. Hypothyroidism was reported, however, at a relatively low rate of 10%, as determined by an elevated thyroid-stimulating hormone (TSH), indicating that thyroid blockade during the treatment interval was effective in most patients.

A major concern has been related to possible long-term effects of radiation to other tissues, especially the induction of secondary malignancies. Myelodysplasia or acute leukaemia was reported in 35 of 995 patients treated with ^{131}I-tositumomab subsequent to previous chemotherapy [19]. The annualised incidence was between 1 and 2%, not unlike that expected for chemotherapy alone. After blinded review of reported cases, 40%

were diagnosed prior to receiving RIT, 8% had no pathological or clinical evidence to support such a diagnosis and 52% were confirmed to have developed treatment-related myelodysplastic syndrome/acute myelogenous leukaemia (tMDS/tAML) following RIT. Cytogenetic analyses consistently revealed abnormalities of chromosomes 5 and 7, typical of alkylating agent exposure. Interestingly, with a median follow-up approaching 5 years, no MDS or AML was reported in any of the 76 patients treated with front-line ^{131}I-tositumomab therapy [19]. As for other secondary cancers, the rates so far do not appear to exceed those expected in the patient population studied. However, longer follow-up will be essential to better define these risks.

To determine whether ^{131}I-tositumomab therapy poses any risk to household members and caregivers, a dosimetry study has been conducted at the University of Nebraska to monitor the radiation exposure from 22 patients treated with ^{131}I-tositumomab (35–70 cGy TBD) [20]. None of the family members of any of the patients has been exposed to more than 500 mrem, which is the upper limit of radiation exposure recommended by the Nuclear Regulatory Commission (NRC). The average corrected total dose of radiation to family members in this study was 168 mrem (range, 27–451), despite the fact that some patients reported spending significant amounts of time at distances of 3–4 feet from family members during the first few days after therapy.

SUMMARY

Anti-CD20 RIT clearly has a role in the management of low-grade and transformed follicular lymphoma. Future studies should be aimed at further defining this role relative to the plethora of other available choices of therapy. RIT has also shown activity in other B-cell histologies, but relatively few patients have been studied. For instance, ongoing or projected studies should clarify its role in the management of diffuse large B-cell lymphoma, Waldenstrom's macroglobulinaemia, mantle cell lymphoma and multiple myeloma. In addition, future directions include incorporation of either standard or high dose of ^{131}I-tositumomab to stem cell transplant preparative regimens. A recent Phase I study showed that ^{131}I-tositumomab (up to 0.75 Gy), when used in combination with BEAM (carmustine, etoposide, cytarabine and melphalan) followed by autologous stem cell transplant (ASCT) does not significantly add to toxicity of BEAM alone and shows promising efficacy in chemotherapy-resistant or refractory NHL [21]. Patients with relapsed/refractory follicular lymphoma treated with high dose of ^{131}I anti-CD20 prior to ASCT experienced improved survival when retrospectively compared to patients treated with standard high-dose chemotherapy [22]. Treatment planning has been established to determine limits on radiation dose absorbed to critical non-haematopoietic organs [23], providing methodology for future studies with high-dose ^{131}I-tositumomab.

REFERENCES

1. Kaminski MS, Fig LM, Zasadny KR *et al*. Imaging, dosimetry, and radioimmunotherapy with iodine 131-labeled anti-CD37 antibody in B-cell lymphoma. *J Clin Oncol* 1992; 10:1696–1711.
2. Buchsbaum DJ, Wahl RL, Normolle DP *et al*. Therapy with unlabeled and ^{131}I-labeled pan-B-cell monoclonal antibodies in nude mice bearing Raji Burkitt's lymphoma xenografts. *Cancer Res* 1992a; 52:6476–6481.
3. Kaminski MS, Estes J, Zasadny KR *et al*. Radioimmunotherapy with iodine I 131 tositumomab for relapsed or refractory B-cell non-Hodgkin's lymphoma: updated results and long-term follow-up of the University of Michigan experience. *Blood* 2000; 96:1259–1266.
4. Buchsbaum DJ, Wahl RL, Glenn SD *et al*. Improved delivery of radiolabeled anti-B1 monoclonal antibody to Raji lymphoma xenografts by predosing with unlabeled anti-B1 monoclonal antibody. *Cancer Res* 1992b; 52:637–642.

5. Wahl RL. The clinical importance of dosimetry in radioimmunotherapy with tositumomab and iodine I 131 tositumomab. *Semin Oncol* 2003; 30:31–38.

6. Zelenetz A, Wahl R, Kaminski M *et al*. Individualized patient dosing prevents underdosing and overdosing of patients with non-Hodgkin's lymphoma (NHL). *Proc Am Soc Clin Oncol* 2001; 20:(#1145):287a.

7. Vose JM, Wahl RL, Saleh M *et al*. Multicenter Phase II study of iodine I 131 tositumomab for chemotherapy-relapsed/refractory low-grade and transformed low-grade B-cell non-Hodgkin's lymphomas. *J Clin Oncol* 2000; 18:1316–1323.

8. Davis TA, Kaminski MS, Leonard JP *et al*. The radioisotope contributes significantly to the activity of radioimmunotherapy. *Clin Cancer Res* 2004; 10:7792–7798.

9. Kaminski MS, Zelenetz AD, Press OW *et al*. Pivotal study of Bexxar (Iodine I 131 tositumomab) for chemotherapy-refractory low-grade or transformed low-grade B-cell non-Hodgkin's lymphoma. *J Clin Oncol* 2001; 19:3908–3911.

10. Horning SJ, Younes A, Jain V *et al*. Efficacy and safety of tositumomab and iodine-131 tositumomab (Bexxar) in B-cell lymphoma, progressive after rituximab. *J Clin Oncol* 2005; 23:712–719.

11. Dosik A, Hack S, Navarro M *et al*. Cytotoxic chemotherapy for non-Hodgkin's lymphoma can be safely administered following relapse from iodine 131 tositumomab (Bexxar). *Proc Am Soc Clin Oncol* 2002; 21:267a (#1065).

12. Ratanatharathorn V, Uberti JP, Ayash L *et al*. Hematopoietic stem cell transplantation (HSCT) in lymphoma patients receiving prior therapy with tositumomab and iodine I 131 tositumomab (Bexxar). Proceedings of American Society of Hematology 43rd Annual Meeting, December 2001, *Blood* 2001; 98:200a (#836).

13. Kaminski MS, Knox SJ, Redford J *et al*. Re-treatment with tositumomab and iodinated I 131 tositumomab (the Bexxar therapeutic regimen) in patients with non-Hodgkin's lymphoma (NHL) with a previous response to Bexxar therapeutic regimen. Proc American Society of Hematology 45th Annual Meeting, December 2003. *Blood* 2003; 102:407a (#1478).

14. Davies AJ, Rohatiner AZS, Howell S *et al*. Tositumomab and Iodine I 131 tositumomab for recurrent indolent and transformed B-cell non-Hodgkin's lymphoma. *J Clin Oncol* 2004; 22:1469–1479.

15. Kaminski MS, Tuck M, Estes J *et al*. 131I-tositumomab therapy as initial treatment for follicular lymphoma. *N Engl J Med* 2005; 352:441–449

16. Press OW, Unger JM, Brazil RM *et al*. A phase 2 trial of CHOP chemotherapy followed by tositumomab/iodine I 131 tositumomab for previously untreated follicular non-Hodgkin lymphoma: Southwest Oncology Group Protocol S9911. *Blood* 2003; 102:1606–1612.

17. Leonard JP, Coleman M, Kostakoglu L *et al*. Durable remissions from fludarabine followed by the iodine 131I tositumomab Bexxar therapeutic regimen for patients with previously untreated follicular non-Hodgkin's lymphoma. *Proc Am Soc Clin Oncol* 2004; 23:560 (#6518).

18. Link B, Kaminski MS, Coleman M *et al*. Phase II study of CVP followed by tositumomab and iodine I 131 tositumomab (Bexxar therapeutic regimen) in patients with untreated follicular non-Hodgkin's lymphoma. *Proc* 2004; 23:560 (#6520).

19. Bennett JM, Kaminski MS, Leonard JP *et al*. Assessment of treatment-related myelodysplastic syndromes and acute myeloid leukemia in patients with non-Hodgkin's lymphoma treated with Tositumomab and Iodine-131 Tositumomab (Bexxar®). *Blood* 2005 Feb 24; [Epub ahead of print].

20. Rutar FJ, Augustine SC, Colcher D *et al*. Outpatient treatment with (131) I-anti-B1 antibody: radiation exposure to family members. *J Nucl Med* 2001; 42:907–915.

21. Vose JM, Bierman PJ, Enke C *et al*. Phase I trial of iodine-131 tositumomab with high-dose chemotherapy and autologous stem-cell transplantation for relapsed non-Hodgkin's lymphoma. *J Clin Oncol* 2005; 23:461–467.

22. Gopal AK, Gooley TA, Maloney DG *et al*. High-dose radioimmunotherapy versus conventional high-dose therapy and autologous hematopoietic stem cell transplantation for relapsed follicular non-Hodgkin lymphoma: a multivariable cohort analysis. *Blood* 2003; 102:2351–2357.

23. Rajendran JG, Fisher DR, Gopal AK *et al*. High-dose (131) I-tositumomab (anti-CD20) radioimmunotherapy for non-Hodgkin's lymphoma: adjusting radiation absorbed dose to actual organ volumes. *J Nucl Med* 2004; 45:1059–1064.

13

CD52 as a target for immunotherapy

M. J. S. Dyer

INTRODUCTION – ASSEMBLING AN ATOMIC BOMB

That antibodies have the specificity necessary to deliver targeted therapy was realised shortly after their discovery in the 1890s [1]. During subsequent years, however, it has proved difficult to produce antibody constructs that destroy tumour cells effectively *in vivo*.

Following the introduction of monoclonal antibodies (MAbs) in the 1970s, several conditions necessary for effective antibody-mediated tumour cell lysis have been identified [2]. These conditions include correct choice of immunoglobulin isotype to activate natural effector mechanisms (including complement-dependent cytotoxicity (CDC) and antibody-dependent cellular cytotoxicity (ADCC)), correct choice of target antigen as well as other factors described below.

Despite these advances, as single agents, the effects of most MAbs in oncology are often only modest, and with the possible exception of anti-immunoglobulin idiotypic MAbs, none are curative. Consequently, the use of MAbs labelled with radioisotopes, drugs or with potent toxins is being investigated [3; chapters 9–13 in this book]. However, since it is possible to eradicate disease in animals with passive antibody therapy using relatively small doses of MAbs [4], confidence remains high that it should be possible to do the same in man.

Identified barriers to effective antibody therapy with unconjugated MAbs include:

a. **Circulating free antigen.** All cell surface antigens will be found in the circulation at low levels, but high levels will preclude tumour cell uptake. CD23, for example, is shed into the circulation in high quantities in patients with advanced chronic lymphocytic leukaemia (CLL). This problem can be overcome by using higher doses of MAb, but at a potential risk of immune complex disease.

b. **Cell surface antigenic modulation and internalisation.** Many cell surface molecules rapidly 'cap' and then internalise in the presence of bivalent MAb. This process can occur very rapidly (within minutes) and effectively renders a cell antigen negative – reappearance of cell surface antigen on the other hand may take several hours. Internalisation of MAbs conjugated with either toxins or radioisotopes is necessary, or at least desirable, for efficacy. In contrast, efficacy of most unconjugated MAbs demands the maintained presence of intact MAb at the cell surface (however, if continued signalling *via* a cell surface molecule is necessary for survival, then removal *via* modulation might be advantageous) [5]. Modulation limits the number of molecules that can be successfully targeted using

Martin J. S. Dyer, MA, DPhil, FRCP, FRCPath, Professor of Haemato-Oncology, MRC Toxicology Unit / Leicester University, Leicester, UK.

regular bivalent MAbs, although this problem may be circumvented by generating monovalent MAbs, either by cell fusion or by genetic manipulation [6].

c. **Low cell surface antigen density.** It is widely believed that high antigen density is necessary for effective MAb action. A certain level of antigen density may be necessary to elicit antibody-mediated cross-linking of the target antigen. However, the empirical evidence for the necessity of high antigen density is lacking and it is clear from the doses of alemtuzumab that are routinely used clinically that clearance of cells from the peripheral blood at least occurs at subsaturating amounts of MAb. Also, under certain circumstances, for example, in the case of tumour necrosis factor-related apoptosis-inducing ligand (TRAIL) receptor MAbs, tumour cell lysis can occur *via* induction of apoptosis in the presence of barely detectable levels of cell surface antigen [7; unpublished observations].

d. **Selection of the correct immunoglobulin isotype to activate natural effector mechanisms (see below).**

e. **The nature of the target epitope.** Not all non-secreted high-abundance non-modulating cell surface antigens make good targets for therapy. CD45 for example is expressed at high abundance on most lymphoid cells, but MAbs against this molecule do not activate CDC or ADCC. Precisely what makes an antigen a good target for therapy is not clear – it may be necessary to generate MAbs that recognise epitopes that are immediately adjacent to the cell surface membrane.

f. **The nature of the target cell.** This area has received less attention than it merits, but it appears that some cell types are inherently more sensitive to MAb-mediated lysis than others. In terms of alemtuzumab this is best exemplified in T-cell prolymphocytic leukaemia (T-PLL), where most patients will enter remission despite extremely high tumour burdens [8]. Whether this relates to expression of complement regulatory protein such as decay-accelerating factor (DAF) and CD59 etc., as has been suggested for CD20, is controversial [9].

The alemtuzumab (Campath-1) antigen, CD52, is a highly expressed cell surface molecule that is not secreted to any appreciable level and does not modulate either *in vitro* or *in vivo*. All of these features contribute to making it a good target for therapy. Against this must be placed its broad distribution, which leaves patients profoundly immunosuppressed for a period of time.

However, it is likely that the clinical success of the Campath-1 series of MAbs at eradicating lymphocytes both *in vitro* for depletion of T-cells prior to stem cell transplantation and *in vivo* arises primarily from the fact that these MAbs were initially selected for their ability to elicit CDC of human lymphocytes with human complement. It should however be noted that CDC of tumour cells does not occur to any appreciable extent *in vivo*; complement activation is necessary but not sufficient in this regard. How the Campath-1 (CD52) antigen facilitates CDC remains unclear, but probably relates to the structure of the antigen as described below. Similarly, how the Campath-1H MAb kills cells *in vivo* remains unknown.

The factors that make CD52 a good target for immunotherapy, as well as some of its limitations, will be reviewed below.

THE CD52 FAMILY OF MABs – SELECTION OF THE CORRECT IMMUNOGLOBULIN ISOTYPE FOR TUMOUR CELL LYSIS

The CD52 molecule was defined by a series of MAbs isolated by Herman Waldmann and his group in Cambridge UK in 1979 [reviewed in 10]. The aim of these experiments was to derive MAbs that would deplete T-cells from bone marrow samples in order to abrogate graft vs. host disease (GvHD). From a rat immunised with human lymphocytes, spleen cells were fused with the rat myeloma cell line Y3 and 7 independent clones were isolated that lysed T cells with human complement. The choice of rat antibodies was fortuitous since rat MAbs are better at eliciting lysis with human complement than the equivalent mouse MAbs. All 7 MAbs were eventually shown to bind to the same antigen, CD52. With one exception, these MAbs were of IgM or IgG2c isotypes. YTH34.5 was an IgG2a and from this both IgG1 and IgG2b class switch variants were selected *in vitro* by immunoglobulin class-switching. Whilst all of the MAbs were lytic with human complement against human normal and malignant lymphocytes, only the IgG2b MAb (Campath-1G) was able to interact with human Fc receptors and thus elicit ADCC.

This collection of rat MAbs with identical specificity but varying isotype has proved very useful both in *in vitro* and *in vivo* studies and allowed the correct choice of immunoglobulin isotype for MAb therapy to be defined [11, 12]. Comparison of the IgM and the IgG2b CD52 MAbs in patients with high white cell count B-CLL or B-PLL showed profound differences between the two MAbs. Infusion of the IgM MAb showed rapid depletion of cells from the peripheral blood but equally rapid reappearance once the infusion stopped. Disappearance of cells from the circulation was associated with massive intravascular complement activation and depletion. However, it seems likely that this only resulted in sequestration of malignant cells rather than lysis, since repeated administration of the IgM MAb failed to make any impact on the disease. In contrast, the IgG2b MAb (subsequently developed as Campath-1G) resulted in depletion of cells from blood, bone marrow and spleen. This occurred without significant activation of complement, as has been seen with the human IgG1 MAb.

Together, these data indicate that Campath-1 MAbs that are able to interact successfully with human Fc receptors to activate ADCC are able to deplete cells *in vivo*. Complement activation is necessary but on its own is insufficient to deplete.

A panel of human CD52 MAbs of differing isotypes was subsequently engineered [13]. The IgG1 isotype was selected for therapeutic development as this isotype demonstrates optimal activation of CDC and ADCC *in vitro*. The importance of optimising the interaction of therapeutic MAb with the Fc receptors is underlined by the observation that efficacy of some therapeutic MAbs depends on the affinity of the interaction with the Fc receptors [14]

A genetically reshaped human IgG1 CD52 MAb (Campath-1H) was produced by grafting the three complementarity-determining regions (CDRs) from YTH34.5 to a human IgG1 gene [15]. This MAb was first used to treat 2 patients with B-cell non-Hodgkin's lymphoma in leukaemic phase [16]. Despite having bulk disease, both patients entered a remission with very small doses of MAb (96 and 126 mg each – most of the MAb available at that time!), much less than used nowadays to treat patients with CLL. The Campath-1H used in these experiments was not in fact identical to that used in the clinic today. Initial batches of Campath-1H were manufactured in rat Y0 myeloma cells. The yields of MAb produced were only low, and therefore, for commercial production, the Chinese Hamster ovary cell line (CHO) was used. This Campath-1H is not glycosylated with the same pattern as native human antibodies and this may have a major impact on efficacy [17].

A human IgG4 CD52 MAb has also been produced. On the basis of its activities *in vitro*, it would be predicted that this MAb would not activate CDC and also not bind so effectively to Fc receptors and thus not deplete so effectively as the IgG1 MAb. Consequently, this MAb (and other IgG4 MAbs) might have applications in radioimmunotherapy, since the uptake in liver and spleen should be less, and more MAb might be taken up specifically by the tumour. Somewhat surprisingly though, when tested in man, the IgG4 MAb resulted in lymphocyte depletion although a formal comparison with the IgG1 MAb has not been made [18].

THE CD52 MOLECULE

The CD52 molecule is fascinating in several ways and is a most unlikely target for any form of therapy! The entire structure of the molecule has been determined but its functions remain unknown. For several years, the nature of the molecule remained elusive. However, chloroform/methanol extraction, along with conventional cDNA/genomic cloning and some elegant glycobiology experiments allowed the nature of the protein and the associated carbohydrate to be determined [19; reviewed in 10].

The human CD52 gene maps on chromosome 1p36. It is a small gene consisting of only two small exons and spanning only 3 kb of genomic DNA. It is transcribed from a TATA-box-less promoter as an RNA transcript of 430 bp. The resulting protein is initially 61 amino acids in length but this is processed by removal of a leader sequence and trimming of the carboxy terminus to produce a mature protein of only 12 amino acids. Despite the short length of the protein, there are two common allelic forms. Whether these alleles are associated with differences in function is not known. Interestingly, the sequence of the processed protein (like the extracellular loop of CD20) is not conserved between species. The closest homologue to CD52 is CD24, which is broadly expressed in haemopoietic and non-haemopoietic cells and is a ligand for P-selectin. Interestingly, CD24 is also thought to play a role in B-cell activation and differentiation.

The CD52 molecule is heavily glycosylated *via* a single, complex N-linked oligosaccharide; the structure of the carbohydrate moiety has been completely determined [19]. Given the lack of conservation of the processed protein sequences, it is likely that the highly negatively charged oligosaccharide plays the most significant role in interactions with other molecules and cells. The oligosaccharide is not necessary for the antigenic epitope for most CD52 MAbs. This epitope is mimicked by short peptides from the carboxy terminus of the mature peptide. Thus it is likely that the CD52 epitope is very close to the cell surface membrane. Whether this feature contributes to the success of CD52 MAbs at inducing cell lysis is not clear. However, it is interesting to note that two other MAbs that have found application in oncology, namely CD20 MAbs in lymphoma and HER2 MAbs in breast cancer, similarly recognise epitopes adjacent to the cell surface [20, 21].

Unlike CD20, which is a tetraspan transmembrane protein, CD52 is only tethered to the cell surface membrane *via* a glycosylphosphatidylinositol (GPI) linker. There are two forms of the phosphatidylinositol linker; again, whether these are associated with functional differences is not clear. The GPI linker of CD52 might have implications therapeutically since cell-cell transfer of GPI-linked molecules can occur [22]. This happens with CD52 in the male reproductive tract. CD52 is produced by cells in the epididymis and seminal vesicles from where it is shed into the seminal fluid and acquired by sperm. 'Free' CD52 has been detected in the serum of patients with CLL although the clinical significance of this observation is uncertain [23]. It is unlikely though that this poses a major barrier to therapy in most cases.

Despite being linked to the membrane *via* a GPI structure, the CD52 antigen does not appear to modulate or internalise when cross-linked by bivalent MAb either *in vitro* or *in vivo* at least in mature lymphoid malignancies. The lack of modulation *in vivo* was demonstrated most clearly when Campath-1G was administered intrathecally to a patient with B-PLL with leukaemic infiltration of the CSF; one day after injection, all of the cells were brightly stained with an anti-rat immunoglobulin antibody [11].

CD52 EXPRESSION

CD52 is broadly expressed among cells of the lymphoid and monocytic lineages. Expression outside of the haemopoietic compartment is limited to cells of the male reproductive tract. Among mature lymphoid cells, the molecule is expressed at very high density, with about 500,000 molecules per cell. The high abundance with the associated high negative charge has lead to the suggestion that the molecule might have a role in preventing adhesion, but this has not been tested.

In the mature B-cell malignancies, CD52 expression is seen in all cases of CLL and B-cell non-Hodgkin's lymphoma, and therefore routine testing of expression does not appear to be necessary before starting alemtuzumab therapy for CLL. However, even among these malignancies, levels of CD52 expression do vary considerably, and it is not clear in CLL whether this has a bearing on eventual clinical outcome with Campath-1H therapy [24]. It has been suggested in T-PLL that higher levels of CD52 expression may be associated with improved clinical responses [25].

Few studies have been performed on mature T-cell malignancies. All T-PLL have been positive at diagnosis, although the antigen appears to be lost on some T-cell NHL. Following initial Campath-1H therapy some cases of CD52-negative relapse of T-cell malignancies have been reported [26], but this has not been observed with B-cell CLL. However, most cases retain CD52 antigen expression at relapse, and it has been possible to re-treat one patient successfully on four separate occasions with Campath-1H [Dyer MJS, unpublished observations].

Levels of CD52 expression tend to be lower at both the early and late stages of lympho-cyte differentiation. Thus, both normal and malignant plasma cells tend to be CD52 nega-tive, as they are for most B-cell differentiation antigens. Recent studies have indicated that some cases of myeloma may express CD52, which might allow therapeutic attempts with alemtuzumab [27]. Whether the myeloma 'stem cell' population expresses CD52 is not known. Lower levels of CD52 are usually seen in B-cell precursor and T-cell precursor acute lymphoblastic leukaemias and some cases may be negative. Alemtuzumab has been reported to have activity in these diseases although its role remains to be defined.

Myeloid cells are usually CD52 negative, the major exception being eosinophils [28]. Alemtuzumab has been used to treat idiopathic hypereosinophilic syndrome (HES) [29]. Marked induction of CD52 expression in the acute pro-myelocytic leukaemic cell line NB4 has also been reported following exposure to all-trans retinoic acid – whether comparable induction in patient cells has not been reported [30]. In contrast, most mature monocytic cells are CD52 positive and may be depleted by Campath-1H therapy along with lymphocytes, although subsets of these cells appear to be resistant.

A variety of assays have indicated that human stem cells are CD52 negative [31]. For example, patients undergoing allogeneic stem cell transplantation can have Campath-1 anti-bodies infused around the time of the transplant, or even mixed in with the stem cells, with little or no effect on engraftment. Thus, the myelosuppressive effects of Campath-1H on neutrophils and platelets frequently seen in patients with CLL are likely to be indirect either through loss of necessary T cells or dendritic cells or through release of myelosuppressive cytokines during lysis of CLL cells. Aplasia is occasionally seen, usually in patients with T-PLL and often after the recovery of normal haemopoiesis; the mechanism of this is not known.

HOW DOES ALEMTUZUMAB KILL LYMPHOCYTES?

The English footballer Len Shackleton [32] once famously wrote an illuminating chapter on the knowledge of soccer club directors about the beautiful game: it was a blank page! I am tempted to do the same here! Although we know that alemtuzumab and other therapeutic MAbs depend on Fc binding for efficacy, the precise mechanism(s) are not known [33]. The problem is particularly acute for alemtuzumab, since this MAb depletes most of the known effector mechanisms including T cells, natural killer (NK) cells and monocytes, leaving only neutrophils and platelets as possible cellular effectors. The nature of the crucial effector cells is of central importance, as it may be possible to augment activity by simple means such as concurrent use of growth factors.

Several mechanisms probably operate. Early in the course of treatment, cells are proba-bly cleared from the blood by opsonisation by reticuloendothelial cells within the liver, spleen and lungs. The process can be extremely rapid in patients with high white cell counts and yet, unlike rituximab, has not been associated with tumour lysis syndrome, implying that once opsonised, cells are killed only slowly.

Precisely how these cells are killed and removed is not clear thereafter. Understanding this point is vital since we need to determine why alemtuzumab does not usually deplete cells from lymph nodes – is this a problem with antibody access (which potentially could be circumvented by giving larger doses) and/or is there a lack of effector cells at these sites? Studies with radiolabelled Campath-1H would help greatly to address this point [34].

Rituximab induces a low level of apoptosis in some B-NHL cell lines and some primary tumour samples; the clinical relevance of this effect is not clear [35]. Similar remarks may apply to alemtuzumab, although alemtuzumab-induced apoptosis has been reported to be caspase independent. Studies on cell lines are more difficult with this MAb since most cell lines lose expression of CD52 with prolonged culture. Overall, it seems unlikely that apoptosis induction is a major means of inducing cell death for both alemtuzumab and rituximab.

SUMMARY

On the basis of the broad cellular distribution of the target antigen, CD52 MAbs would not be a first choice candidate for therapeutic development. The loss of T cells as well as malignant B cells remains a significant clinical problem, as does the lack of efficacy against nodal masses. Nevertheless, through the rational development and clinical assessment of a series of CD52 MAb constructs, much has been learnt about optimal MAb design. There has also been considerable clinical benefit for patients not only with fludarabine-resistant CLL and T-PLL but also for patients undergoing allogeneic stem cell transplantation and for a variety of autoimmune diseases.

Important questions remain about optimal design of antibody construct and which cell surface molecule(s) to target. Progress may come in at least three different ways. Firstly, improved antibodies can be engineered. For unconjugated MAbs, the human IgG1 molecule is preferred for activating both CDC and ADCC. 'Second generation' CD20 MAbs have been engineered with enhanced CDC and are currently undergoing trials in CLL [36, www.genmab.com]. Glycoengineered CD52 MAbs will begin trials in early in 2005 [www.glycart.com].

Secondly, better target antigens and epitopes may be defined. New cell surface molecules continue to be defined using proteomic analysis [37]. Functional analysis of these molecules may allow new therapeutic approaches. It is likely that cell surface molecules that transduce apoptotic signals will be good targets, so long as they can be made tumour-cell specific.

Finally, as with chemotherapy, it is likely that synergistic combinations of MAbs, targeting different antigens or different epitopes on the same antigens, will be used rather than as single agents. Bi-specific reagents capable of targeting two signalling pathways may be advantageous since these could deliver simultaneously synergistic effects.

REFERENCES

1. Silverstein AM. Labeled antigens and antibodies: the evolution of magic markers and magic bullets. *Nat Immunol* 2004; 5:1211–1217.
2. Dyer MJS. A history of the use of antibodies in the treatment of malignancy. In Cheson BD (ed), *Monoclonal Antibody Therapy of Hematologic Malignancies.* Darwin Scientific Publishing, Abingdon, UK, 2001, pp 1–12.
3. Payne G. Progress in immunoconjugate cancer therapeutics. *Cancer Cell* 2003; 3:207–212.
4. Bernstein ID, Tam MR, Nowinski RC. Mouse leukemia: therapy with monoclonal antibodies against a thymus differentiation antigen. *Science* 1980; 207:68–71.
5. Kelm S, Gerlach J, Brossmer R *et al*. The ligand-binding domain of CD22 is needed for inhibition of the B cell receptor signal, as demonstrated by a novel human CD22-specific inhibitor compound. *J Exp Med* 2002; 195:1207–1213.

6. Clark M, Bindon C, Dyer MJS *et al*. The improved lytic function and *in vivo* efficacy of monovalent monoclonal CD3 antibodies. *Eur J Immunol* 1989; 19:381–388.

7. Inoue S, Macfarlane M, Harper N *et al*. Histone deacetylase inhibitors potentiate TNF-related apoptosis-inducing ligand (TRAIL)-induced apoptosis in lymphoid malignancies. *Cell Death Differ* 2004; 11(suppl 2):S193–S206.

8. Dearden CE, Matutes E, Cazin B *et al*. High remission rate in T-cell prolymphocytic leukemia with CAMPATH-1H. *Blood* 2001; 98:1721–1726.

9. Golay J, Lazzari M, Facchinetti V *et al*. CD20 levels determine the *in vitro* susceptibility to rituximab and complement of B-cell chronic lymphocytic leukemia: further regulation by CD55 and CD59. *Blood* 2001; 98:3383–3389.

10. Hale G. CD52 (CAMPATH1). *J Biol Regul Homeost Agents* 2001; 15:386–391.

11. Dyer MJS, Hale G, Hayhoe FG, Waldmann H. Effects of CAMPATH-1 antibodies *in vivo* in patients with lymphoid malignancies: influence of antibody isotype. *Blood* 1989; 73:1431–1439.

12. Dyer MJS, Hale G, Marcus RE, Waldmann H. Remission induction in patients with lymphoid malignancies using unconjugated CAMPATH-1 monoclonal antibodies. *Leuk Lymphoma* 1990; 2:179–190.

13. Bindon CI, Hale G, Bruggemann M, Waldmann H. Human monoclonal IgG isotypes differ in complement activating function at the level of C4 as well as C1q. *J Exp Med* 1988; 168:127–142.

14. Cartron G, Dacheux L, Salles G *et al*. Therapeutic activity of humanized anti-CD20 monoclonal antibody and polymorphism in IgG Fc receptor FcγRIIIa gene. *Blood* 2002; 99:754–758.

15. Riechmann L, Clark M, Waldmann H, Winter G. Reshaping human antibodies for therapy. *Nature* 1988; 332:323–327.

16. Hale G, Dyer MJS, Clark MR *et al*. Remission induction in non-Hodgkin lymphoma with reshaped human monoclonal antibody CAMPATH-1H. *Lancet* 1988; 2:1394–1399.

17. Lifely MR, Hale C, Boyce S *et al*. Glycosylation and biological activity of CAMPATH-1H expressed in different cell lines and grown under different culture conditions. *Glycobiology* 1995; 5:813–822.

18. Isaacs JD, Wing MG, Greenwood JD *et al*. A therapeutic human IgG4 monoclonal antibody that depletes target cells in humans. *Clin Exp Immunol* 1996; 106:427–433.

19. Treumann A, Lifely MR, Schneider P, Ferguson MA. Primary structure of CD52. *J Biol Chem* 1995; 270:6088–6099.

20. Polyak MJ, Deans JP. Alanine-170 and proline-172 are critical determinants for extracellular CD20 epitopes; heterogeneity in the fine specificity of CD20 monoclonal antibodies is defined by additional requirements imposed by both amino acid sequence and quaternary structure. *Blood* 2002; 99:3256–3262.

21. Cho HS, Mason K, Ramyar KX *et al*. Structure of the extracellular region of HER2 alone and in complex with the Herceptin Fab. *Nature* 2003; 421:756–760.

22. Ilangumaran S, Robinson PJ, Hoessli DC. Transfer of exogenous glycosylphos-phatidylinositol (GPI)-linked molecules to plasma membranes. *Trends Cell Biol* 1996; 6:163–167.

23. Albitar M, Do KA, Johnson MM *et al*. Free circulating soluble CD52 as a tumor marker in chronic lymphocytic leukemia and its implication in therapy with anti-CD52 antibodies. *Cancer* 2004; 101:999–1008.

24. Rossmann ED, Lundin J, Lenkei R *et al*. Variability in B-cell antigen expression: implications for the treatment of B-cell lymphomas and leukemias with monoclonal antibodies. *Hematol J* 2001; 2:300–306.

25. Ginaldi L, De Martinis M, Matutes E *et al*. Levels of expression of CD52 in normal and leukemic B and T cells: correlation with *in vivo* therapeutic responses to Campath-1H. *Leuk Res* 1998; 22:185–191.

26. Birhiray RE, Shaw G, Guldan S *et al*. Phenotypic transformation of CD52(pos) to CD52(neg) leukemic T cells as a mechanism for resistance to CAMPATH-1H. *Leukemia* 2002; 16:861–864.

27. Kumar S, Kimlinger TK, Lust JA *et al*. Expression of CD52 on plasma cells in plasma cell proliferative disorders. *Blood* 2003; 102:1075–1077.

28. Elsner J, Hochstetter R, Spiekermann K, Kapp A. Surface and mRNA expression of the CD52 antigen by human eosinophils but not by neutrophils. *Blood* 1996; 88:4684–4693.

29. Sefcick A, Sowter D, DasGupta E *et al*. Alemtuzumab therapy for refractory idiopathic hypereosinophilic syndrome. *Br J Haematol* 2004; 124:558–559.

30. Li SW, Tang D, Ahrens KP *et al*. All-trans-retinoic acid induces CD52 expression in acute promyelocytic leukemia. *Blood* 2003; 101:1977–1980.

31. Gilleece MH, Dexter TM. Effect of Campath-1H antibody on human hematopoietic progenitors *in vitro. Blood* 1993; 82:807–812.

32. Shackleton L. 'The Clown Prince of Soccer'. Virgin Books, London, 1958.

33. Clynes RA, Towers TL, Presta LG, Ravetch JV. Inhibitory Fc receptors modulate *in vivo* cytoxicity against tumor targets. *Nat Med* 2000; 6:443–446.

34. Hutchins JT, Kull FC, Jr, Bynum J *et al.* Improved biodistribution, tumor targeting, and reduced immunogenicity in mice with a gamma 4 variant of Campath-1H. *Proc Natl Acad Sci USA* 1995; 92:11980–11984.

35 Manches O, Lui G, Chaperot L *et al. In vitro* mechanisms of action of rituximab on primary non-Hodgkin lymphomas. *Blood* 2003; 101:949–954.

36. Teeling JL, French RR, Cragg MS *et al.* Characterization of new human CD20 monoclonal antibodies with potent cytolytic activity against non-Hodgkin lymphomas. *Blood* 2004; 104:1793–1800.

37. Boyd RS, Adam PJ, Patel S *et al.* Proteomic analysis of the cell-surface membrane in chronic lymphocytic leukemia: identification of two novel proteins, BCNP1 and MIG2B. *Leukemia* 2003; 17:1605–1612.

14

Relapsed and refractory CLL: a clinical challenge

K. R. Rai, N. Driscoll, D. M. Janson, D. V. Patel

AFTER FLUDARABINE HAS FAILED, WHAT NEXT?

The majority of patients with chronic lymphocytic leukemia (CLL) who achieve remission following fludarabine treatment are known to suffer a relapse after a median of 20–30 months [1]. CLL often becomes refractory to repeated courses of treatment with the same drug. For patients who become refractory or who demonstrate a primary resistance to fludarabine, the prognosis is generally poor. Resistance to the purine analogues is emerging as a major problem in the management of patients with CLL. In addition to fludarabine or any other purine analogues, many of these patients have also already been exposed to (and may be resistant to) alkylating agents. The most effective salvage regimens are considered to be combinations of purine analogues and cyclophosphamide [2]. The use of alternative nucleoside analogues, such as cladribine or pentostatin, has been studied in the setting of fludarabine-refractory CLL. Response rates with these drugs have been reported to be modest (32%) with accompanying toxicities of grade 3–5 neutropaenia (75%), thrombocytopaenia (68%) and infections (43%) [3]. Alternative therapies are needed for such patients, preferably using agents whose mechanisms of action do not overlap with those of prior chemotherapies. The use of monoclonal antibodies offers such an approach. Alemtuzumab is a humanised monoclonal antibody directed against CD52 that has been approved for the treatment of CLL that is refractory to fludarabine. This article will review the development and role of alemtuzumab for the treatment of relapsed/refractory CLL.

EARLY TRIALS OF CAMPATH-1H IN LYMPHOPROLIFERATIVE DISEASES

Alemtuzumab, also called Campath-1H, was initially investigated in three multi-centre Phase I trials in non-Hodgkin lymphoma (NHL) at doses ranging up to 240 mg per week. Prophylactic pre-medications were not allowed during these trials and infusion related toxicities (rigors, fever, hypotension, rash) were common. Following these early NHL trials, two multi-centre Phase II trials (Protocol 125-K32–005 and 125-K32–009) were conducted in Europe and the USA, respectively. These trials treated a total of 149 patients with a variety of lymphoproliferative diseases.

Osterborg and colleagues [4] published a report on a subset of 29 of the patients treated on study 125-K32–005, who had CLL and who had relapsed after an initial response to

Kanti R. Rai, MD, Chief, Division of Haematology and Oncology, Long Island Jewish Medical Center, New York, USA.

N. Driscoll, Division of Haematology and Oncology, Long Island Jewish Medical Center, New York, USA.

Dale M. Janson RPA-C, MBA, Division of Haematology and Oncology, Long Island Jewish Medical Center, New York, USA.

D. V. Patel, Division of Haematology and Oncology, Long Island Jewish Medical Center, New York, USA.

chemotherapy (n = 8) or who were refractory to chemotherapy (n = 21). Of interest is that only 3 of these 29 patients had previously been treated with fludarabine. This was due primarily to the fact that fludarabine was not available in Europe until 1994. All patients were treated with Campath-1H at a dose of 30 mg intravenously over 2 h three times per week (TIW) for a maximum of 12 weeks.

Osterborg and co-workers reported that 3 of 8 patients (38%) with relapsed and 9 of 21 (43%) with refractory disease were able to achieve a response using Campath-1H. It was also shown that CLL cells were rapidly eliminated from blood in 97% of the patients and a bone marrow complete response (CR) was achieved in 36% while splenomegaly resolved in 32% of patients. By contrast, lymphadenopathy resolved in only 2 of 29 (7%) of patients. The median response duration was 12 months (range, 6–25+). While World Health Organization (WHO) grade 4 neutropaenia and thrombocytopaenia developed in 3 (10%) and 2 patients (7%), respectively, these toxicities resolved in most responding patients during continued Campath-1H treatment. Profound lymphopaenia ($<0.5 \times 10^3/\mu$) occurred in all patients and 2 patients developed opportunistic infections (OIs). Four patients had bacterial septicaemia.

Twenty-four patients with B-cell CLL (n = 23) or T-cell prolymphocytic leukaemia (n = 1) were included in the U.S. phase II trial 125-K32-009 [5]. These patients were treated at six U.S. centres with a target dose of 30 mg TIW for up to 16 weeks. Unlike the European trial, all of these patients were previously treated with fludarabine and 71% had either not responded to fludarabine or had responded initially but relapsed within 6 months of treatment. The other 29% of patients had initially been sensitive to fludarabine but had relapsed and had not responded to subsequent chemotherapy regimens. In this study, 8 of 24 (33%) of patients achieved a major response (all partial remissions; PR) with a median time to response of 3.9 months (range, 1.6–5.3 months) and a median duration of response of 15.4 months (range, 4.6–38.0 months). Median time to disease progression was 19.6 months (range, 7.7–42.0 months) and the median survival time was 35.8 months (range, 8.8 to $\geq$47.1 months).

In the U.S. phase II 125-K32-009 trial, while infusion-related reactions were the most common toxicities seen with rigors and fever occurring in 92 and 100% of patients, respectively, infectious toxicities were also observed at a fairly high rate. Due to the fact that prophylactic antibiotics were not mandated in the study, OIs occurred in 10 of 24 (41.7%) of patients, with pulmonary infections being the most common. There were 3 proven cases and one suspected case of *pneumocystis carinii* pneumonia (PCP) and one case of candida/aspergillus infection. OIs were more common among those patients who did not have a clinical beneficial response to alemtuzumab. Two of the 8 responders developed OIs, whereas 8 of 16 non-responders suffered from some form of OI. All cases of proven or suspected PCP were in patients who did not receive prophylactic trimethoprim/sulfamethoxazole (TMP/SMZ).

ALEMTUZUMAB IN B-CELL CLL PATIENTS AFTER FLUDARABINE FAILURE: THE 'PIVOTAL' STUDY

The largest study to date of alemtuzumab in previously treated patients with CLL was published in 2002 by Keating and colleagues [6]. In that study, a total of 93 patients with B-cell CLL, 92 of whom had failed prior fludarabine, were treated with intravenous alemtuzumab at a target dose of 30 mg TIW for up to 12 weeks. Also required for entry into this study was prior treatment with an alkylating agent. These were a group of heavily pretreated patients with the median number of prior regimens being three (range, 2–7) while 46% of the patients had received multiple fludarabine treatments. Almost half of the patients (48%) had never responded to any nucleoside analogue-based regimen.

Responses were assessed according to the NCI Working Group (NCI-WG) criteria [7]. The overall response rate was 33% (31/93) with 29 of 31 PR and 2 of 31 CR. Of the PRs, 6 of the 29 patients had clearing of disease from all sites which might have qualified them as CR but had persistent anaemia or thrombocytopaenia which rendered them PR by the NCI-WG criteria.

Responses in the blood and bone marrow in the Keating study were impressive, with median peripheral blood CD19+/CD5+ cells in 89 patients studied declining from $33.6 \times 10^3/\mu$ at baseline to $0.003 \times 10^3/\mu$ at week 4 of alemtuzumab therapy. Seventy-eight patients had peripheral lymphocytosis at baseline with 67 of these patients evaluable at the last assessment. Of these, 65 (83%) had complete resolution and 2 (2.6%) had >50% improvement of the peripheral lymphocytosis. Bone marrow involvement was present at baseline in 85 patients and was evaluable in 62 patients after therapy. There were 22 patients (26%) who achieved complete clearance of bone marrow disease as assessed in biopsy specimens while another 16 patients (19%) had >50% clearance of the marrow. If one looks at the 31 patients who had a response (CR or PR), the results are even more impressive, with 15 of 31 (48%) achieving complete clearance of bone marrow and another 7 of 31 (23%) showing >50% clearance.

Also of interest in the pivotal study was the assessment of clinical benefit, defined as resolution of B symptoms or fatigue, resolution of massive splenomegaly, improvement in WHO performance status or improvement in anaemia. Of the 31 patients who responded to treatment, resolution of B symptoms was seen in all 17 patients who exhibited these symptoms at baseline. Overall, 59 patients had complaints of fever, night sweats or weight loss at baseline and 31 of these patients (52.5%) had complete resolution of these troubling complaints. In addition, there were improvements in the median chemotherapy-free periods among the responders (n = 31), increasing from 4.0 months after a therapeutic regimen prior to alemtuzumab to 12.4 months following response with alemtuzumab treatment. Massive splenomegaly (>6 cm) resolved in 90% of responders and 25% overall.

Unlike the early studies with alemtuzumab in CLL cited above, prophylaxis against viral infections and PCP was required in this larger pivotal trial and made a considerable difference to the incidence of PCP infections. Only one case of PCP was reported and this occurred in a patient who did not receive prophylaxis as outlined in the study. Overall, 11 patients developed OIs during the treatment period and another 7 patients developed OIs in the post-treatment follow-up period. The most commonly reported OI was reactivation of cytomegalovirus (CMV) with 7 cases reported, all occurring during the treatment period. Five of the cases resolved and 2 resulted in discontinuation of alemtuzumab with subsequent withdrawal from the study.

Again in this study, infusion-related events were the most common reported adverse events (AEs) with fevers and/or rigors occurring in about 90% of patients. This was similar to the results seen in the Osterborg [4] and Rai [5] studies. As will be seen, these common and very bothersome toxicities have prompted investigation into the alternative route of administration of alemtuzumab by subcutaneous injection.

In 2003, Ferrajoli and colleagues [8], reported on 78 patients with a variety of advanced or refractory chronic lymphoproliferative disorders. Alemtuzumab was given at 30 mg TIW intravenously for a minimum of 4 weeks and a maximum of 12 weeks, depending on response. Pre-medication with acetaminophen and diphenhydramine was required prior to each infusion and all patients were given prophylactic antibiotic coverage with TMP/SMZ and valacyclovir.

CLL was the most common (n = 42) diagnosis in this series of 78 heavily pre-treated patients who had received a median of three (range, 1–9) prior therapies. Amongst these 42 patients with CLL, 19 were considered sensitive to, while 23 patients were considered refractory to, fludarabine. Among the subgroup of patients with CLL, there was a 31% (13/42) overall response rate with CR occurring in 2 patients (5%), PR in 10 patients (24%) and nodular PR in one patient (2%). Of the 19 patients with CLL that were 'fludarabine sensitive', 2 CRs and 5 PRs were achieved for an overall response rate of 37%. In those 23 patients who were considered 'fludarabine resistant', there were no CRs and 6 PRs for an overall response rate of 26%.

As in previous studies, clearance of blood lymphocytosis was achieved in a large proportion (84%) of the total patient population while nearly half of the patients (49%) achieved resolution of bone marrow disease. A decrease in the size of enlarged spleen and liver by 50% or more occurred in 56 and 59% of patients, respectively, while lymphadenopathy decreased by at least 50% in 39% of patients.

Seventy-one percent of the CLL patients developed proven or clinically suspected infection. CMV reactivation was the most common viral infection, occurring in 29% of 42 CLL patients. All of these patients responded to intravenous ganciclovir or foscarnet. Other infectious toxicities reported for the entire group of 78 patients were 17 episodes of bacteraemia in 11 patients, eleven episodes of pneumonia in 10 patients, 3 cases of herpes virus infections and one case of invasive aspergillosis.

Despite the pre-medication requirement, infusion-related AEs were common with fever occurring in 85% and rigors in 42% of patients. Other immediate events included rash (42%), nausea (35%), dyspnoea (31%), hypotension (18%) and headache (7%). Cardiovascular toxicity was seen in 3 patients, all of whom had T-cell malignancies. Haematological toxicities included grade 3 (19%) and grade 4 (15%) neutropaenia while grade 3 and grade 4 thrombocytopaenia occurred in 28 and 13%, respectively. Persistent lymphopaenia resulted in all patients.

Moreton and colleagues [*J Clin Oncol*, in press] have recently reported their experience of alemtuzumab in 91 patients with relapsed and refractory CLL. Eighty-eight of the patients had been previously treated with purine analogues and a half of these were refractory to their latest purine-analogue-containing regime. The aim of therapy for this series of patients was to eradicate CLL to below detectable levels of minimal residual disease (MRD) using a highly sensitive flow cytometric assay (see Chapter 16). The overall response rate in this series of patients was 55% with 36% of these achieving a CR and 20% having no detectable MRD at the end of therapy. The strongest predictor of response was whether patients had grossly enlarged lymphadenopathy – only one patient of 11 with single lymph nodes of greater than 5 cm achieved a PR with no CR or MRD-negative patients. In contrast, the overall response rate in 33 patients without significant lymphadenopathy was 87% (29/33) with 24 (73%) of 33 achieving CR and 39% having eradication of detectable MRD. Patients who had a CR had prolonged survival compared to the non-CR patients. The 20% of patients who became MRD negative had a far superior survival, with 83% surviving 5 years.

Rigors and fever were the most common adverse events occurring in 76% of patients and were more frequently grade 1 or 2 in severity. Less frequent AEs included fatigue (11%), dyspnoea (4%), headache (4%), dizziness (3%), bronchospasm (2%) and diarrhoea (2%). AEs declined in frequency by the end of week 3 of therapy. Neutropaenia below $1.0 \times 10^9/l$ occurred in 43 (48%) patients and below $0.5 \times 10^9/l$ in 27 (30%). Granulocyte colony-stimulating factor (G-CSF) was administered to 18 (20%) patients with a median neutrophil count of $0.35 \times 10^9/l$ (range, 0.02–0.6) and the neutrophil count rose to a median of $1.15 \times 10^9/l$ (range, 0.5–9.2). Thrombocytopaenia occurred in 65 (73%) and was less than $50 \times 10^9/l$ in 41 (46%). Thirty-nine patients (43%) experienced one or more infections during or within one month of completing alemtuzumab therapy. There were 19 mild (grade 1 or 2) infectious episodes and 33 severe (grade 3 or 4) episodes. A total of 8 (8%) patients developed CMV reactivation at a median of 34 days after the start of therapy (range, 14–58). One patient died from CMV pneumonitis and after this, screening with pre-emptive therapy for CMV reactivation was instituted. All cases of CMV reactivation detected on screening resolved on anti-viral therapy. There were 31 documented infections in the period following alemtuzumab amongst 21 (23%) patients (excluding infections occurring during neutropaenia following subsequent stem cell transplantation). Infections following the cessation of alemtuzumab in non-MRD-negative CR patients occurred after a median of 9 months (range, 1–41) and in the MRD-negative patients after a median of 3 months (range, 1–12).

SUBCUTANEOUS ALEMTUZUMAB

Because of the virtual certainty of infusion-related reactions which occur at a very high frequency, even when patients are pre-treated with antihistamines and acetaminophen, investigators have embarked upon studies to determine if alemtuzumab can be made more user-friendly when it is administered *via* the subcutaneous route.

In a Phase II trial by Lundin and co-workers [9], 41 previously untreated CLL patients were given subcutaneous alemtuzumab at a dose of 30 mg TIW for a maximum of 18 weeks. Dose escalation, from 3 to 10 to 30 mg as tolerated, over a period of 1–2 weeks was used in the event of local skin erythema or oedema. After the dose-escalation phase and the disappearance of 'first-dose' skin reactions, almost all patients self-administered alemtuzumab. The overall clinical response rate was 87%, with 19% of patients achieving a CR. While 66% of the patients achieved CR or nodular PR in the bone marrow, only 29% of patients had complete resolution of lymphadenopathy. The median time to treatment failure was more than 18 months. Of note is that infusion-related reactions such as rigors, rash, nausea, dyspnoea and hypotension were rare, although transient injection site skin reactions were seen in 90% of patients.

The German CLL Study Group initiated the CLL2H trial to evaluate the subcutaneous application of Campath-1H 30 mg TIW for a maximum of 12 weeks in fludarabine-refractory CLL patients [10]. An intravenous dose-escalation schedule of 3, 10 and 30 mg was used and patients were then switched to the subcutaneous route of administration. This trial essentially duplicated the 'pivotal' trial conducted by Keating and colleagues [6] but replaced the intravenous route with the subcutaneous route of administration. In an interim analysis of the first 50 patients enrolled, there were 4% CR, 33% PR, 44% stable disease and 18% progressive disease. The median overall survival at the time of the report was 17.4 months and median progression-free survival was 10.8 months. These results compare favourably to the Keating trial. Response rates similar to the overall study population were observed in patients with poor-prognostic genetic subtypes (i.e. deletions of 17p, 11q and unmutated V_H genes).

Hale and colleagues [11] studied the blood concentrations of alemtuzumab as well as anti-globulin responses following intravenous or subcutaneous routes of administration in CLL patients. Subcutaneous alemtuzumab yielded serum concentrations similar to those achieved with intravenous alemtuzumab, although this was achieved with slightly higher cumulative doses. The dominant factor influencing biodistribution and pharmacokinetics appears to be the extent of tumour burden. Subcutaneous alemtuzumab is more convenient and better tolerated but may be associated with formation of anti-alemtuzumab antibodies, particularly in those patients who were previously untreated. The 2 of 31 patients who demonstrated anti-alemtuzumab antibody on subcutaneous treatment, unlike the other patients, did not show significant reductions in lymphocyte counts but had marked local skin reactions which did not diminish with continued therapy.

These studies demonstrate that subcutaneous alemtuzumab, a more convenient alternative to intravenous, is safe and appears to have similar efficacy and an improved side-effect profile compared with intravenous alemtuzumab (Table 14.1). In addition, according to Lundin *et al.* [9], the subcataneous route of administration may reduce healthcare costs.

CYTOMEGALOVIRUS REACTIVATION

The infectious toxicities of alemtuzumab have been well documented and are generally prevented with appropriate prophylactic medications. One topic of continued interest and

Table 14.1.   Responses to alemtuzumab in relapsed/refractory CLL

Author/Year	n	Overall response rate %	Complete response rate %	Partial response rate %	Route of administration	Prior fludarabine Yes/No
Osterborg et al. [4]	29	42	4	38	iv	No*
Rai et al. [5]	24	33	0	33	iv	Yes
Keating et al. [6]	93	33	2	31	iv	Yes
Stilgenbauer et al. [10]	50	37	4	33	sc	Yes

*3/29 patients had received prior fludarabine.
iv = Intravenous infusion; sc = subcutaneous injection.

Table 14.2.   Prevalance of CMV reactivation in CLL patients treated with alemtuzumab

Author/Year	Disease status	Cases of CMV/ patients treated	Prevalence %	Organ involvement Yes/No	Rx with ganciclovir	Resolution of symptoms Yes/No	Taken off study
Keating et al. [6]	Rel/Ref	7/93	7.5	No	NA	Yes	2/7
Nguyen et al. [12]	Rel/Ref	5/34	14.7	No	Yes	Yes	NA
Lundin et al. [9]	1st line	4/41	9.7	No	Yes (3/4)	Yes	2/4
Wendtner et al. [13]	Consolidation after 1st line	4/11	36.3	Yes (2/4)	Yes	Yes	NA

Rel/Ref = Relapsed or refractory disease; NA = not available.

concern is the issue of CMV reactivation (Table 14.2). In the pivotal trial by Keating and colleagues [6], in relapsed or refractory CLL patients, CMV reactivation occurred in 7.5% of patients. The typical presentation was fever and antigenaemia. Organ involvement did not occur and there were no deaths. The Stanford group had a similar experience [12]. Five out of 34 patients with relapsed and refractory CLL treated with alemtuzumab developed fever and CMV antigenaemia. All patients had resolution of fever and antigenaemia after therapy with ganciclovir. None of the 5 patients developed symptoms or findings suggestive of a CMV-associated clinical syndrome. Lundin and co-workers [9] reported CMV reactivation (verified by polymerase chain reaction) following alemtuzumab therapy among 4 out of 41 (10%) previously untreated CLL patients. All 4 had fever without pneumonitis. These events occurred after 4, 5, 11 and 12 weeks of alemtuzumab therapy, respectively. Three patients received intravenous ganciclovir treatment and responded promptly. One patient recovered spontaneously. In 2 of these 4 cases, alemtuzumab treatment was restarted while the patient received oral ganciclovir prophylaxis without further CMV problems. The German CLL Study Group studied consolidation with alemtuzumab in patients with CLL in first remission in a Phase III randomised trial [13]. After a median of 4 weeks, alemtuzumab treatment was interrupted due to serious infections in 7 of 11 patients. Four patients showed CMV reactivation detected by CMV-specific PCR and required intravenous ganciclovir treatment because of rising viral load combined with fevers or because of CMV pneumonia. CMV pneumonia was diagnosed in 2 patients who had increased CMV titre by CMV-specific PCR, positive CMV antigen, radiological signs of pneumonia and clinical findings of fever, dyspnoea and coughing. Ganciclovir resolved the CMV symptoms and CMV-DNA declined to baseline levels by week 8 in all treated patients. The clinical significance of detection of CMV by plasma DNA PCR in patients with CLL treated with alemtuzumab remains uncertain, but this test provides an objective measure of CMV activity and may be diagnostic in patients with unexplained fever.

SUMMARY

Therapy with alemtuzumab offers an alternative, more effective option compared to combination chemotherapy for treatment of patients with CLL who have relapsed or who are refractory to the nucleoside analogues. Although there are significant potential toxicities associated with alemtuzumab, such as the infusional reactions and the risk of CMV reactivation, most are manageable. Despite these side-effects, the response rates are sufficient to justify the use of this humanised monoclonal antibody in refractory CLL. Pre-treatment anti-pyretics and anti-histamines are recommended to prevent or mitigate the acute infusional reactions associated with intravenous infusion. Recent use of alemtuzumab *via* the subcutaneous route has been shown to be well tolerated and has yielded similar response rates as the infusional method of administration. Prophylaxis with TMP/SMZ as well as valacyclovir or a similar anti-viral can prevent many of the OIs seen in early trials. Reactivation of CMV infection remains a challenge but can be effectively managed with diligent monitoring and early treatment. Future areas of research will include the use of alemtuzumab in combination with other monoclonal antibodies and or other targeted therapies.

ACKNOWLEDGEMENTS

This work was supported by a grant from the Peter Jay Sharp Foundation, Chemotherapy Foundation, Joel Finkelstein Cancer Foundation, the Tebil Foundation and the Horace W. Goldsmith Foundation.
Dr. Rai is the recipient of a research grant from Berlex Laboratories.

REFERENCES

1. Rai KR, Peterson BL, Appelbaum FR *et al*. Fludarabine compared with chlorambucil as primary therapy for chronic lymphocytic leukemia. *N Engl J Med* 2000; 343:1750–1757.
2. Keating MJ, O'Brien S, Kontoyiannis D *et al*. Results of first salvage therapy for patients refractory to a fludarabine regimen in chronic lymphocytic leukemia. *Leuk Lymphoma* 2002; 43:1755–1762.
3. Byrd J, Stilgenbauer S, Flinn I. Chronic lymphocytic leukemia. *Hematology* 2004:163–183.
4. Osterborg A, Dyer MJ, Bunjes D *et al*. Phase II multicenter study of human CD52 antibody in previously treated chronic lymphocytic leukemia. European Study Group of CAMPATH-1H Treatment in chronic lymphocytic leukemia. *J Clin Oncol* 1997; 15:1567–1574.
5. Rai KR, Freter CE, Mercier RJ *et al*. Alemtuzumab in previously treated chronic lymphocytic leukemia patients who also had received fludarabine. *J Clin Oncol* 2002; 20:3891–3897.
6. Keating MJ, Flinn I, Jain V *et al*. Therapeutic role of alemtuzumab (Campath-1H) in patients who have failed fludarabine: results of a large international study. *Blood* 2002; 99:3554–3561.
7. Cheson BD, Bennett JM, Grever M *et al*. National Cancer Institute-sponsored Working Group guideline for chronic lypmphocytic leukemia: revised guidelines for diagnosis and treatment. *Blood* 1996; 87:4990–4997.
8. Ferrajoli A, O'Brien SM, Cortes JE *et al*. Phase II study of alemtuzumab in chronic lymphoproliferative disorders. *Cancer* 2003; 98:773–778.
9. Lundin J, Kimby E, Bjorkholm M *et al*. Phase II trial of subcutaneous alemtuzumab (Campath-1H) as first-line treatment for patients with B-cell chronic lymphocytic leukemia (B-CLL). *Blood* 2002; 100:768–773.
10. Stilgenbauer S, Winkler D, Krober A *et al*. Subcutaneous Campath-1H (alemtuzumab) in fludarabine-refractory CLL; interim analysis of the CLL2H Study of the German CLL Study Group (GCLLSG). *Blood* 2004; 104:478a.

11. Hale G, Rebello P, Brettman LR *et al*. Blood concentrations of alemtuzumab and antiglobulin responses in patients with chronic lymphocytic leukemia following intravenous or subcutaneous routes of administration. *Blood* 2004; 104:948–955.
12. Nguyen DD, Cao TM, Dugan K *et al*. Cytomegalovirus viremia during CAMPATH-1H therapy for relapsed and refractory chronic lymphocytic leukemia and prolymphocytic leukemia. *Clin Lymphoma* 2002; 3:105–110
13. Wendtner CM, Ritgen M, Schweighofer CD *et al*. Consolidation with alemtuzumab in patients with chronic lymphocytic leukemia in first remission- experience on safety and efficacy within a randomized multicenter phase III trial of the German CLL Study Group (GCLLSG). *Leukemia* 2004; 18:1093–1101.

15

Optimising the use of alemtuzumab in CLL: new therapeutic end points, disease stratification and therapy earlier in the disease course

P. Hillmen

INTRODUCTION

Chronic lymphocytic leukaemia (CLL) is the most common form of leukaemia in adults in the Western world. Conventionally, the mainstays of therapy for CLL have been the alkylating agents, such as chlorambucil and cyclophosphamide, and purine analogues, such as fludarabine and cladrabine. Although the overall response rates (ORR) to these therapies are reasonably high, it is unusual to obtain complete remissions (CR; up to 10% with chlorambucil and 25% with single-agent fludarabine) [1]. In studies comparing fludarabine with chlorambucil, a prolongation in survival has not been observed despite the better response rates seen with fludarabine. There are several reasons for this apparent failure to prolong survival in randomised trials of purine analogues compared to alkylating agents: (1) when patients are randomised between chlorambucil and fludarabine the actual question being addressed is whether fludarabine as first-line therapy is better than fludarabine as second-line therapy because almost a half of patients (46% in the largest study reported [1]) who fail or relapse after chlorambucil will respond to second-line fludarabine; (2) the majority of the responses to fludarabine monotherapy are partial remissions; and (3) the National Cancer Institute (NCI) response criteria which were published in 1996 [2] have a relatively liberal definition of CR (Table 15.1) in that patients achieving a CR can have up to 5% CLL cells in the marrow when sensitive detection methods are applied. The lack of improved overall survival in these studies and the availability of newer therapeutic approaches, such as monoclonal antibodies alone (alemtuzumab) or in combination (rituximab or alemtuzumab), stem cell transplantation (SCT; reduced intensity conditioning allogeneic transplantation or autologous transplantation) and combination chemotherapies (such as fludarabine, cyclophosphamide and mitoxantrone; FCM) has been the stimulus for the development of sensitive assays to minimal residual disease (MRD) in CLL. These assays can detect extremely low levels of CLL (down to a single CLL cell in 100,000 leucocytes) which can be routinely used to improve the depth of remission obtained with these newer therapeutic approaches [3]. The *eradication of detectable MRD* is possible in a significant proportion of patients with CLL but such intensification of therapy carries with it an increased risk of treatment-related toxicity.

Peter Hillmen, Department of Haematology, Pinderfields Hospital, Wakefield, UK.

Table 15.1. Definition of a complete remission by National Cancer Institute-criteria

Parameter	Outcome 2 months after end of therapy
Symptomatology	None
Total lymphocytes	$\leq 4000/\mu l$
Lymph nodes (physical examination only)	Not palpable
Liver and spleen	Not palpable
Neutrophils*	$\geq 1500/\mu l$
Platelets*	$>100,000/\mu l$
Haemoglobin*	$>110\,g/l$
Bone marrow (morphology)	$<30\%$ lymphocytes; no nodules on trephine biopsy**

*If counts recover beyond 2 months after the completion of chemotherapy then the response is still a partial remission even if there is no detectable CLL present.
**Can amount to as many as 5% CLL cells by flow cytometry (personal observation).

It is apparent that the clinical behaviour and outcome varies markedly between individual patients. Several recently described biological markers allow the separation of good-risk from poor-risk disease. For example, patients with CLL in which the immunoglobulin gene of the tumour contains somatic mutations, indicating that the B cell from which the tumour originates had already passed through a germinal centre, have a very good prognosis such that the vast majority will not die from their disease. In marked contrast, patients with unmutated (germ-line) immunoglobulin genes will almost all rapidly progress to require therapy, and have a high probability of dying as a direct result of their CLL [4, 5]. This finding suggests that the approach to treatment for these two subtypes of CLL should be different – a more intensive approach with its incumbent risks is probably justified for unmutated CLL but may not be for most patients with mutated CLL.

The other important advance in our understanding of CLL has been the observation that cytogenetic abnormalities, in particular, the loss of 17p (the location of the p53 gene) or 11q (the location of the ataxia telangiectasia mutated (ATM) gene) are associated with a significantly worse response to therapy and prognosis [6]. The importance of this observation has been explained by the observation that both of these abnormalities disrupt the p53 pathway which is fundamental to the activity of both alkylating agents and purine analogues [7, 8]. This information indicates that the time has come to consider whether patients should be stratified at diagnosis to the most appropriate therapy (*disease stratification*).

Patients with relapsed and resistant CLL have an extremely poor prognosis when treated with conventional combination chemotherapy with a median survival of 10 months and a 5-year survival of around 10% [9]. It is also well described that the risk of therapy in these patients is extremely high regardless of the therapy given. In a large series of patients with CLL presented by Molteni and colleagues [10] at the European Haematology Association Meeting in 2003 one third of all patients with CLL experienced opportunistic infections (mainly bacterial). Patients who had received more than one prior therapy had a three-fold increase in infection rate. Perkins and co-workers [11] reported that 24 of 27 patients with refractory CLL treated with combination chemotherapy experienced grade 3 or 4 infections with a median number of two hospital admissions with infections per patient during their next therapy. Considering such a high incidence of serious infections, it is not surprising that a high incidence of infection is seen with alemtuzumab when used in refractory disease and in fact, the number of infections seen in the alemtuzumab pivotal studies is not excessive compared with similar refractory populations [12]. However, there are clearly some infections, such as the reactivation of cytomegalovirus (CMV), which occur at an increased frequency during alemtuzumab treatment and are a direct result of the immune suppression associated with the drug. However, CMV reactivation can be successfully managed with appropriate screening and pre-emptive therapy of early reactivation. This raises the possibility that the use of alemtuzumab earlier in the patient's disease course might optimise the beneficial effects of the drug whilst reducing the possible complications. Therefore, *alemtuzumab earlier in the disease course*, such as consolidation or front-line therapy, should be considered at least for selected patients.

ASSESSMENT AND ERADICATION OF MINIMAL RESIDUAL DISEASE IN CLL

The current response criteria for CLL were published in 1996 [2] and although the definition of a CR did require examination of the bone marrow, no assessment of residual disease was required. It is clear from most series that, regardless of the therapy employed, patients achieving an NCI CR have a better progression-free survival (PFS) than non-responders [13]. However, in many studies, this improved PFS has not translated into improved overall survival as patients may be effectively treated with salvage therapy. In addition, no plateau in the overall survival curve is seen, even for patients in CR. This finding and the development of therapies which are much more effective at eradicating residual disease such as combination chemotherapy (FCM [14]), autologous SCT [15, 16], allogeneic SCT [17], fludarabine plus cyclophosphamide plus rituximab (FCR) [18, 19] and alemtuzumab [20], have driven the development of assays which will detect extremely low levels of residual CLL.

Methods of detecting MRD in CLL depend upon either flow cytometry or the polymerase chain reaction (PCR). The use of low-sensitivity techniques, such as flow cytometry for CD5 and CD19 co-expressing cells or PCR with consensus primers to the immunoglobulin heavy chain, is relatively insensitive in the presence of polyclonal B cells. Unfortunately, at the end of therapy, the time point when MRD assessment is most important, there is often a brisk increase in normal B cells, and thus these low-sensitivity tests are of very limited value. High-sensitivity flow cytometric assays (or 'MRD Flow') [3] utilise the disease-specific phenotype to identify CLL cells (Figure 15.1). These assays can be applied to all patients, and reliably detect CLL cells if they represent over 1% of total B cells, or over 0.01% of total leucocytes. One of the principle advantages of MRD flow is that results are generated rapidly so that they can be used to guide therapy in real time, enabling continued treatment until the patient has reached an MRD-negative response. The validity of this approach has recently been demonstrated in patients receiving alemtuzumab [20]. Allele-specific oligonucleotide PCR (ASO-PCR) is a slightly more sensitive method for the detection of residual disease enumerating CLL cells accurately when they represent over 0.01% of leucocytes. However, ASO-PCR requires the design and validation of a patient-specific PCR primer for every patient, which is time consuming and only possible in approximately 90% of patients. The results are generated more slowly than flow cytometric approaches, but can be performed retrospectively. Therefore, ASO-PCR is rarely used in routine practice due to the technical complexity of the assay.

The availability of assays that can detect low levels of CLL and the advent of therapeutic approaches that can eradicate detectable CLL in a proportion of patients provide the tools with which to address whether the therapeutic target in CLL should be the eradication of MRD rather than simply achieving an NCI CR. Moreton and colleagues [20] reported in 2005 that over 50% of patients with relapsed/refractory CLL achieve an NCI response following alemtuzumab. The aim of therapy was to achieve the deepest possible remission, including the eradication of MRD in responding patients. Eradication of detectable CLL from the blood and marrow using MRD flow was achieved in 18 (20%) of the 91 patients treated. In addition, of the remaining patients who failed to respond to alemtuzumab alone, MRD negativity was established with either combined alemtuzumab and fludarabine (n = 2) or following autologous SCT utilising stem cells collected after alemtuzumab therapy (n = 4). Therefore,

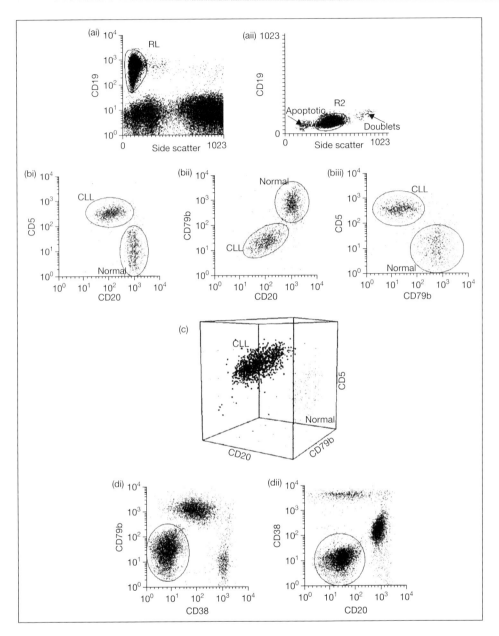

Figure 15.1. Highly sensitive MRD assessment using multi-parameter flow cytometry (gating strategy for specific identification of CLL cells). (a) Total B cells were identified using 2 regions: (i) CD19 and side scatter, to exclude granular cells showing non-specific CD19 binding; and (ii) forward and side scatter, to exclude apoptotic cells and doublets. (b) CLL cells were separated from normal B cells according to their CD5, CD20 and CD79b. CLL cells could be separated from normal B cells using (i) CD5 vs. CD20 in 82% of cases; (ii) CD79b vs. CD20 in 35% of cases; and (iii) CD5 vs. CD79b in 88% of cases. (c) To separate CLL cells from normal B cells, all three antigens must be assessed on gated B cells. (d) To separate CLL cells from normal B cells and normal B progenitors in the bone marrow in all cases, CD38 is included; this requires two tests: (ii) CD19 vs. CD5 vs. CD38 vs. CD79b. (ii) CD19 vs. CD5 vs. CD38 vs. CD20; and (Reproduced courtesy of *Blood* [(Rawstron *et al.* Blood 2001; 98:29–35)].

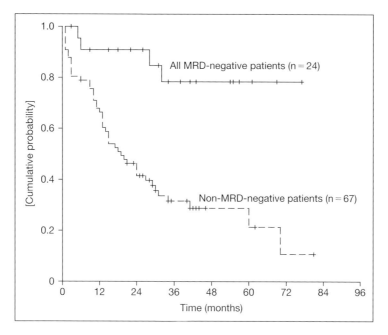

Figure 15.2. Kaplan Meier Survival Plot of survival of the 24 patients achieving an MRD-negative CR following alemtuzumab (alone [n = 18], combined with fludarabine [n = 2] or followed by autologous stem cell transplantation [n = 4]) compared to those patient who remained MRD-positive (n = 67). The median survival for MRD negative responders has not been reached. The median survival of patients who did not achieve an MRD-negative CR was 19 months: 95% CI (12.0–26.0) (Reproduced courtesy of *J Clin Oncol*).

a total of 24 (26%) out of 91 of patients achieved an MRD-negative CR with alemtuzumab and these patients had a significantly longer overall survival (approximately 80 v. 30% at 3 years, respectively; Figure 15.2). Therefore alemtuzumab can be used to eradicate detectable MRD in CLL – probably a desirable end point of therapy in refractory CLL. The next logical question is whether selected patients could be treated earlier in their disease, when they might either have lower bulk disease, when the efficacy of and complications associated with the drug might be optimised. One possibility is the use of alemtuzumab after an MRD-positive response to conventional chemotherapy. Alternatively alemtuzumab might be safer and more effective if used as the first therapy when the patient's disease is probably most sensitive to therapy (see below).

DISEASE STRATIFICATION AND THE USE OF ALEMTUZUMAB IN P53 DYSFUNCTIONAL CLL

One of the recurring cytogenetic abnormalities observed in CLL is deletion of the short arm of chromosome 17 when analysed by FISH (17p−). This abnormality indicates the loss of one p53 allele and is often associated with mutation of the other p53 allele [21]. Therefore, the patient's CLL has dysfunction of the p53 pathway and this confers resistance to conventional chemotherapy, such as alkylating agents or purine analogues. The 17p− abnormality is relatively infrequent in patients presenting with CLL, occurring in 5–10% of patients. However, 17p− and p53 dysfunction is increasingly common in patients who are refractory to fludarabine. The reason for this resistance is that both alkylating agents (by damaging DNA) and purine analogues (by interfering with DNA repair) utilise the p53 pathway to drive the CLL cells into cell cycle arrest and/or apoptosis. Therefore, these agents effectively damage DNA but the cell is unable to apoptose and, since the DNA damage may occur in tumour suppressor genes or oncogenes, may be detrimental, effectively 'creating' chemotherapy resistance. It is probable that treatment with conventional p53-dependent therapies creates a selective advantage for p53 dysfunctional subclones of the CLL clone. In addition, deletion of the long arm of chromosome 11 (11q−) is also a poor prognostic finding and, at least in a proportion of patients, this involves loss of one allele of the ATM gene. In some patients 11q− is associated with somatic mutation of the other ATM allele [22]. Remarkably, the ATM protein is part of the p53 pathway and therefore abnormalities of ATM will potentially disrupt the p53 pathway again explaining the poor prognosis of 11q− CLL. This information is more than of only academic interest as p53 dysfunction will confer resistance to conventional chemotherapy and there is now convincing evidence indicating that therapies which do not utilise the p53 pathway for their function may be more effective. The two principle therapies which are effective in p53 dysfunctional CLL are monoclonal antibodies, particularly alemtuzumab, and high-dose steroids. The logical approach for patients with predominantly blood and bone marrow disease with no or only small lymph nodes is to use alemtuzumab. However, patients with large-volume lymph nodes are unlikely to respond to alemtuzumab alone and in these patients, a strategy of controlling the lymph nodes with high-dose steroids such as high-dose methyl prednisolone ($1 \, g/m^2/day$ for 5 days repeated every 4 weeks) [23] followed by consolidation with alemtuzumab to eradicate blood and bone marrow disease, can be effective. Therefore, specific knowledge of the genetic abnormalities in a patient's CLL, particularly of those affecting the p53 pathway, allows the selection of appropriate therapies and sequencing of these therapies in order to reduce the damage caused by ineffective chemotherapy and to treat patients most effectively.

ALEMTUZUMAB EARLIER IN THE DISEASE COURSE

The improvement in our understanding of CLL and, in particular, the identification of patients with a poor prognosis at diagnosis, will result in the stratification of patients according to the biological characteristics of their disease. It is therefore likely that patients with mutated CLL or with isolated 13q deletion will be managed with therapies which reduce the potential complications rather than attempt to eradiate detectable MRD. However, this conservative approach to treating patients with poor-risk disease, p53 dysfunctional or unmutated CLL, will only lead to short remissions and probably to increasing resistance to salvage therapies. In this poor-risk disease, the use of monoclonal antibodies as consolidation, to eradicate detectable MRD, or even as front-line therapy, is worthy of consideration.

CONSOLIDATION THERAPY WITH ALEMTUZUMAB

One of the major problems in the treatment of poor-risk CLL is the early relapse of patients who have achieved a response to therapy [24]. Analysis for MRD in these patients demonstrates that few patients have no detectable CLL after 'induction' therapy, and therefore it is very likely that the progression of the disease results from expansion of this residual disease. Moreover, it is likely that the small proportion of cells that remain after initial chemotherapy are a more resistant subpopulation of the CLL clone which probably explains why relapse is usually less responsive to therapy. In addition, the pharmacokinetics of a monoclonal antibody are intimately related to the amount of target antigen which, in the case of alemtuzumab, is related to tumour bulk. Pharmacological studies have demonstrated that the volume of distribution for alemtuzumab is related to disease bulk and the time to detectable plasma levels of alemtuzumab is related to number of circulating tumour cells and the route of administration, in that intravenous dosing is more efficient than sub-cutaneous dosing, whereas the latter is far better tolerated [25]. A compromise may be to give subcutaneous alemtuzumab for 18 weeks rather than the convention of 12 weeks of intravenous alemtuzumab. The terminal half-life of alemtuzumab is, not surprisingly, the same regardless of the route of administration used. Therefore, a good argument could be made that the optimal place to use alemtuzumab is as consolidation therapy to eradicate MRD after induction therapy in patients in poor-risk CLL.

There has been a single randomised trial of alemtuzumab consolidation following initial therapy with purine-analogue-based treatment which was performed by the German CLL Study Group and reported in 2004 [26]. Patients were treated to maximum response with fludarabine or fludarabine plus cyclophosphamide and were then randomised to alem-tuzumab at the standard dose (30 mg three times a week for 12 weeks). Alemtuzumab was given intravenously and at a median of 2 months following the 'induction' therapy. This trial was stopped prematurely after 21 patients were entered (11 receiving alemtuzumab and 10 watch and wait) because of the high infection rate in the alemtuzumab arm – 7 of the 11 patients experienced grade 3 or 4 infections and although no patient died, a number of patients were very unwell. Four patients in the alemtuzumab group experienced CMV reactivation and all responded to ganciclovir therapy. However, despite the very small number of patients, this trial showed a significant improvement in PFS for patients receiv-ing alemtuzumab consolidation with no patient progressing compared to a median PFS of 24.7 months in the 'watch and wait' arm. This study demonstrated that alemtuzumab con-solidation is likely to have a major impact on the treatment of CLL if a better-tolerated regime can be developed. The features of the regimen that probably contributed to the tox-icity in this study were the dose of alemtuzumab used, the route of administration and the interval from completion of induction chemotherapy to starting consolidation.

Three other non-randomised series of patients treated with consolidation alem-tuzumab have been reported. O'Brien [27, 28] from the MD Anderson Cancer Center pre-sented data on 58 patients who received alemtuzumab consolidation at a median of 6 months (range: 1–40) from a fludarabine-containing induction therapy. The first 24 patients received 10 mg of intravenous alemtuzumab three times a week for 4 weeks fol-lowed by an interval for assessment and were then scheduled to receive a further 4 weeks at 30 mg three times a week. However, relatively few patients received the second block of alemtuzumab, and therefore the protocol was modified so that the remaining 34 patients received 30 mg three times a week. In this series of patients, 26 (53%) of the 58 patients had an improvement in remission status with alemtuzumab, although the impact on PFS could not be assessed.

Rai and colleagues [29] reported 80 patients who received alemtuzumab consolidation therapy 2 months after an abbreviated course of induction therapy with fludarabine (patients received 4 rather than the conventional 6 cycles of fludarabine). This was not a randomised trial but the first cohort of 56 patients received 30 mg alemtuzumab three times a week intravenously, whereas the remaining 24 patients had the same dose given subcutaneously. Unfortunately, the response rate to initial fludarabine was markedly dif-ferent between the two cohorts of patients, making a comparison impossible. The majority of patients improved their remission status; however, one patient died from CMV pneu-monitis (subsequent patients were screened for CMV reactivation and of the 10 who had CMV reactivation all were managed successfully). Once again, there was a significant improvement in response rate with alemtuzumab (ORR from 56 to 92% for the intravenous cohort and from 36 to 66% for the subcutaneous cohort). The effect on PFS could not be assessed.

Montillo and co-workers [30, 31] have reported 30 patients who have been treated a median of 5 months following fludarabine-based therapy with a smaller dose (10 mg three times a week) of alemtuzumab given subcutaneously. This dose, route and interval from flu-darabine were well tolerated with 16 (53%) of the 30 patients improving their remission sta-tus. Only low-sensitivity MRD assessment (consensus primer PCR) has been reported and 16 (53%) of the 30 patients converted from a clonal B-cell population to a normal polyclonal pattern. Fifteen of the 30 patients had CMV reactivation by CMV PCR, all were treated with oral ganciclovir and the CMV reactivation resolved with no patient developing sympto-matic CMV disease. Although this is a safe regimen, it might be anticipated that a higher dose would have a greater effect.

Therefore, it appears that consolidation with alemtuzumab after response to conven-tional therapy offers the possibility of deepening remissions, and therefore eradicating detectable MRD from a proportion of patients with a high probability of improved PFS. There is, however, some risk and expense to this approach, and it is therefore likely that this approach should be reserved for patients with poor-risk CLL, such as those with unmutated CLL. The optimal regime for alemtuzumab as a consolidation has not been established, but it is likely that the interval between completion of chemotherapy and alemtuzumab is criti-cal and should probably be in the region of 6 months. In addition, the route of alemtuzumab is not defined but the subcutaneous route has a lot of attractions. Finally, the dose has not been formally established.

ALEMTUZUMAB AS INITIAL THERAPY FOR CLL

It appears that alemtuzumab is the most efficacious single agent in CLL but that there are concerns about its toxicity in use. However, it is also clear that the greatest concern is when alemtuzumab (or any other drug) is used in refractory CLL, at which time the risk of opportunistic infections is high. A logical move would be to consider the use of alem-tuzumab as the initial therapy for poor-risk CLL.

In 1996 Osterborg and colleagues [32] reported the use of alemtuzumab as front-line ther-apy in 9 patients with CLL. The patients received 30 mg three times a week with 4 having subcutaneous and 5 intravenous therapy for up to 18 weeks. Three patients achieved a CR and a further 5 a partial remission giving an ORR of 89%. Apart from a single patient who developed CMV pneumonitis, the side-effects observed were mild. Building upon this expe-rience, the same group reported a further 41 patients with CLL who were treated with sub-cutaneous alemtuzumab as first-line therapy at a dose of 30 mg three times a week for a total of 18 weeks [33]. The ORR on an intent-to-treat basis was 81%. Three patients were removed from the study in the first week of treatment because of local pain at the injection site, fever and fatigue. Thirty-eight patients received at least 4 weeks of therapy and of these, 19% achieved a CR and 68% a partial remission. The median time to treatment failure had not been reached at the time of publication (18+ months; range, 8–44+ months). Transient injection site skin reactions were seen in 90% of patients and transient grade 4 neutropaenia developed in 21% of the patients. Other side-effects, including infections, were rare except that 10% of patients developed CMV reactivation. These patients rapidly responded to intravenous ganciclovir [33]. Therefore, alemtuzumab is an active therapy in previously untreated patients with CLL and appears to have an improved toxicity com-pared with its use in relapsed and refractory disease. Recently, an international randomised controlled trial comparing chlorambucil with intravenous alemtuzumab (CAM307) as front-line therapy for CLL has completed recruitment. In this trial a total of 297 untreated patients were randomised between chlorambucil and alemtuzumab with the preliminary safety results being presented in abstract form in 2004 [34]. Adverse events occurring in over 10% of alemtuzumab patients included pyrexia, rigors, dermatitis, urticaria, headache, hyper-tension, hypotension ('infusion reactions'), CMV antigen reactivation, nausea and neu-tropaenia. In chlorambucil patients, adverse events occurring in over 10% of patients included nausea and vomiting. A total of 7 deaths were reported, 2 in the alemtuzumab arm and 5 in the chlorambucil arm. Preliminary analysis indicated that 22 of 149 (15%) patients treated with alemtuzumab developed symptomatic CMV reactivation. In 14 of 22 (64%) cases, mild to moderate fever was the only clinical symptom. All symptomatic CMV reactivations resolved promptly with ganciclovir and most patients were able to complete alemtuzumab therapy as planned. No symptomatic CMV reactivations were reported in the chlorambucil arm. Thus the toxicity profile of alemtuzumab in previously untreated patients appears to be acceptable with no increased treatment-related mortality compared with chlorambucil in this randomised trial. The efficacy results from this trial are eagerly awaited. ([34]; ASH 2004, CAM307)

SUMMARY

There have been massive strides in our understanding of the biology of CLL as well as a rapid expansion of the treatment options for the disease. The wide range of therapies with increased efficacy promises to completely alter the approach to therapy for patients with CLL. The robustness of the new biological prognostic markers in CLL will allow a change in the indications for the initiation of therapy from purely clinical to biologically-based criteria. For example, it is very likely in the future that when a patient presents with early stage CLL, he or she will have their biological parameters studied and the 'good risk' patients will be reassured and seen infrequently in the clinic, whereas the 'poor risk' patients will be offered intensive, probably targeted therapy, with the intent of eradicating detectable CLL. In addition, certain categories of patients, such as those with p53 pathway abnormalities, are highly likely to be identified at diagnosis and then to receive specific therapy targeted at their genetic abnormality.

An important part of this revolution in the management of CLL will be played by therapeutic monoclonal antibodies. It appears very likely that the most effective 'induction' therapy for poor-risk CLL will be combination therapy, including a purine analogue and monoclonal antibody, such as FCR. It is likely that consolidation therapy with alemtuzumab will then be used to eradicate MRD after completion of induction therapy, although the most appropriate regimen, including dose, dosing frequency, route of administration and interval after induction therapy, has yet to be established.

The future of the management of patients with CLL will involve the selection of patients at diagnosis for appropriate therapy, whether that is dose intensifying in poor-risk disease or minimising therapy, and therefore complications, in good-risk patients. In selected patients, the aim of therapy for CLL will undoubtedly move in the foreseeable future towards 'curative intent'.

REFERENCES

1. Rai *et al.* Fludarabine compared with chlorambucil as primary therapy for chronic lymphocytic leukemia. *N Engl J Med* 2000; 343:1750–1757.
2. Cheson *et al.* *J Clin Oncol* 1996; 87:4990–4997.
3. Rawstron *et al.* Quantitation of minimal disease levels in chronic lymphocytic leukemia using a sensitive flow cytometric assay improves the prediction of outcome and can be used to optimize therapy. *Blood* 2001; 98:29–35.
4. Damle *at al.* Ig V gene mutation status and CD38 expression as novel prognostic indicators in chronic lymphocytic leukemia. *Blood* 1999; 94:1840–1847.
5. Hamblin *et al.* Unmutated Ig V(H) genes are associated with a more aggressive form of chronic lymphocytic leukemia. *Blood* 1999; 94:1848–1854.
6. Dohner *et al.* Genomic aberrations and survival in chronic lymphocytic leukemia. *N Engl J Med* 2000; 343:1910–1916.
7. Pettitt *et al.* Mechanism of action of purine analogues in chronic lymphocytic leukaemia. *Br J Haematol* 2003; 121:692–701.

8.   Pettitt *et al*. p53 dysfunction in B-cell chronic lymphocytic leukemia: inactivation of ATM as an alternative to TP53 mutation. *Blood* 2001; 98:814–822.
9.   Keating MJ *et al*. Results of first salvage therapy for patients refractory to a fludarabine regimen in chronic lymphocytic leukemia. *Leuk Lymphoma* 2002; 43:1755–1762.
10. Molteni *et al*. European Hematology Association; 2003. Abstract 619.
11. Perkins SJ *et al*. Frequency and type of serious infections in fludarabine-refractory B-cell chronic lymphocytic leukemia and small lymphocytic lymphoma: implications for clinical trials in this patient population. *Cancer* 2002; 94:2033–2099.
12. Keating M *et al*. Therapeutic role of alemtuzumab (Campath-1H) in patients who have failed fludarabine: results of a large international study. *Blood* 2002; 99:3554–3561.
13. Keating *et al*. Long-Term Follow-Up of Patients With Chronic Lymphocytic Leukemia (CLL) Receiving Fludarabine Regimens as Initial Therapy. *Blood* 1998; 92:1165–1171.
14. Bosch F *et al*. Fludarabine, cyclophosphamide and mitoxantrone in the treatment of resistant or relapsed chronic lymphocytic leukaemia. *Br J Haematol* 2002; 119:976–984.
15. Dreger *et al*. The prognostic impact of autologous stem cell transplantation in patients with chronic lymphocytic leukemia: a risk-matched analysis based on the V_H gene mutational status. *Blood* 2004; 103:2850–2858.
16. Milligan *et al*. Results of the MRC pilot study show autografting for younger patients with chronic lymphocytic leukemia is safe and achieves a high percentage of molecular responses. *Blood* 2005; 105:397–404.
17. Moreno *et al*. *J Clin Oncol* 2005; 23:in press.
18. Keating MJ *et al*. *J Clin Oncol*; in press (20/6/05).
19. Wierda W *et al*. *J Clin Oncol;* in press (20/6/05).
20. Moreton *et al*. *J Clin Oncol;* in press (1/5/05).
21. Dohner *et al*. p53 gene deletion predicts for poor survival and non-response to therapy with purine analogs in chronic B-cell leukemias. *Blood* 1995; 85:1580–1589.
22. Austen *et al*. *Blood,* 2004; 104(suppl 1). Abstract 774.
23. Thornton *et al*. High dose methyl prednisolone in refractory chronic lymphocytic leukaemia. *Leuk Lymphoma* 1999; 34:167–170.
24. Ritgen *et al*. Unmutated immunoglobulin variable heavy-chain gene status remains an adverse prognostic factor after autologous stem cell transplantation for chronic lymphocytic leukemia. *Blood* 2003; 101:2049–2053.
25. Hale *et al*. Blood concentrations of alemtuzumab and antiglobulin responses in patients with chronic lymphocytic leukemia following intravenous or subcutaneous routes of administration. *Blood* 2004; 104:948–955**.**
26. Wendtner *et al*. Consolidation with alemtuzumab in patients with chronic lymphocytic leukemia (CLL) in first remission—experience on safety and efficacy within a randomized multicenter phase III trial of the German CLL Study Group (GCLLSG). *Leukemia* 2004; 18:1093–1101.
27. O'Brien SM *et al*. Alemtuzumab as treatment for residual disease after chemotherapy in patients with chronic lymphocytic leukemia. *Cancer* 2003 Dec 15; 98:2657–63.
28. O'Brien S *et al*. *Blood* 2003; 102(suppl 1):371a.
29. Rai K *et al*. *Blood* 2003; 102(suppl 1):2506a.
30. Montillo *et al*. Safety and efficacy of subcutaneous Campath-1H for treating residual disease in patients with chronic lymphocytic leukemia responding to fludarabine. *Haematologica* 2002; 87:695–700.
31. Montillo M *et al*. European Hematology Association; 2004. Abstract 594.
32. Osterborg A *et al*. Humanized CD52 monoclonal antibody Campath-1H as first-line treatment in chronic lymphocytic leukaemia. *Br J Haematol* 1996; 93:151–153.
33. Lundin J *et al*. Phase II trial of subcutaneous anti-CD52 monoclonal antibody alemtuzumab (Campath-1H) as first-line treatment for patients with B-cell chronic lymphocytic leukemia (B-CLL). *Blood* 2002; 100:768–73.
34. Hillmen *et al*. *Blood* 2004; 104(suppl 1):2505a.

16

Alemtuzumab in combination with other therapies in B-cell lymphoproliferative disorders

K. W. L. Yee, S. M. O'Brien

INTRODUCTION

Alemtuzumab (Campath-1H) is a humanised unconjugated monoclonal antibody directed against the CD52 antigen, which is located on lymphocytes at various stages of differentiation, monocytes, macrophages and eosinophils [1–3]. Hematopoietic stem cells, erythrocytes and platelets do not express CD52. The highest levels are expressed on cells from T-cell prolymphocytic leukaemia (T-PLL), followed by B-CLL, with the lower levels on normal` B cells [4]. High expression of CD52 is also present on cells from most B-cell lymphomas, including high-grade non-Hodgkin's lymphoma (NHL) and mantle cell lymphoma (MCL) [3, 5], hairy cell leukaemia [6] and Waldenstrom's macroglobulinaemia [7–10]. In contrast, lower or no expression is seen in multiple myeloma and plasma cell dyscrasias [10–14], and acute lymphoblastic leukaemia (ALL) [15–17]. Postulated mechanisms of action of alemtuzumab include complement-dependent cytolysis, antibody-dependent cellular cytotoxicity (ADCC) and direct induction of apoptosis [18–21].

CHRONIC LYMPHOCYTIC LEUKAEMIA (CLL)

Alemtuzumab has appreciable activity in fludarabine (F)-refractory CLL, including in those patients with p53 mutations and/or deletions [22–31]. However, responses were less likely to be observed in patients with advanced disease (Rai stage IV), significant adenopathy or poor performance status [23–25]. Therefore, in patients with advanced disease and/or significant adenopathy alemtuzumab may have greater efficacy when administered in combination with other cytoreductive agents or as consolidation therapy, in an attempt to eradicate residual disease.

PREVIOUSLY TREATED PATIENTS

Alemtuzumab-containing induction regimens
Exposure of primary CLL cells to alemtuzumab in combination with rituximab or purine analogues (such as F and cladribine) resulted in a significantly higher degree of apoptosis

Karen W. L. Yee, MD, Fellow, Department of Leukemia, University of Texas M.D. Anderson Cancer Center, Houston, Texas, USA.

Susan M. O'Brien, MD, Professor, Department of Leukemia, University of Texas M.D. Anderson Cancer Center, Houston, Texas, USA.

than produced by either agent given alone [21]. This improved efficacy may be due to up-regulation of pro-apoptotic Bax expression or down-regulation of the anti-apoptotic proteins FLIP and bcl-2. Therefore, in an attempt to improve upon response rates and to prevent the development of resistance, alemtuzumab has been combined with purine analogues and/or monoclonal antibodies.

Fludarabine and alemtuzumab (FCam)

The combination of alemtuzumab (30 mg three times a week continuous; 12 doses every 4 weeks) with F (FCam) has shown to be efficacious in patients with refractory CLL [32] (Table 16.1). All 6 patients treated with this combination were refractory to single-agent alemtuzumab and 5 of 6 patients were refractory to single-agent F. The overall response (OR) rate was 83% (complete response (CR) 16%; partial response (PR) 67%) with 2 of 5 patients having no detectable marrow disease by high-sensitivity flow cytometry (MRD Flow). Two patients underwent stem cell harvest followed by autologous stem cell transplantation. Toxicity was acceptable with 1 patient requiring hospitalisation for pneumonia during neutropaenia and 2 patients requiring granulocyte colony-stimulating factor (G-CSF) for neutropaenia. There were no cases of cytomegalovirus (CMV) reactivation.

An alternative schedule for the combination of F and alemtuzumab, where patients received fewer doses of alemtuzumab each month, has been investigated in the treatment of patients with relapsed CLL [33, 34] (Table 16.1). Thirty-four patients were evaluable for response. Treatment consisted of F 30 mg/m^2 IV days 1–3 followed by alemtuzumab 30 mg IV days 1–3 of each 28-day cycle for 6 cycles. Median age was 61 years (range, 38–80), and 76% of patients had Binet stage C disease. The median number of prior therapies was 2 (range, 1–8) and included prior F, rituximab and alemtuzumab. CMV reactivation occurred in 2 patients: one of whom died from *E. coli* sepsis. Two patients with refractory disease developed fungal pneumonia. The OR rate was 85% (CR 29%; PR 56%) with 15 of 34 patients (44%) having no detectable disease in the peripheral blood as determined by flow cytometry. Of note, 7 patients with active autoimmune haemolytic anaemia and/or autoimmune thrombocytopaenia at study entry were successfully treated with FCam. A phase III multicentre randomised study evaluating FCam compared to F alone as second-line therapy in patients with relapsed or refractory CLL is ongoing.

Rituximab and alemtuzumab (RCam)

The efficacy and safety of alemtuzumab combined with rituximab (RCam) has been assessed in patients with relapsed or refractory CLL [35–37]. The rationale for the combination was based on the following: (1) CD20 and CD52 antigens are co-expressed on the leukaemic cells, and (2) efficacy of single-agent alemtuzumab is limited in patients with significant organomegaly and lymphadenopathy. Three studies were conducted using different dosing schedules of RCam [35–37]; one study used higher weekly doses of rituximab (i.e. 375 mg IV on week 1, then 500 mg IV on weeks 2–4) and continuous infusion of alemtuzumab for 6 consecutive days followed by subcutaneous alemtuzumab twice a week [37] and a second study administered standard-dose alemtuzumab intravenously only twice a week [36] (Table 16.1). Lower response rates (OR 9%; CR 0% with 1 PR lasting 10 weeks) were observed in the study by Nabhan and colleagues [35] study than in the two other RCam studies (OR 63–67%; CR 6–44%) [36, 37] and with single-agent alemtuzumab therapy (OR 31–52%; CR 0–26%) [22–26, 29–31]. This difference may be due to the lower doses of alemtuzumab administered to 6 of 12 patients and only a 4-week course of therapy being administered [35]. No study reported overall survival (OS). In general, a higher frequency and severity of adverse events were seen with alemtuzumab than rituximab. Most non-haematological toxicities were infusion-related (<Grade 2) [35–37]. Bacterial infections occurred in 17–44% of patients and fevers of unknown origin in 13% [36, 37]. CMV

Table 16.1 Alemtuzumab-containing induction regimens in previously treated CLL patients

Regimen	Patient characteristics				Median	Response			Reference
	Median age (range, y)	N (evaluable)	Rai/Binet stage (%)	Prior F (%)	F/U (months)	Response rate (%)	Disease control (median, months)	Overall survival (median, months)	
Fludarabine and alemtuzumab (FCam)									
F 25 mg/m² IV D1–3 + **Cam** 3 mg escalating to 30 mg IV, then 30 mg IV tiw q28d	52 (40–71)	6	B 50; C 50	83	12	OR 83 CR 16; PR 67	NR	NR	[32]
F 30 mg/m² IV D1–3 followed by **Cam** 3 mg escalating to 30 mg IV, then 30 mg IV D1–3 q28d × 6	61 (38–80)	37 (34)	C 76	NR	NR	OR 85 CR 29; PR 56	NR	NR	[33, 34]
Rituximab and alemtuzumab (RCam)									
R 375 mg/m² IV week 1, 3, 4 and 5 + **Cam** 3, 10, or 30 mg IV tiw week 2–5	69.5 (53–73)	12 (11)	IV 75	92	NR	OR 9 CR 0; PR 9	2.5	NR	[35]
R 375 mg/m² IV × 4 weeks (1st dose divided into 100 mg/m² IV D1 and 275 mg/m² IV D2 for WBC >50000/μl) + **Cam** 3 mg escalating to 30 mg IV D1–3 week 1, then 30 mg IV D3 and 5 weeks 2–4; repeat q28d × 1	62 (44–79)[a]	48[a]	III–IV 79	54+[a]	6.5	OR 63[b] CR 6; NPR 7; PR 50[b]	TTP 6 months[a]	11 months[a]	[36]
R 375 mg/m² IV D1, then 500 mg/m² IV D8, 15 and 22 + **Cam** 15 mg ci D2–7 week 1, then 30 mg sc D3 and 5 weeks 2–4 q28d × 3 (**Cam** given by sc, only cycles 2 and 3)	57 (42–78)[c]	14 (9)[c]	III–IV 44[c]	44+	NR	OR 67[c] CR 44; PR 23	NR	NR	[37]

Table 16.1 Continued

Regimen	Patient characteristics				Median F/U (months)	Response			Reference
	Median age (range, y)	N (evaluable)	Rai/Binet stage (%)	Prior F (%)		Response rate (%)	Disease control (median, months)	Overall survival (median, months)	
Fludarabine, cytarabine, mitoxantrone, dexamethasone and alemtuzumab (FAND/Cam)									
FAND (i.e. **F** 25 mg/m² IV at 0, 24 and 48 h, **Ara-C** 700 mg/m² IV at 4, 28 and 52 h, **mito** 10 mg/m² IV at 6 h and **dexa** 20 mg IV D1–3) × 2, *then* **FAND/Cam** (with **Cam** 30 mg IV × 3 doses) × 2, *then observed 1 month followed by* **Cam** 30 mg IV tiw × 4weeks for residual disease	50	7 (4)	NR	100	NR	OR 100 CR 75; PR 25	NR	NR	[39]
Cyclophosphamide, fludarabine, alemtuzumab and rituximab (CFAR)									
C 250mg/m2 IV D3–5, **F** 25mg/m² IV D3–5, **Cam** 30mg IV D1, 3 and 5 and **R** 375 or 500mg/m2 IV D2 q28d 3 × 6 cycles	58 (46–79)	38 (31)	II/IV 61	100	9	OR 55 CR 23; PR 35	TTP not reached	14	[42]

a includes CLL (n = 32), CLL/PLL (n = 9), PLL (n = 1), MCL (n = 4), and RS (n = 2) patients; b for CLL patients only; c includes CLL (n = 12) and CLL/SLL (n = 2) patients. A = Cytarabine; C = cyclophosphamide; Cam = alemtuzumab; ci = continuous infusion; dexa = dexamethasone; F = fludarabine; mito = mitoxantrone; R = rituximab; TTP = time to progression; OR = overall response; CR = complete response; PR = partial response; NPR = nodular PR; NR = not reported reactivation occurred in up to 27% of patients [36, 37]. Myelosuppression was seen in up to two thirds of patients (usually ≤Grade 2) [36]. Therefore, therapy with RCam is feasible; no unexpected toxicities were seen when the two monoclonal antibodies were combined in patients with advanced stage disease.

Fludarabine, cytarabine, mitoxantrone, dexamethasone and alemtuzumab (FAND/Cam)
Treatment of relapsed or refractory patients with CLL with F, cytarabine, mitoxantrone and dexamethasone (FAND) chemotherapy yielded OR rates of 68% (CR 58%) [38]. Alemtuzumab was added to the FAND regimen in an effort to improve efficacy [39] (Table 16.1). Seven patients with previously treated, advanced CLL were treated with 2 courses of FAND (i.e. F 25 mg/m^2 IV at 0, 24 and 48 h, cytarabine 700 mg/m^2 IV at 4, 28 and 52 h, mitoxantrone 10 mg/m^2 IV at 6 h and dexamethasone 20 mg IV days 1–3) followed sequentially by 2 courses of FAND/alemtuzumab (i.e. FAND followed by 3 administrations of alemtuzumab 30 mg IV) and 4 weeks of standard-dose schedule alemtuzumab post-induction for patients with evidence of residual disease. Median age was 50 years; median number of prior treatments was 3 (range, 2–5). All 4 evaluable patients responded (CR 75%; PR 25%), with no residual disease detected by immunophenotyping in 3 patients; one of whom achieved a molecular remission. Toxicities included grade 3 or 4 neutropaenia and thrombocytopaenia, CMV reactivation, and bacterial pneumonia.

Fludarabine, cyclophosphamide, alemtuzumab and rituximab (CFAR)
Similarly, in an attempt to improve upon results obtained with chemoimmunotherapy combining F with cyclophosphamide and rituximab (FCR) in previously treated patients (OR 72%; CR 28%; nodular PR (NPR) 14%; PR 30%) [40, 41], MD Anderson investigators have added alemtuzumab to the FCR regimen (CFAR) [42, personal communication] (Table 16.1). The CFAR regimen consists of alemtuzumab 30 mg IV days 1, 3 and 5, rituximab 375 or 500 mg/m^2 IV day 2, cyclophosphamide 250 mg/m^2 IV and F 25 mg/m^2 IV days 3–5 of each 28-day cycle for 6 cycles. Thirty-one patients with relapsed/refractory CLL were evaluable for response. Median age was 58 years (range, 46–79) and median number of prior treatments was 4 (range, 1–9). Fifty-five percent and 42% of patients were refractory to alkylating agents and F, respectively. Ten percent had undergone prior autologous or allogeneic stem cell transplant. Grade 3 or 4 haematological toxicities included neutropaenia (23 and 74% of >70 evaluable courses, respectively) and thrombocytopaenia (26 and 32% of >70 evaluable courses, respectively). Grade 3 or 4 non-haematological toxicities included nausea and/or vomiting, fever and/or chills, fatigue, mucositis, constipation, arthralgia, pneumonia and dyspnoea. CMV reactivation occurred in 5 patients; all responded to therapy. There was 1 death within the first 3 cycles of therapy. Late complications included the development of acute myelogenous leukaemia and myelodysplasia in one patient each; the first patient had been heavily pre-treated with alkylating-agent-based chemotherapies and the second had undergone an autologous stem cell transplant and had complex cytogenetics, including deletions 5 and 7, prior to CFAR therapy. Myelosuppression (n = 10) and disease progression (n = 6) were the most common reasons for early discontinuation of therapy. The OR rate was 55% (CR 23%; PR 35%). Six of 7 patients achieving a CR and 9 of 11 patients achieving a PR (i.e. no disease but persistent thrombocytopaenia and anaemia) had no detectable disease by flow cytometry. The median time to progression (TTP) has not been reached after a median follow-up of 9 months. The median OS was 14 months and 18 of 31 patients were alive at the time of reporting. Although the response rates were lower and the incidence of myelosuppression was higher in patients receiving CFAR than in those receiving FCR chemoimmunotherapy, patients treated with CFAR had received more prior therapies compared to patients treated with FCR [41]. Therefore, CFAR has significant activity in this heavily pre-treated group of

patients. The incidence of neutropaenia may be reduced with the administration of growth factors. The study is ongoing.

Single-agent alemtuzumab consolidation therapy

Consolidation with single-agent alemtuzumab has been able to improve responses obtained with F in patients with CLL [43–46] (Table 16.2). Thirty-five patients (at least 3 of whom have been previously treated) who achieved a PR or better after F therapy (10 CR, 11 NPR and 14 PR) received alemtuzumab 10 mg subcutaneously tiw for 6 weeks [43, 44]. Alemtuzumab was administered a median of 5 months (range, 2–11) after F therapy. Alemtuzumab was able to convert 9 patients starting in NPR to CR (with 5 achieving a molecular CR), 12 in PR to either a NPR (2) or CR (10) (with 6 achieving a molecular CR) and 7 in CR to a molecular CR. No serious bacterial infections were reported. Although there were no cases of CMV disease, oral ganciclovir was used to treat CMV reactivation in 15 (57%) patients.

The efficacy of alemtuzumab for the treatment of minimal residual disease after chemotherapy has been further evaluated in 58 patients with CLL [45, 46] (Table 16.2). Patients achieving a PR (n = 32), NPR (n = 19) or CR with evidence of disease by immunophenotyping (n = 7) after any type of chemotherapy were eligible. Patients had received a median of 2 regimens (range, 1–7). Alemtuzumab was administered a median of 6 months (range, 1–40) after the last chemotherapy at a dose of 10 mg IV tiw for 4 weeks for the initial 24 patients. In an attempt to improve responses, the subsequent 34 patients received alemtuzumab at a dose of 30 mg IV tiw for 4 weeks. Patients who had received alemtuzumab at a dose of 10 mg, and had residual disease after a 4-week observation period, could be re-treated with alemtuzumab for another 4 weeks at a dose of 30 mg IV tiw. Forty-nine patients were evaluable. The OR rate was 53% (OR 39% at the 10 mg dose vs. 65% at the 30 mg dose; p = 0.066). Forty-seven percent of patients starting in NPR achieved CR and 46% starting in PR achieved NPR or CR. Residual bone marrow disease cleared in most patients with 11 of 29 patients (38%) achieving a molecular remission. The major reason for failure to improve response was the presence of adenopathy. Median TTP has not been reached in responders after a median follow-up of 24 months. Subgroup analysis indicated a trend for a longer TTP in patients with no detectable disease by molecular analysis after a median follow-up of 18 months. Grade 1 to 2 infusion-related events were commonly observed. Infections occurred in 15 patients (3 bacterial and 12 CMV reactivation). Two patients had fever of unknown origin. There was 1 death from pneumonia and 3 patients developed EBV-positive large cell lymphoma (all resolved: 2 spontaneously and 1 after treatment with cidofovir and immunoglobulin). It is unclear whether immunosuppression related to alemtuzumab therapy (which depletes both T- and B cells) and/or preceding therapy with other therapeutic agents, such as purine analogues, may have resulted in the proliferation of EBV-positive cells [47–51]; the large cell lymphoma resolved spontaneously in 2 patients with further time elapsing after treatment with alemtuzumab.

A smaller study evaluated the role of alemtuzumab consolidation after F and cyclophosphamide (FC) chemotherapy as second-line therapy in patients with CLL [52] (Table 16.2). Nine patients with advanced, progressive CLL who had received only one prior treatment were enrolled onto the study. Treatment consisted of 4 cycles of FC chemotherapy administered every 4 weeks followed by alemtuzumab. Alemtuzumab was given 2 months after FC chemotherapy at standard dose schedule to a maximum response (planned duration of 4–8 weeks). Median age was 60 years (range, 50–65); 67% of patients had received prior alkylating agents and 33% prior F. Five patients completed the treatment and were evaluable for response. CMV reactivation was noted in 4 of 5 patients. Infusion-related symptoms were mild, and no other major toxicities or infections were reported. After FC chemotherapy, OR rate was 80% (CR 20%; PR 60%; Stable disease (SD) 20%). With the addition of alemtuzumab, improvement in responses was observed in all 5 patients (CR 80%; PR 20%). After FC chemotherapy, minimal residual disease as

Table 16.2 Single-agent alemtuzumab consolidation in CLL patients

Regimen	Patient characteristics				Median	Response			Reference
	Median age (range, y)	N (evaluable)	Rai/Binet stage (%)	Prior F (%)	F/U (months)	Response rate (%)	Disease control (median, months)	Overall survival (median, months)	
No Prior Therapy									
F 25 mg/m² IV D1–5 q28d × 4 followed by observation × 2 months, then responders (≥SD), **Cam** 3 mg escalating to 30 mg IV then 30 mg IV tiw × 6 weeks	NR	57 (56)	NR	0	10	OR 92 CR 42; PR 50	NR	OS 10 months 87%	[65]
F 25 mg/m² IV D1–5 q28d × 4 followed by observation × 2 months, then responders (≥SD), **Cam** 3 mg escalating to 30 mg sc then 30 mg sc tiw × 6 weeks	60 (41–74)	28	NR	0	NR	OR 66 CR 22; PR 44	NR	NR	[66]
F 25 mg/m² IV D1–5 q28d × 6 or F 30 mg/m² IV D1–3 + C 250 mg/m² IV D1–3 q28d × 6 (**FC**) followed by randomisation to either observation only or **Cam** 3 mg escalating to 30 mg IV then 30 mg IV tiw × 12 weeks[a]	60 (37–66)	23 (21)	III–IV 14	0	21.4	OR 70 vs. 100 CR 20 vs. 27	PFS no progression vs. 24.7[b]	No difference	[68]
Prior therapy									
F (schedule NS), then responders (≥PR), **Cam** 10 mg sc tiw × 6 weeks	55 (41–62)	12	NR	NR	NR	OR 75 CR 75	NR	NR	[44]

Table 16.2 Continued

Regimen	Patient characteristics				Median F/U (months)	Response			Reference
	Median age (range, y)	N (evaluable)	Rai/Binet stage (%)	Prior F (%)		Response rate (%)	Disease control (median, months)	Overall survival (median, months)	
Chemotherapy NS, *then* responders (≥PR), **Cam** 10 or 30 mg IV tiw × 4–8 weeks	60 (44–79)	58 (49)	NR	41+	24	OR 53 CR 47; NPR/CR 46	TTP not reached	NR	[45, 46]
F 25 mg/m² IV D1–3 + **C** 250 mg/m² IV D1–3 q28d × 4 (**FC**) *followed by* observation × 2 months, *then* **Cam** 30 mg IV tiw × 4–8 weeks	60 (50–65)	9 (5)	B 78; C 11	33	NR	OR 100 CR 80; PR 20	NR	NR	[52]

aRandomised trial terminated early due to increased grade 3–4 infectious toxicities in alemtuzumab arm; b p = 0.036.
C = Cyclophosphamide; Cam = alemtuzumab; F = fludarabine; NPR = nodular PR; NR = not reported; NS = not specified; OR = overall response; OS = overall survival; CR = complete response; PR = partial response; SD = stable disease.

determined by flow cytometry was detectable in 4 of 5 of patients compared with 0 of 2 patients assessed after alemtuzumab.

PREVIOUSLY UNTREATED PATIENTS

Single-agent alemtuzumab consolidation therapy
Similarly, alemtuzumab has been administered to F-responsive patients in an attempt to improve the quality of responses obtained with single-agent F (OR 63–89%; CR 9–40%) [53–58] and F-based regimens (OR 80–100%; CR 21–80%) [57, 59–64] in previously untreated patients. Preliminary results of two phase II trials evaluating alemtuzumab consolidation therapy following F in previously untreated CLL patients have been reported [65, 66] (Table 16.2). Standard dose/schedule F was administered for 4 months. After a 2-month observation period to allow for haematological recovery and assessment of response, patients achieving SD or better (i.e. CR and PR) received standard-dose/schedule alemtuzumab intravenously [65] or subcutaneously [66] for 6 weeks. The subcutaneous route was used in an attempt to decrease the infusional toxicities observed with intravenous alemtuzumab [24, 29, 67]. Response rates after F were lower than what has been reported (OR 36–56% with CR 4%), possibly because only 4 courses of F were administered [53–58, 65, 66] All 36 and 18 of 24 eligible patients received alemtuzumab, respectively. Grade 3 or 4 toxicities included infections in 12 (33%) patients receiving intravenous alemtuzumab. CMV reactivation and/or disease occurred in 22% (with 1 fatality and 1 persistent disease despite therapy) and 17% of patients receiving intravenous or subcutaneous alemtuzumab, respecti-vely. No grade ≥ 2 injection site reactions were observed in patients receiving subcutaneous alem-tuzumab. A significant proportion of patients with SD or PR after F had an improvement in their remission status following alemtuzumab consolidation to PRs and/or CRs (OR 66–92%; CR 22–42%). There is insufficient data to determine whether higher response rates are achieved after intravenous compared with subcutaneous administration of alem-tuzumab as lower response rates were observed with F treatment in the patients who received alemtuzumab subcutaneously than those who received intravenous alemtuzumab.

The German CLL Study Group (GCLLSG) assessed the safety and efficacy of alem-tuzumab consolidation in patients with CLL in first remission (i.e. $\geq$PR) [68] (Table 16.2). Twenty-three patients responding to first-line therapy with either F alone or FC were ran-domised to either standard dose alemtuzumab for 12 weeks or observation only 2 months after completion of chemotherapy. Patients were balanced with respect to age, disease stage, response to F or FC, IgV$_H$ mutational status and cytogenetic abnormalities. Of the 21 evaluable patients, 11 were randomised to the alemtuzumab arm before the study was stopped due to grade 3–4 infections occurring in 7 (64%) patients (i.e. 1 pulmonary aspergillosis, 4 CMV reactivations requiring treatment, 1 pulmonary tuberculosis and 1 herpes zoster) and grade 4 haematological toxicities in the alemtuzumab arm (36%), occurring at a median of 4 weeks. Only 2 of 11 patients completed all 12 weeks of therapy with alemtuzumab. Six months after randomisation, 2 patients (in PR after F or FC ther-apy) in the alemtuzumab arm converted to a CR, while 3 patients in the observation arm progressed. Five of six patients in the alemtuzumab arm achieved a molecular remission in the peripheral blood compared to 0 of 3 patients in the observation arm (p = 0.048). After a median follow-up of 21.4 months, all patients were alive. However, progression-free survival (PFS) was superior in the alemtuzumab arm compared to the observation arm (i.e. no progression vs. 24.7 months, respectively, p = 0.036). The increased incidence of non-CMV infections observed in the GCLLSG [68] and the Cancer and Leukemia Group B (CALGB) [65] studies compared with the Italian [43, 44] and MD Anderson [45, 46] stud-ies (i.e. 27 and 33% vs. <10%, respectively) may be due to the shorter interval between chemotherapy and alemtuzumab administration (i.e. 2 months compared to 5–6 months, respectively).

A phase II study evaluating induction therapy with F and rituximab followed by consolidation with alemtuzumab therapy in previously untreated patients with CLL is currently enrolling patients. At this time, the results of alemtuzumab consolidation are promising, but an optimal regimen remains to be determined. The optimal induction therapy prior to administration of consolidation therapy with alemtuzumab, the route of administration (intravenous vs. subcutaneous), as well as the dose and scheduling of alemtuzumab is unclear.

PROLYMPHOCYTIC LEUKAEMIA (PLL)

Data on the use of alemtuzumab in patients with PLL is limited. Of 9 previously treated patients with B-cell PLL who received alemtuzumab, responses were seen in 6, including 3 PRs and 3 CRs [24, 69, 70]. One relapsed/refractory patient with PLL received therapy with RCam and achieved a CR [36].

B-CELL NON-HODGKIN'S LYMPHOMA

Single-agent alemtuzumab has little activity in previously treated patients with advanced indolent and high-grade B-cell lymphomas (OR 0–43%; CR 0–28%) [24, 71–75]. As in CLL, activity appeared greater in the blood and bone marrow than in nodal disease, suggesting that alemtuzumab may be more effective in patients with NHL with disease predominantly in the bone marrow or minimal disease. However, the results of trials of single-agent alemtuzumab in previously treated patients with non-bulky or minimal residual NHL were disappointing (OR 17%; CR 11%) [76]. Excessive infectious complications were observed, leading to early termination of the study; this may have been due to the lack of anti-viral and anti-bacterial prophylaxis.

Preclinical data has demonstrated that co-administration of RCam significantly increased the amount of apoptosis in primary NHL cells compared with either agent alone [77]. Therefore, a phase I/II study evaluating RCam in patients with relapsed or refractory low-grade B-cell NHL is currently accruing patients.

The safety and efficacy of alemtuzumab administered in combination with either rituximab [36] or high-dose cytarabine and mitoxantrone [78] has been evaluated in a small series of patients with MCL [36, 78] and Richter's syndrome [36]. No responses were observed in patients with MCL or Richter's syndrome after treatment with RCam [36]. In contrast, the OR rate was 100% (CR 78%; PR 22%) in the 9 patients with MCL treated with high-dose cytarabine, mitoxantrone and alemtuzumab [78]. Median age was 60 years (range, 48–65); 89% had advanced stage disease (stage III–IV) and 56% had received prior therapy. Significant induction therapy toxicities included neutropaenia (100%), CMV reactivation (44%) and fungal infection (11%). Two patients withdrew from the study (1 for severe infection and another for constitutional decline) and died within 4 months of study withdrawal. The remaining 7 patients went on to autologous stem cell transplant. With a median follow-up of 7 months, duration of CR was 1–16 months.

HAIRY CELL LEUKAEMIA

Experience with single-agent alemtuzumab has been limited to anecdotal reports [24, 79]. No studies have been published evaluating alemtuzumab in combination with other agents in this disease.

WALDENSTROM'S MACROGLOBULINAEMIA

Preliminary reports of two phase II studies assessing alemtuzumab monotherapy in a small series of previously treated patients with Waldenstrom's macroglobulinaemia have indicated that OR rates of 43–71% (CR 0–14%) can be achieved [9, 80]. Serious infectious complications were observed in one trial [9]. An NCI-sponsored phase II study evaluating single-agent alemtuzumab in this patient population is also underway. No studies have evaluated alemtuzumab in combination with other agents.

MULTIPLE MYELOMA AND PLASMA CELL DYSCRASIAS

Exposure to alemtuzumab can inhibit cell growth and induce apoptosis in CD52-expressing multiple myeloma cell lines and/or primary cells and prolong survival of mouse myeloma xenografts [14, 81, 82]. It is unclear whether CD52 is expressed on the clonogenic cells of myeloma, which may be a reason for the apparent lack of activity of alemtuzumab in this disease. Single-agent subcutaneously administered alemtuzumab has minimal activity in heavily pre-treated patients with multiple myeloma (OR 11%; PR 11%) [83]. There are no data available on the efficacy of alemtuzumab administered in conjunction with other agents or at earlier stages of disease.

ACUTE LYMPHOBLASTIC LEUKAEMIA (ALL)

Alemtuzumab monotherapy has been administered to 12 patients with ALL [84–87]. A complete remission without platelet recovery (CRp) and PR was achieved in 2 patients. In addition, several patients had clearance of peripheral blood blasts and/or reduction in bone marrow blasts [84, 86, 87]. The safety and efficacy of alemtuzumab in combination with different chemotherapeutic agents is currently being evaluated in several studies: (1) with hyperCVAD (hyperfractionated cyclophosphamide, vincristine, doxorubicin and dexamethasone alternating with high-dose methotrexate (MTX) and cytarabine) chemotherapy [88] in adult patients with aggressive CD52+ lymphoproliferative disorders, including relapsed ALL, CLL and Richter's transformation, (2) with MTX and mercaptopurine in paediatric and young adult patients with relapsed ALL and (3) as post-remission intensification in patients with previously untreated ALL.

SUMMARY

Although approved as single-agent treatment of refractory patients with (CLL), alemtuzumab's specific role in the treatment of hematological malignancies, including CLL, is under active investigation. At this time, several questions remain unanswered. What is the optimal timing of alemtuzumab administration? Will better results be obtained when alemtuzumab is given as part of an induction regimen or as consolidative therapy? In either of these scenarios, which cytoreductive agents should be used? If given as consolidation therapy, what period of time should elapse between induction therapy and initiation of treatment with alemtuzumab? Will the route of administration (i.e. intravenous vs. subcutaneous) affect efficacy? Because of the significant myelosuppression, will there be an increased occurrence of opportunistic infections, other than those currently reported, or secondary malignancies? Other than bulky nodal disease, and potentially, advanced disease stage in CLL, are there any other predictors of response to alemtuzumab? Which patients will develop resistance to alemtuzumab? Trials are underway that address some of these issues and will help clarify alemtuzumab's efficacy and toxicities.

REFERENCES

1. Elsner J, Hochstetter R, Spiekermann K, Karp A. Surface and mRNA expression of the CD52 antigen by human eosinophils but not by neutrophils. *Blood* 1996; 88:4684–4693.
2. Hale G, Bright S, Chumbley G *et al*. Removal of T cells from bone marrow for transplantation: a monoclonal antilymphocyte antibody that fixes human complement. *Blood* 1983; 62:873–882.

3.   Salisbury JR, Rapson NT, Codd JD *et al*. Immunohistochemical analysis of CDw52 antigen expression in non-Hodgkin's lymphomas. *J Clin Pathol* 1994; 47:313–317.
4.   Ginaldi L, De Martinis M, Matutes E *et al*. Levels of expression of CD52 in normal and leukemic B and T cells: correlation with *in vivo* therapeutic responses to CAMPATH-1H. *Leuk Res* 1998; 22:185–191.
5.   Bass AJ, Gong J, Nelson R, Rizzieri DA. CD52 expression in mantle cell lymphoma. *Leuk Lymphoma* 2002; 43:339–342.
6.   Quigley MM, Bethel KJ, Sharpe RW, Saven A. CD52 expression in hairy cell leukemia. *Am J Hematol* 2003; 74:227–230.
7.   Treon SP, Kelliher A, Keele B *et al*. Expression of serotherapy target antigens in Waldenstrom's macroglobulinemia: therapeutic applications and considerations. *Semin Oncol* 2003; 30:248–252.
8.   Santos DD, Hatjiarissi E, Tournilhac O *et al*. CD52 is expressed on human mast cells and is a therapeutic target for anti-CD52 monoclonal antibody Campath-1H in Waldenstrom's macroglobulinemia and mast cell disorders. *Blood* 2004; 104:304b.
9.   Owen RG, Rawstron AC, Osterborg A *et al*. Activity of alemtuzumab (Mabcampath) in relapsed/refractory Waldenström's macroglobulinemia. *Blood* 2003; 102:664a–665a.
10. Rawstron AC, Laycock-Brown G, Davies FE *et al*. CD52 expression patterns in normal and neoplastic B-cells: myeloma is an unlikely target for single agent alemtuzumab therapy. *Blood* 2004; 104:303b.
11. Kumar S, Kimlinger TK, Lust JA *et al*. Expression of CD52 on plasma cells in plasma cell proliferative disorders. *Blood* 2003; 102:1072–1077.
12. Lin P, Owens R, Tricot G, Wilson CS. Flow cytometric immunophenotypic analysis of 306 cases of multiple myeloma. *Am J Clin Pathol* 2004; 121:482–488.
13. Singhal S, Goolsby C, Taylor R *et al*. Identifying novel therapeutic targets in myeloma: CD20, CD25 and CD52 expression on malignant plasma cells. *Blood* 2003; 102:373b.
14. Carlo-Stella C, Di Nicola M, Longoni P *et al*. Primary plasma cells expressing CD52 are efficiently targeted *in vivo* by alemtuzumab. *Blood* 2004; 104:943a.
15. Jagoda K, Giebel S, Stella-Holowiecka B *et al*. CD52 and CD20 as potential targets for anti-leukemic immunotherapy in adult acute lymphoblastic leukemia. *Blood* 2004; 104:184b.
16. Dyer MJ, Hale G, Hayhoe FG, Waldmann H. Effects of CAMPATH-1 antibodies *in vivo* in patients with lymphoid malignancies: influence of antibody isotype. *Blood* 1989; 73:1431–1439.
17. Gupta S, Lamanna N, Rose R *et al*. CD52 expression in acute leukemia and advanced MDS: 118 cases at Memorial Sloan-Kettering Cancer Center. *Blood* 2003; 102:876a–877a.
18. Crowe JS, Hall VS, Smith MA *et al*. Humanized monoclonal antibody CAMPATH-1H: myeloma cell expression of genomic constructs, nucleotide sequence of cDNA constructs and comparison of effector mechanisms of myeloma and Chinese hamster ovary cell-derived material. *Clin Exp Immunol* 1992; 87:105–110.
19. Rowan W, Tite J, Topley P, Brett SJ. Cross-linking of the CAMPATH-1 antigen (CD52) mediates growth inhibition in human B- and T-lymphoma cell lines, and subsequent emergence of CD52-deficient cells. *Immunology* 1998; 95:427–436.
20. Stanglmaier M, Reis S, Hallek M. Rituximab and alemtuzumab induce a nonclassic, caspase-independent apoptotic pathway in B-lymphoid cell lines and in chronic lymphocytic leukemia cells. *Ann Hematol* 2004; 83:634–645.
21. Smolewski P, Szmigielska-Kaplon A, Cebula B *et al*. Proapoptotic activity of alemtuzumab alone and in combination with rituximab or purine nucleoside analogues in chronic lymphocytic leukemia cells. *Leuk Lymphoma* 2005; 46:87–100.
22. Kennedy B, Rawstron A, Haynes A *et al*. Eradication of detectable minimal disease with Campath-1H therapy results in prolonged survival in patients with refractory B-CLL. *Blood* 2001; 98:367a.
23. Keating MJ, Flinn I, Jain V *et al*. Therapeutic role of alemtuzumab (Campath-1H) in patients who have failed fludarabine: results of a large international study. *Blood* 2002; 99:3554–3561.
24. Ferrajoli A, O'Brien SM, Cortes JE *et al*. Phase II study of alemtuzumab in chronic lymphoproliferative disorders. *Cancer* 2003; 98:773–778.
25. Rai KR, Freter CE, Mercier RJ *et al*. Alemtuzumab in previously treated chronic lymphocytic leukemia patients who also had received fludarabine. *J Clin Oncol* 2002; 20:3891–3897.
26. Rai KR, Keating MJ, Coutre S *et al*. Patients with refractory B-CLL and T-PLL treated with alemtuzumab (Campath®) on a compassionate basis. A report on efficacy and safety of CAM 511 trial. *Blood* 2002; 100:802a.
27. Ciolli S, Gigli F, Marinelli F *et al*. High response rates and reduced first-dose reactions with subcutaneous alemtuzumab in patients with relapsed and refractory CLL. *Blood* 2003; 102:357b.

28. Stilgenbauer S, Dohner H. Campath-1H-induced complete remission of chronic lymphocytic leukemia despite p53 gene mutation and resistance to chemotherapy. *New Engl J Med* 2002; 347:452–453.
29. Stilgenbauer S, Winkler D, Kröber A *et al*. Subcutaneous Campath-1H (alemtuzumab) in fludarabine-refractory CLL: interim analysis of the CLL2h study of the German CLL Study Group (GCLLSG). *Blood* 2004; 104:140a.
30. Lozanski G, Heerema NA, Flinn IW *et al*. Alemtuzumab is an effective therapy for chronic lymphocytic leukemia with p53 mutations and deletions. *Blood* 2004; 103:3278–3281.
31. Osuji N, Del Giudice I, Matutes E *et al*. Alemtuzumab for chronic lymphocytic leukemia with and without p53 deletions. *Blood* 2004; 104:688a.
32. Kennedy B, Rawstron A, Carter C *et al*. Campath-1H and fludarabine in combination are highly active in refractory chronic lymphocytic leukemia. *Blood* 2002; 99:2245–2247.
33. Elter T, Bochmann P, Schulz H *et al*. FluCam – a new, 4-weekly combination of fludarabine and alemtuzumab for patients with relapsed chronic lymphocytic leukemia. *Blood* 2004; 104:690a.
34. Elter T, Bochmann P, Schulz H *et al*. Results of a phase II trial of fludarabine with concomitant application of alemtuzumab in a four-weekly schedule (FluCam) in patients with relapsed CLL. 2nd interim analysis. *J Clin Oncol* 2004; 22:605s.
35. Nabhan C, Patton D, Gordon LI *et al*. A pilot trial of rituximab and alemtuzumab combination therapy in patients with relapsed and/or refractory chronic lymphocytic leukemia (CLL). *Leuk Lymphoma* 2004; 45:2269–2273.
36. Faderl S, Thomas DA, O'Brien S *et al*. Experience with alemtuzumab plus rituximab in patients with relapsed and refractory lymphoid malignancies. *Blood* 2003; 101:3413–3415.
37. Faderl S, Albitar M, Wierda W *et al*. Continuous I.V. infusion (c.i.) followed by subcutaneous (s.c.) alemtuzumab plus rituximab is active in patients with relapsed/refractory chronic lymphoproliferative disorders (LPD). *Blood* 2003; 102:676a.
38. Mauro FR, Foa R, Meloni G *et al*. Fludarabine, ara-C, novantrone and dexamethasone (FAND) in previously treated chronic lymphocytic leukemia patients. *Haematologica* 2002; 87:926–933.
39. Mauro FR, Gentile M, Giammartini E *et al*. FAND/Alemtuzumab (Campath®, Mabcampath®) therapy for the treatment of patients with poor-prognosis chronic lymphocytic leukemia. *Blood* 2003; 102:355b.
40. Wierda W, O'Brien S, Wen S *et al*. Chemoimmunotherapy with fludarabine, cyclophosphamide and rituximab for relapsed and refractory chronic lymphocytic leukemia. *J Clin Oncol* 2005; Mar 14 [Epub ahead of print].
41. Wierda W, O'Brien S, Faderl S *et al*. Improved survival in patients with relapsed – refractory chronic lymphocytic leukemia (CLL) treated with fludarabine, cyclophosphamide, and rituximab (FCR) combination. *Blood* 2003; 102:110a.
42. Wierda W, Faderl S, O'Brien S *et al*. Combined cyclophosphamide, fludarabine, alemtuzumab, and rituximab(CFAR) is active for relapsed and refractory patients with CLL. *Blood* 2004; 104:101a.
43. Montillo M, Cafro AM, Tedeschi A *et al*. Safety and efficacy of subcutaneous Campath-1H for treating residual disease in patients with chronic lymphocytic leukemia responding to fludarabine. *Haematologica* 2002; 87:695–700.
44. Montillo M, Tedeschi A, Rossi V *et al*. Alemtuzumab as consolidation after a response to fludarabine is effective to purge residual disease in patients with chronic lymphocytic leukemia. *Blood* 2004; 104:140a.
45. O'Brien SM, Kantarjian HM, Thomas DA *et al*. Alemtuzumab as treatment for residual disease after chemotherapy in patients with chronic lymphocytic leukemia. *Cancer* 2003; 98:2657–2663.
46. O'Brien SM, Gribben JG, Thomas DA *et al*. Alemtuzumab for minimal residual disease in CLL. *Blood* 2003; 102:109a.
47. Hale G, Waldmann H for CAMPATH Users. Risks of developing Epstein-Barr virus-related lymphoproliferative disorders after T-cell-depleted marrow transplants. *Blood* 1998; 91:3079–3083.
48. Curtis RE, Travis LB, Rowlings PA *et al*. Risk of lymphoproliferative disorders after bone marrow transplantation: a multi-institutional study. *Blood* 1999; 94:2208–2216.
49. Abruzzo LV, Rosales CM, Medeiros LJ *et al*. Epstein-Barr virus-positive B-cell lymphoproliferative disorders arising in immunodeficient patients previously treated with fludarabine for low-grade B-cell neoplasms. *Am J Surg Pathol* 2002; 26:630–636.
50. Rizzieri DA, Weitman S, Vaughn DM. An EBV-positive lymphoproliferative disorder after therapy with alemtuzumab. *N Engl J Med* 2003; 349:2570–2572.
51. Cheson BD, Vena DA, Barrett J, Freidlin B. Second malignancies as a consequence of nucleoside analog therapy for chronic lymphoid leukemias. *J Clin Oncol* 1999; 17:2454–2460.

52. Vitolo U, Orsucci L, Di Celle PF *et al.* Alemtuzumab (Campath®, MabCampath®) consolidation after fludarabine phosphate and cyclophosphamide second-line chemotherapy for progressive chronic lymphocytic leukemia. *Blood* 2003; 102:356b.

53. Johnson S, Smith AG, Löffler H *et al.* Multicentre prospective randomized trial of fludarabine versus cyclophosphamide, doxorubicin, and prednisone (CAP) for treatment of advanced-stage chronic lymphocytic leukaemia. *Lancet* 1996; 347:1432–1438.

54. Rai KR, Peterson BL, Appelbaum FR *et al.* Fludarabine compared with chlorambucil as primary therapy for chronic lymphocytic leukemia. *N Engl J Med* 2000; 343:1750–1757.

55. Leporrier M, Chevret S, Cazin B *et al.* Randomized comparison of fludarabine, CAP, and ChOP in 938 previously untreated stage B and C chronic lymphocytic leukemia patients. *Blood* 2001; 98:2319–2325.

56. Eichhorst BF, Busch R, Stauch M *et al.* Fludarabine (F) induces higher response rates in first line therapy of older patients (pts) with advanced chronic lymphocytic leukemia (CLL) than chlorambucil: interim analysis of a phase III study of the German CLL Study Group (GCLLSG). *Blood* 2003; 102:109a.

57. Eichhorst BF, Busch R, Hopfinger G *et al.* Fludarabine plus cyclophosphamide (FC) induces higher remission rates and longer progression free survival (PFS) than fludarabine (F) alone in first line therapy of advanced chronic lymphocytic leukemia (CLL): results of a phase III study (CLL4 protocol) of the German CLL Study Group (GCLLSG). *Blood* 2003; 102:72a.

58. Rummel MJ, Gamm H, Rost A *et al.* Fludarabine versus fludarabine plus epirubicin in the treatment of chronic lymphocytic leukemia – results of a randomized phase-III multicenter study. *Blood* 2003; 102:437a.

59. Flinn IW, Byrd JC, Morrison C *et al.* Fludarabine and cyclophosphamide with filgrastim support in patients with previously untreated indolent lymphoid malignancies. *Blood* 2000; 96:71–75.

60. Hallek M, Schmitt B, Wilhelm M *et al.* Fludarabine plus cyclophosphamide is an efficient treatment for advanced chronic lymphocytic leukaemia (CLL): results of a phase II study of the German CLL Study Group. *Br J Haematol* 2001; 114:342–348.

61. Schiavone EM, De Simone M, Palmieri S *et al.* Fludarabine plus cyclophosphamide for the treatment of advanced chronic lymphocytic leukemia. *Eur J Haematol* 2003; 71:23–28.

62. O'Brien SM, Kantarjian HM, Cortes J *et al.* Results of the fludarabine and cyclophosphamide combination regimen in chronic lymphocytic leukemia. *J Clin Oncol* 2001; 19:1414–1420.

63. Gonzalez H, Maloum K, Tezenas du Montcel S *et al.* Fludarabine + cyclophosphamide in chronic lymphoproliferative disorders. *Blood* 2003; 102:357b.

64. Keating MJ, O'Brien S, Lerner S *et al.* Chemoimmunotherapy with fludarabine (F), cyclophosphamide (C), and rituximab (R) improves complete response (CR), remission duration and survival as initial therapy of chronic lymphocytic leukemia (CLL). *J Clin Oncol* 2004; 22:573s.

65. Rai KR, Byrd JC, Peterson BL *et al.* A phase II trial of fludarabine followed by alemtuzumab (Campath-1H) in previously untreated chronic lymphocytic leukemia (CLL) patients with active disease: Cancer and Leukemia Group B (CALGB) Study 19901. *Blood* 2002; 100:205a.

66. Rai KR, Byrd JC, Peterson BL *et al.* Subcutaneous alemtuzumab following fludarabine for previously untreated patients with chronic lymphocytic leukemia (CLL): Cancer and Leukemia Group B (CALGB) Study 19901. *Blood* 2003; 102:676a.

67. Hale G, Rebello P, Brettman LR *et al.* Blood concentrations of alemtuzumab and antiglobulin responses in patients with chronic lymphocytic leukemia following intravenous or subcutaneous routes of administration. *Blood* 2004; 104:948–955.

68. Wendtner CM, Ritgen M, Schweighofer CD *et al.* Consolidation with alemtuzumab in patients with chronic lymphocytic leukemia (CLL) in first remission – experience on safety and efficacy within a randomized multicenter phase III trial of the German CLL Study Group (GCLLSG). *Leukemia* 2004; 18:1093–1101.

69. McCune SL, Gockerman JP, Moore JO *et al.* Alemtuzumab in relapsed or refractory chronic lymphocytic leukemia and prolymphocytic leukemia. *Leuk Lymphoma* 2002; 43:1007–1011.

70. Bowen AL, Zomas A, Emmett E *et al.* Subcutaneous CAMPATH-1H in fludarabine-resistant/relapsed chronic lymphocytic and B-prolymphocytic leukaemia. *Br J Haematol* 1997; 96:617–619.

71. Lundin J, Österborg A, Brittinger G *et al.* CAMPATH-1H monoclonal antibody in therapy for previously treated low-grade non-Hodgkin's lymphomas: a phase II multicenter study. European Study Group of CAMPATH-1H Treatment in Low-Grade Non-Hodgkin's Lymphoma. *J Clin Oncol* 1998; 16:3257–3263.

72. Tang SC, Hewitt K, Reis MD, Berinstein NL. Immunosuppressive toxicity of CAMPATH1H monoclonal antibody in the treatment of patients with recurrent low grade lymphoma. *Leuk Lymphoma* 1996; 24:93–101.

73. Lim SH, Davey G, Marcus R. Differential response in a patient treated with Campath-1H monoclonal antibody for refractory non-Hodgkin lymphoma. *Lancet* 1993; 341:432–433.

74. Hale G, Dyer MJ, Clark MR *et al*. Remission induction in non-Hodgkin lymphoma with reshaped human monoclonal antibody CAMPATH-1H. *Lancet* 1988; 2:1394–1399.

75. Uppenkamp M, Engert A, Diehl V *et al*. Monoclonal antibody therapy with CAMPATH-1H in patients with relapsed high- and low-grade non-Hodgkin's lymphomas: a multicenter phase I/II study. *Ann Hematol* 2002; 81:26–32.

76. Khorana A, Bunn P, McLaughlin P *et al*. A phase II multicenter study of CAMPATH-1H antibody in previously treated patients with nonbulky non-Hodgkin's lymphoma. *Leuk Lymphoma* 2001; 41:77–87.

77. Gazitt Y, Akay C, Doxey D *et al*. Synergy between CD52 and CD20 antibody-induced apoptosis correlates with the extent of co-expression of CD20 and CD52 antigens on mononuclear cells derived from chronic lymphocytic leukemia (CLL) and non-Hodgkin's lymphoma (NHL) patients: implications to antibody-based therapy. *Blood* 2004; 104:287b–288b.

78. Wanko SO, Gocherman JP, Moore JO *et al*. Multimodal dose dense therapy for mantle cell lymphoma. *Blood* 2004; 104:329a.

79. Fietz T, Rieger K, Schmittel A *et al*. Alemtuzumab (Campath 1H) in hairy cell leukaemia relapsing after rituximab treatment. *Hematol J* 2004; 5:451–452.

80. Hunter ZR, Branagan AR, Treon SP. Campath-1H in Waldenström's macroglobulinemia. *Blood* 2004; 104:313b.

81. Gasparetto C, Rooney BJ, Houser L *et al*. Multiple myeloma cells express CD52 and are sensitive to treatment with CAMPATH-1H. *Blood* 2002; 100;812a.

82. Matsui W, Huff CA, Wang Q *et al*. Multiple myeloma stem cells and plasma cells display distinct drug sensitivities. *Blood* 2004; 104:679a.

83. Gasparetto C, Horowitz ME, Gockerman JP *et al*. Campath-1H may have activity in the treatment of multiple myeloma. *Blood* 2004; 104:314b.

84. Kolitz JE, O'Mara V, Willemze R *et al*. Treatment of acute lymphoblastic leukemia (ALL) with Campath-1H: initial observations. *Blood* 1994; 84:301a.

85. Faderl S, Kantarjian HM, O'Brien S *et al*. A broad exploratory trial of Campath-1H in the treatment of acute leukemias. *Blood* 2000; 96:324a.

86. Piccaluga PP, Martinelli G, Malagola M *et al*. Anti-leukemic and anti-GVHD effects of campath-1H in acute lymphoblastic leukemia relapsed after stem-cell transplantation. *Leuk Lymphoma* 2004; 45:731–733.

87. Laporte JP, Isnard F, Garderet L *et al*. Remission of adult acute lymphocytic leukaemia with alemtuzumab. *Leukemia* 2004; 18:1557–1558.

88. Kantarjian HM, O'Brien S, Smith TL *et al*. Results of treatment with Hyper-CVAD, a dose-intensive regimen, in adult acute lymphoblastic leukemia. *J Clin Oncol* 2000; 18:547–561.

17

The role of alemtuzumab in allogeneic stem cell transplantation

K. S. Peggs

INTRODUCTION

Two of the major obstacles to further improvement in allogeneic haematopoietic stem cell transplantation (HSCT) outcomes are the toxicity associated with the development of graft-versus-host disease (GvHD) and the propensity for malignant disease to relapse, which are both influenced by a number of transplant- and disease-related factors. To some degree, the two are interlinked. The immune-mediated allogeneic effect that is responsible for GvHD also appears to be responsible, at least in part, for the graft-versus-tumour activity of HSCT that is most notably demonstrated by the ability of donor lymphocyte infusions (DLIs) to mediate anti-tumour responses in patients relapsing following transplantation [1]. In accordance with the theory that the effectors causing GvHD are the donor T cells, the most efficient method for prevention of GvHD following HSCT is T-cell depletion of the graft. This can be achieved by a number of techniques falling within three broad categories: physical methods (e.g. counterflow centrifugal elutriation, E-rosette depletion), immunological methods (e.g. monoclonal antibody (anti-CD6, -CD8, or -TCRαβ) and rabbit complement, Campath-1 antibodies *in vitro* or *in vivo*, immunotoxins), and combined physical/immunologic methods (selection for cells expressing CD34 by immunoadsorption columns, immunomagnetic beads). The concurrent T-cell depletion of the recipient that can be achieved with *in vivo* Campath antibodies that activate antibody-dependent cell-mediated cytotoxicity (ADCC) facilitates engraftment and limits the requirement for escalation of the intensity of conditioning that is otherwise often required to prevent an increased incidence of graft rejection (Figure 17.1). However, donor lymphocytes contribute an anti-leukaemia effect and lymphocyte depletion may exacerbate problems with immune reconstitution resulting in increased risks of both infection and relapse. Thus there is a fine balance between the risks of GvHD and host-versus-graft reactions, relapse and infection.

Although initially developed as T-cell depleting antibodies that would activate human effector systems (such as complement), and that could be used to reduce GvHD following allogeneic transplantation, the more widespread distribution of the target antigen on haematopoietic cells led to another potential application, which became more fully realised once the IgG2b class-switch variant (Campath-1G), which binds human Fc receptors to activate ADCC, and the humanised equivalent (Campath-1H or alemtuzumab) were developed [2]. The humanisation of monoclonal antibodies potentially reduces immune responses

Karl S. Peggs, BM, BCh, MA, MRCP, MRCPath, Senior Lecturer in Bone Marrow Transplantation, Department of Haematology, University College Hospital, Royal Free and University College London Medical School, London, UK.

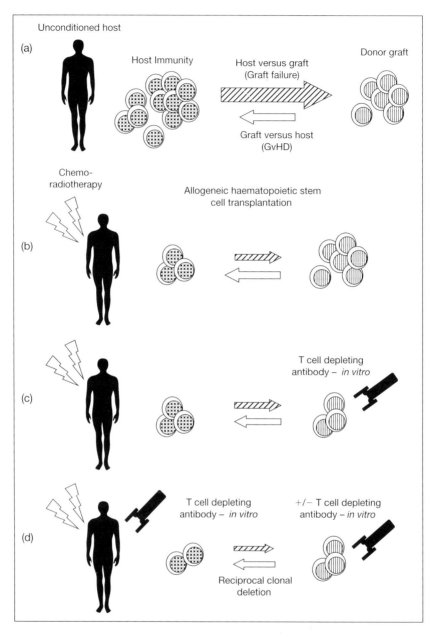

Figure 17.1 The balance of host and donor immunity determines the outcome of opposing host-versus-graft (HvG) and graft-versus-host (GvH) reactions. In the unconditioned host (a) the graft will be rejected. Conditioning with chemo-radiotherapy (b) reduces host immunity sufficiently to allow donor engraftment, but immune cells in the graft can now mediate graft-versus-host disease (GvHD). T-cell depletion of the graft with monoclonal antibody *in vitro* (c) is an effective means of reducing GvHD. The opposing immunological processes will be more balanced, leading to an increased risk of graft failure. Further immune suppression of the host will reduce this risk. This can be achieved by increasing the intensity/immunosuppressive capacity of the chemo-radiotherapy or by depleting the host of T cells with *in vivo* monoclonal antibodies (d). This can be combined with *in vitro* T-cell depletion of the graft but the long half-life of alemtuzumab obviates this requirement.

directed towards the antibody, allowing repeated dosing and further evaluation of activity as a direct anti-tumour agent in lymphoid malignancies. Initially, interest focused on its use in chronic lymphocytic leukaemia or CLL (at least partially because early studies had suggested that activity may be greater against blood and bone marrow disease but less marked against solid masses/nodal disease [2]), but reports of its use in a variety of other B- and T-cell disorders have followed. Thus the incorporation of alemtuzumab in transplantation protocols for lymphoid malignancies has the dual benefits of reducing GvHD and effecting direct anti-tumour responses.

PHARMACOLOGY AND PHARMACOKINETICS

Alemtuzumab (Campath-1H) is a humanised IgG1 monoclonal antibody with specificity for the CD52 antigen, which is widely expressed at high density on all human lymphoid cells (except plasma cells) as well as eosinophils, monocytes, dendritic cells and macrophages [3]. The half-life of alemtuzumab is dependent on the amount of target CD52 antigen in the patient and is therefore affected by the amount of residual disease for tumours that express CD52. Following an *in vivo* dose of 20 mg/day for 5 days (day −8 to day −4) prior to allogeneic transplantation, there is persistence of alemtuzumab *in vivo* past day 0 sufficient to cause T-cell lysis by complement fixation and ADCC, and significant levels of antibody persist up to day +28 post-transplant (Figure 17.2) [4]. Alternative dosing schedules have also been reported. Patients receiving an *in vivo* dose of 10 mg/day from day −5 to day +4 (total dose 100 mg), or from day −10 to day −6 (total dose 50 mg), achieved peak antibody concentrations of 6.1 µg/ml and 2.5 µg/ml, respectively [5]. Campath-1H could be detected for 23 days post-transplant in the former group, and 11 days in the latter. This data contrasts somewhat with the inability to detect Campath-1H at day −1 in 11 patients receiving 10 mg/day from day −7 to day −3 as part of an alternate conditioning regimen [6]. The estimated terminal half-life of 15–21 days contrasts with the half-life of <1 day previously estimated for the rat monoclonal antibody Campath-1G [7]. Administration to the recipient as part of the conditioning regimen results in effective recipient T-cell and dendritic cell depletion in the peripheral blood [8] but it remains unknown whether alemtuzumab leads to depletion of tissue dendritic cells that might initiate GvHD [9]. In addition, if sufficient antibody is circulating on the day of transplantation the graft will also be depleted of T cells,

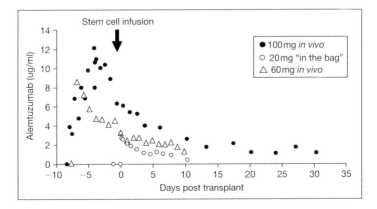

Figure 17.2 Mean alemtuzumab levels according to different dosing schedules. Filled circles show the profile for 20 mg × 5 doses *in vivo* (day −8 to −4), open triangles for 30 mg × 2 doses *in vivo* (day −8 and −7), and open circles for 20 mg added to the graft *in vitro* 30 min prior to infusion on day 0. Concentrations as low as 0.1 µg/ml are sufficient to opsonise lymphocytes for ADCC *in vitro*. Hence levels are sufficient to mediate T-cell depletion of the graft following *in vivo* administration to the recipient.

which may contribute to a reduction in the incidence and severity of GvHD. The relative importance of depletion of host antigen-presenting cells and of donor T cells to the reduction in GvHD incidence is currently unclear, and the optimal dose and scheduling of antibody to prevent GvHD and minimise post-transplant immune suppression remains unknown. Delayed clearance of the humanised antibody may impair immune reconstitution, affect rates of viral reactivation and limit efficacy of the donor T-cell-mediated graft-versus-leukaemia (GvL) effect. Lymphocyte reconstitution is reported as slower with higher Campath doses [4, 5], and CD4 counts in particular may remain depressed for extended periods following therapy.

Two major approaches to the integration of Campath antibodies in transplantation protocols have been used. Both appear effective at limiting the incidence of GvHD. Antibody can be mixed with the graft *in vitro* and the whole mixture infused (Figure 17.1c). This approach has mainly been reported in patients with chronic or acute myeloid leukaemia. It results in effective depletion of donor T cells, and excess antibody may be available to deplete recipient cells. Doses of 10–20 mg have generally been used. With the latter, the median peak antibody level was 3.2 μg/ml (range, 1.0–5.0 μg/ml), occurring at 15 min following the infusion of stem cells containing alemtuzumab (Figure 17.2) [4]. By day +10, levels were below the limit of quantitation in the majority of patients. This approach is likely to be more efficient at depleting donor rather than host T cells and may result in increased rates of graft rejection [10]. In addition, the dose administered to the recipient is relatively modest and will have less direct anti-tumour activity in lymphoid malignancies. Both issues can be addressed by either increasing the intensity of host conditioning, although this may result in an attendant increase in transplant-related morbidity and mortality, or by administering Campath antibody to the patient *in vivo* either before the transplant, or before and after the transplant (Figure 17.1d) [10–12]. The latter approach removes the need to treat the graft *in vitro*. Even with the relatively short half-life of Campath-1G, sufficient antibody persists at the time of stem cell infusion to mediate a substantial degree of ADCC following a dose of 10 mg daily from day −5 to day −1 [7], and the rates of GvHD remain low, suggesting that more prolonged administration of higher doses may not be necessary.

REDUCED INTENSITY REGIMENS INCORPORATING ALEMTUZUMAB

Patients with chronic lymphoid disorders undergoing allogeneic transplantation are characterised by an older age and relatively high transplant-related mortality (TRM) rates compared with those with acute leukaemia or chronic myeloid leukaemia. Although Campath-mediated T-cell depletion may reduce TRM and even allow consideration of the application of unrelated donor allogeneic transplantation in these groups [13], the toxicity of conventional myeloablative approaches remains prohibitive for all but a relatively small minority of patients. These patients have, therefore, been the focus for the development of reduced intensity transplantation approaches, characterised by less myelotoxic but more immunosuppressive conditioning protocols. The increased recipient immune suppression enables stable donor engraftment, despite the reduction in cytoreductive capacity. The Campath antibodies are attractive agents for incorporation in such protocols because of the profound recipient immune suppression they cause, with the added possibility of direct anti-tumour activity. The most commonly used regimens combine alemtuzumab with fludarabine and an alkylating agent, usually melphalan or busulphan [14, 15]. Alemtuzumab has also been added to the BEAM (carmustine, etoposide, cytosine arabinoside, and melphalan) regimen and used in reduced intensity conditioning for lymphoma [16]. A partial list of reported regimens containing alemtuzumab or Campath-1G is shown in Table 17.1. These regimens vary in their myeloablative and immunosuppressive properties and it is currently unclear which is optimal for any given clinical scenario. Additional GvHD prophylaxis has varied between studies, ranging from pre-transplant anti-thymocyte globulin

Table 17.1 Alemtuzumab-containing reduced intensity regimens

Conditioning regimen	Reference
Alemtuzumab 100 mg + fludarabine 150 mg/m² + melphalan 140 mg/m²	[14, 15, 26, 31]
Campath-1G 50 mg + BEAM	[7]
Alemtuzumab 50 mg + BEAM	[16]
Fludarabine 180 mg/m² + ATG 40 mg/kg + busulphan 6.4 mg/kg + in vitro T-cell depletion with alemtuzumab 20 mg	[17]
BEAM = Carmustine, etoposide, cytosine arabinoside, and melphalan; ATG = anti-thymocyte globulin.	

(ATG) with no post-transplant prophylaxis [17], to cyclosporin A either alone [14, 15], or in combination with methotrexate [16].

ENGRAFTMENT AND CHIMAERISM

Engraftment is rapid with all of the reduced intensity regimens incorporating alemtuzumab. The median times to neutrophil recovery (0.5×10^9/l) were 10–16 days, and the median times to achieve platelets $>20 \times 10^9$/l were 6–21 days [7, 14, 16, 17]. The incidence of graft rejection was <5% using peripheral blood stem cells from sibling donors [14, 16] and was 6% in the only relatively large reported series of unrelated donor transplants (using bone marrow) [15]. Early chimaerism studies demonstrate most patients to be full donor chimaeras as early as day 7 following the transplant, but 34–65% develop stable mixed chimaerism between 1 and 6 months post-transplant consistent with the establishment of bilateral transplantation tolerance in a proportion of cases [14, 16, 17]. In the majority, the proportion of donor chimaerism remains greater than 80%. Since this approach to transplantation relies heavily on graft-versus-malignancy effects, the development of mixed T-cell chimaerism following transplantation might be associated with a higher incidence of disease relapse and has acted as a trigger for using DLIs in some series [18].

GRAFT-VERSUS-HOST DISEASE

Published results of sibling donor stem cell transplantation using other reduced intensity conditioning regimens have shown a 38–60% incidence of grade II–IV acute GvHD, which is the primary cause of death in some patients. Incorporation of alemtuzumab in the HLA-identical sibling setting reduces GvHD, with acute grade II–IV GvHD in 0–5% [14, 16, 17]. For reduced intensity regimens without alemtuzumab, the experience with unrelated donor transplants using a fludarabine and melphalan protocol is of high rates of severe GvHD, with 1 in 4 patients dying as a direct result of GvHD [19]. A similar regimen containing alemtuzumab was associated with a low incidence of GvHD despite a significant incidence of HLA disparity. Only 6% of patients had grade III–IV and 15% grade II acute GvHD [15].

It is important to remain cognisant of the fact that T-cell depleted approaches that may need to rely on delayed DLI to reconstitute anti-tumour immunity will be associated with a delayed increase in the incidence of GvHD that may not be apparent in early reports. Forty-six of the first 106 patients treated on the fludarabine/melphalan/alemtuzumab protocol at our institution required subsequent DLI for mixed chimaerism or disease control. Twelve (26%) developed grade II–IV GvHD (5/32 sibling donor transplants, 7/14 unrelated donor transplants) [18]. Sixteen of 65 patients treated on the BEAM/alemtuzumab protocol received DLI, and 6 developed grade I–III GvHD [16]. It is currently difficult to be sure of the true incidence of chronic GvHD on these protocols, but it is likely that the eventual incidence of acute GvHD is 10–15% higher than documented in the initial reports for sibling donors, and probably higher for unrelated donors.

INFECTIOUS COMPLICATIONS

The use of alemtuzumab has been associated with delayed immune reconstitution and an increased incidence of viral infections. Pre-emptive anti-cytomegalovirus (anti-CMV) therapy based on PCR-based assays in 101 patients effectively limited the mortality associated with CMV reactivation [20]. The incidence of infection was 84.8% in the 60 high/intermediate risk patients (donor or recipient CMV seropositive). The probability of recurrence of CMV infection was more common in unrelated donor transplant recipients. The median time to a CD4+ T cell >0.2 × 10^9/l was 9 months in the patients studied. In spite of the higher incidence of CMV infection, there was no significant difference in overall survival and non-relapse mortality between CMV-infected and -uninfected patients. Infection rates appeared no less frequent with lower doses of alemtuzumab or with Campath-1G [21]. There also appears to be an increased incidence of adenovirus, respiratory syncytial virus and parainfluenza virus in alemtuzumab-treated patients; however, many of these infections are not associated with serious clinical sequelae [22]. Epstein-Barr virus (EBV)-associated post-transplant lymphoproliferative disorders occur with increased frequency following T-cell depletion but appear less common following Campath compared to ATG, perhaps because of coincident depletion of B cells, the latent reservoir of EBV [23, 24].

Interestingly, registry data detailing myeloablative transplants revealed an unexpected and apparently paradoxical effect of post-transplant cyclosporin, which appeared to reduce the risk of dying from infection after 6 months post-transplantation [25]. Although part of the benefit could be explained by a reduction in GvHD, the effect was still evident when patients with GvHD or graft rejection were excluded from analysis.

DISEASE-SPECIFIC OUTCOMES

NON-HODGKIN'S LYMPHOMA/CHRONIC LYMPHOCYTIC LEUKAEMIA

Eighty-eight patients undergoing reduced intensity transplantation for non-Hodgkin's lymphoma or NHL (low grade NHL (n = 41), follicular lymphoma (n = 29), CLL (n = 9), lymphoplasmacytoid lymphoma (n = 3); high grade NHL (n = 37), diffuse large B cell (n = 22), transformed low grade (n = 11), peripheral T cell (n = 4); and mantle cell lymphoma (n = 10)) with the fludarabine/melphalan/alemtuzumab conditioning regimen were recently reported from the UK collaborative group [26]. Thirty-seven (42%) had undergone prior autologous transplantation. The median number of prior treatment courses was 3 (range 1–6). Those with high-grade disorders had received more prior therapy than those with low-grade diseases. Twenty-one patients were in complete response at the time of transplantation, 57 in chemosensitive partial response, and 10 had refractory or progressive disease. Sixty-five patients received mobilised stem cells from HLA-identical siblings and 23 received bone marrow from matched unrelated donors. Grade III–IV acute GvHD developed in 4 patients and chronic GvHD in 6 patients. With a median follow-up of 36 months (range 18–60), the actuarial overall survival at 3 years was 34% for high-grade NHL, 60% for mantle cell lymphoma and 73% for low-grade NHL (p = <0.001). The 100-day and 3-year TRM (estimated by the Kaplan-Meier method) for patients with low-grade NHL were 2 and 11%, respectively, and were better (p = 0.01) than for patients with high-grade NHL (27 and 38%, respectively). Relapse remained a major problem. Relapse incidences at 3 years, again estimated by the Kaplan-Meier method, were 53% for the high-grade NHL, 50% for the mantle cell lymphoma, and 44% for the low-grade NHL groups. Twenty patients received DLIs for minimal residual disease, persistent disease or relapse and 15 received DLI for mixed haematopoietic chi-maerism. The actuarial current progression-free survival at 3 years, including those who achieved remission following DLI for progression, was 34% for high-grade NHL, 50% for mantle cell lymphoma, and 65% for low-grade NHL (p = 0.002). Similar outcomes have been reported in a group of 65 patients using a regimen containing alemtuzumab and BEAM con-ditioning, although in concert with the more intensive nature of this regimen, the outcomes for those failing a prior autograft or over the age of 46 years were significantly worse [16].

HODGKIN'S LYMPHOMA

The efficacy of allogeneic myeloablative transplantation in Hodgkin's lymphoma remains controversial, particularly because of very high procedural mortality using total body irradi-ation (TBI)-based conditioning regimens. The malignant Reed-Sternberg cells do not express the CD52 antigen [27] and would not be direct targets for alemtuzumab-mediated lysis. However, these tumours are characterised by heavy infiltration with cytokine-secreting inflammatory cells, and an indirect effect mediated by activity against these accessory cells is plausible. The results from 49 reduced intensity transplants performed with the fludarabine/melphalan/alemtuzumab regimen in multiply relapsed Hodgkin's lymphoma patients appear encouraging [28]. Median age was 32 years, number of prior treatment lines 5, and time from diagnosis 4.8 years. Forty-four had progressed following autologous transplantation. Thirty-three were chemo-sensitive at the time of transplantation (8 com-plete response, 25 partial response). Thirty-one had matched related and 18 unrelated donors. Median follow-up is 967 (102–2,232) days. Grade II–IV acute GvHD occurred in 8 patients prior to DLI and chronic GvHD in 7. Sixteen received DLI from 3 months after transplantation for residual disease/progression. Six developed Grade II–IV acute GvHD and 5 chronic GvHD. Nine (56%) demonstrated disease responses following DLI (8 com-plete, 1 partial). Non-relapse mortality (cumulative incidence) was 16.3% at 2 years (7.2% related vs. 34.1% unrelated donors, p = 0.0206). Projected 4-year overall and current pro-gression-free survivals are 55.7 and 39.0%, respectively (62.0 and 41.5% for related donors, respectively). Both were significantly superior for patients in complete remission at the time of transplantation (100%, p = 0.0398 and 83.3%, p = 0.0389).

MULTIPLE MYELOMA

The expression of the CD52 antigen on plasma cells has historically been reported as low or absent and there has therefore been little interest in the use of alemtuzumab as a directly therapeutic agent in multiple myeloma. More recently, this issue has been re-addressed but the level of antigen expression, both in terms of the number of positive cells and the antigenic density, remains controversial [29, 30]. Hence T-cell depletion has generally been performed in an effort to reduce GvHD and the relatively high TRM rates that characterise series of patients transplanted for myeloma, rather than to provide anti-tumour activity. In an effort to enhance graft-versus-myeloma activity, a study of adjuvant dose-escalating DLIs adminis-tered from 6 months post-transplantation was planned in 20 patients with HLA-matched related (n = 12) or unrelated (n = 8) donors and chemotherapy-sensitive disease [31]. Acute GvHD following transplantation was minimal (3 grade II, no grade III/IV). Non-relapse mortality was relatively low (15%) and related mainly to infective causes. Disease responses by 6 months post-transplantation were modest (2 complete, 4 partial, 2 minimal, 6 no change, 3 progressive, 3 not evaluable). Fourteen patients received escalating-dose DLI for resid-ual/progressive disease. Disease responses were more common in those developing GvHD but response durations were disappointing and progression often occurred despite persist-ing full donor chimaerism. Two-year estimated overall and current progression-free survival were 71 and 30%, respectively.

DONOR LYMPHOCYTE INFUSIONS

It is evident that current approaches incorporating alemtuzumab will rely in a proportion of cases on the existence of a therapeutically relevant and clinically exploitable DLI-associated GvL effect for long-term success. The evidence in support of such activity remains relatively scarce in NHL (reviewed in [32]) and Hodgkin's lymphoma [28], whilst in myeloma its existence is well established but its durability unproven [33]. Each dose is associated with a risk of development of GvHD, which is modulated by DLI dose, donor type/HLA disparity, and time from transplantation. A single institution study of dose-escalating DLI in 46 patients following the fludarabine/melphalan/alemtuzumab protocol, who received a total of 109 DLIs (median 2, range 1–6) to treat mixed chimaerism, residual disease or disease progression included mainly patients with myeloma, Hodgkin's lymphoma, and NHL [18]. Thirty-two had an HLA-matched family donor and 14 an unrelated donor. GvHD was more common (p = 0.002), occurred at lower T-cell doses, and was more severe in the unrelated donor cohort. Conversion from mixed to multi-lineage full donor chimaerism occurred in 30 of 35 evaluable patients. Presence or absence of mixed chimaerism in the granulocyte lineage at the time of DLI did not predict for chimaerism response or development of GvHD. Disease responses were documented in 63% myeloma and 70% Hodgkin's lymphoma patients, were limited in degree and durability in the former group, and were not predicted by changes in chimaerism status.

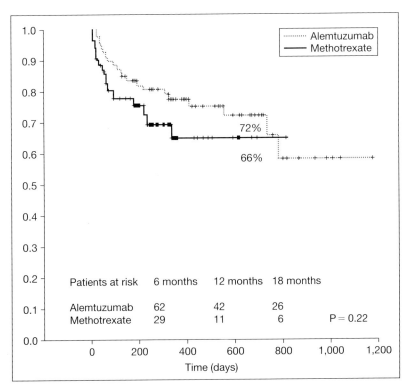

Figure 17.3   Comparison of Kaplan-Meier curves for overall survival of patients with lymphoproliferative disorders undergoing reduced intensity transplantation from sibling donors. Both groups received the same doses of melphalan and fludarabine. One group received cyclosporine and methotrexate as GvHD prophylaxis, and the other received cyclosporine and alemtuzumab [34].

SUMMARY

Alemtuzumab reduces the incidence of acute and chronic GvHD following stem cell transplantation and reduces GvHD-related mortality. Whilst there is a delay in immune reconstitution and an increased incidence of viral infections with the use of alemtuzumab, many of these infections are asymptomatic, and at least in the case of CMV in the sibling setting, do not adversely affect TRM. Disease relapse appears more common but approaches incorporating DLI may offset this tendency in immune responsive malignancies. Delivery of these therapies in a less toxic manner remains a priority for future research. Current evidence suggests that the advantage of reduced GvHD mediated by alemtuzumab may balance the disadvantages of increased infection and disease relapse, so that overall and event-free survival are similar with regimens that use alemtuzumab and those that use methotrexate for GvHD prophylaxis (Figure 17.3) [34]. However, it is important not to underestimate the impact on quality of life achieved by reducing the significant morbidities associated with the development of GvHD. The optimum dosing and scheduling of alemtuzumab remains unknown. De-escalation of the dose may allow more rapid immune reconstitution without compromising anti-GvHD activity. Application earlier in conditioning protocols based on an increasing knowledge of pharmacokinetics may effect similar direct anti-tumour activity and allow discrimination of the relative importance of the depletion of recipient antigen-presenting cells and of donor T cells in GvHD outcomes. Protocols incorporating Campath-1G might help to answer these questions given its shorter half-life *in vivo*. Whilst current approaches require further refinement, they offer a platform on which to build future studies aimed at enhancing immune reconstitution to both tumour- and pathogen-specific targets.

REFERENCES

1. Kolb HJ, Schattenberg A, Goldman JM, Hertenstein B, Jacobsen N, Arcese W *et al*. Graft-versus-leukemia effect of donor lymphocyte transfusions in marrow grafted patients. European Group for Blood and Marrow Transplantation Working Party Chronic Leukemia. *Blood* 1995; 86:2041–2050.
2. Dyer MJ, Hale G, Hayhoe FG, Waldmann H. Effects of CAMPATH-1 antibodies *in vivo* in patients with lymphoid malignancies: influence of antibody isotype. *Blood* 1989; 73:1431–1439.
3. Hale G, Swirsky DM, Hayhoe FG, Waldmann H. Effects of monoclonal anti-lymphocyte antibodies *in vivo* in monkeys and humans. *Mol Biol Med* 1983; 1:321–334.
4. Morris EC, Rebello P, Thomson KJ, Peggs KS, Kyriakou C, Goldstone AH *et al*. Pharmacokinetics of alemtuzumab (CAMPATH-1H) used for *in vivo* and *in vitro* T-cell depletion in allogeneic transplants: relevance for early adoptive immunotherapy and infectious complications. *Blood* 2003; 102:404–406.
5. Rebello P, Cwynarski K, Varughese M, Eades A, Apperley JF, Hale G. Pharmacokinetics of CAMPATH-1H in BMT patients. *Cytotherapy* 2001; 3:261–267.
6. Khouri IF, Albitar M, Saliba RM, Ippoliti C, Ma YC, Keating MJ *et al*. Low-dose alemtuzumab (Campath) in myeloablative allogeneic stem cell transplantation for CD52-positive malignancies: decreased incidence of acute graft-versus-host-disease with unique pharmacokinetics. *Bone Marrow Transplant* 2004; 33:833–837.
7. Cull GM, Haynes AP, Byrne JL, Carter GI, Miflin G, Rebello P *et al*. Preliminary experience of allogeneic stem cell transplantation for lymphoproliferative disorders using BEAM-CAMPATH conditioning: an effective regimen with low procedure-related toxicity. *Br J Haematol* 2000; 108:754–760.
8. Klangsinsirikul P, Carter GI, Byrne JL, Hale G, Russell NH. Campath-1G causes rapid depletion of circulating host dendritic cells (DCs) before allogeneic transplantation but does not delay donor DC reconstitution. *Blood* 2002; 99:2586–2591.
9. Buggins AG, Mufti GJ, Salisbury J, Codd J, Westwood N, Arno M *et al*. Peripheral blood but not tissue dendritic cells express CD52 and are depleted by treatment with alemtuzumab. *Blood* 2002; 100:1715–1720.

10. Hale G, Waldmann H. Control of graft-versus-host disease and graft rejection by T cell depletion of donor and recipient with Campath-1 antibodies. Results of matched sibling transplants for malignant diseases. *Bone Marrow Transplant* 1994; 13:597–611.

11. Jacobs P, Wood L, Fullard L, Waldmann H, Hale G. T cell depletion by exposure to Campath-1G *in vitro* prevents graft-versus-host disease. *Bone Marrow Transplant* 1994; 13:763–769.

12. Spencer A, Szydlo RM, Brookes PA, Kaminski E, Rule S, Van Rhee F *et al*. Bone marrow transplantation for chronic myeloid leukemia with volunteer unrelated donors using *ex vivo* or *in vivo* T-cell depletion: major prognostic impact of HLA class I identity between donor and recipient. *Blood* 1995; 86:3590–3597.

13. Shaw BE, Peggs K, Bird JM, Cavenagh J, Hunter A, Alejandro MJ *et al*. The outcome of unrelated donor stem cell transplantation for patients with multiple myeloma. *Br J Haematol* 2003; 123:886–895.

14. Kottaridis PD, Milligan DW, Chopra R, Chakraverty RK, Chakrabarti S, Robinson S *et al. In vivo* CAMPATH-1H prevents graft-versus-host disease following nonmyeloablative stem cell transplantation. *Blood* 2000; 96:2419–2425.

15. Chakraverty R, Peggs K, Chopra R, Milligan DW, Kottaridis PD, Verfuerth S *et al*. Limiting transplantation-related mortality following unrelated donor stem cell transplantation by using a nonmyeloablative conditioning regimen. *Blood* 2002; 99:1071–1078.

16. Faulkner RD, Craddock C, Byrne JL, Mahendra P, Haynes AP, Prentice HG *et al*. BEAM-alemtuzumab reduced-intensity allogeneic stem cell transplantation for lymphoproliferative diseases: GVHD, toxicity, and survival in 65 patients. *Blood* 2004; 103:428–434.

17. Barge RM, Osanto S, Marijt WA, Starrenburg CW, Fibbe WE, Nortier JW *et al*. Minimal GVHD following *in-vitro* T cell-depleted allogeneic stem cell transplantation with reduced-intensity conditioning allowing subsequent infusions of donor lymphocytes in patients with hematological malignancies and solid tumors. *Exp Hematol* 2003; 31:865–872.

18. Peggs KS, Thomson K, Hart DP, Geary J, Morris EC, Yong K *et al*. Dose-escalated donor lymphocyte infusions following reduced intensity transplantation: toxicity, chimerism, and disease responses. *Blood* 2004; 103:1548–1556.

19. Khouri IF, Keating M, Korbling M, Przepiorka D, Anderlini P, O'Brien S *et al*. Transplant-lite: induction of graft-versus-malignancy using fludarabine-based nonablative chemotherapy and allogeneic blood progenitor-cell transplantation as treatment for lymphoid malignancies. *J Clin Oncol* 1998; 16:2817–2824.

20. Chakrabarti S, Mackinnon S, Chopra R, Kottaridis PD, Peggs K, O'Gorman P *et al*. High incidence of cytomegalovirus infection after nonmyeloablative stem cell transplantation: potential role of Campath-1H in delaying immune reconstitution. *Blood* 2002; 99:4357–4363.

21. Bainton RD, Byrne JL, Davy BJ, Russell NH. CMV infection following nonmyeloablative allogeneic stem cell transplantation using Campath. *Blood* 2002; 100:3843–3844.

22. Chakrabarti S, Avivi I, Mackinnon S, Ward K, Kottaridis PD, Osman H *et al*. Respiratory virus infections in transplant recipients after reduced-intensity conditioning with Campath-1H: high incidence but low mortality. *Br J Haematol* 2002; 119:1125–1132.

23. Ho AY, Adams S, Shaikh H, Pagliuca A, Devereux S, Mufti GJ. Fatal donor-derived Epstein-Barr virus-associated post-transplant lymphoproliferative disorder following reduced intensity volunteer-unrelated bone marrow transplant for myelodysplastic syndrome. *Bone Marrow Transplant* 2002; 29:867–869.

24. Peggs KS, Banerjee L, Thomson K, Mackinnon S. Post transplant lymphoproliferative disorders following reduced intensity conditioning with *in vivo* T cell depletion. *Bone Marrow Transplant* 2003; 31:725–726.

25. Hale G, Cobbold S, Novitzky N, Bunjes D, Willemze R, Prentice HG *et al*. CAMPATH-1 antibodies in stem-cell transplantation. *Cytotherapy* 2001; 3:145–164.

26. Morris E, Thomson K, Craddock C, Mahendra P, Milligan D, Cook G *et al*. Outcomes after alemtuzumab-containing reduced-intensity allogeneic transplantation regimen for relapsed and refractory non-Hodgkin lymphoma. *Blood* 2004; 104:3865–3871.

27. Salisbury JR, Rapson NT, Codd JD, Rogers MV, Nethersell AB. Immunohistochemical analysis of CDw52 antigen expression in non-Hodgkin's lymphomas. *J Clin Pathol* 1994; 47:313–317.

28. Peggs KS, Hunter A, Chopra R, Parker A, Mahendra P, Milligan D *et al*. Clinical evidence of a graft-versus-Hodgkin's lymphoma effect following reduced intensity allogeneic transplantation. *Lancet* 2005; in press.

29. Kumar S, Kimlinger TK, Lust JA, Donovan K, Witzig TE. Expression of CD52 on plasma cells in plasma cell proliferative disorders. *Blood* 2003; 102:1075–1077.
30. Lin P, Owens R, Tricot G, Wilson CS. Flow cytometric immunophenotypic analysis of 306 cases of multiple myeloma. *Am J Clin Pathol* 2004; 121:482–488.
31. Peggs KS, Mackinnon S, Williams CD, D'Sa S, Thuraisundaram D, Kyriakou C et al. Reduced-intensity transplantation with *in vivo* T-cell depletion and adjuvant dose-escalating donor lymphocyte infusions for chemotherapy-sensitive myeloma: limited efficacy of graft-versus-tumor activity. *Biol Blood Marrow Transplant* 2003; 9:257–265.
32. Peggs KS, Mackinnon S, Linch D. The role of allogeneic transplantation in non-Hodgkin's lymphoma. *Br J Haematol* 2005; 128:153–168.
33. Peggs K, Mackinnon S. Graft-versus-myeloma: are durable responses a clinical reality following donor lymphocyte infusion? *Leukemia* 2004; 18:1541–1542.
34. Perez-Simon JA, Kottaridis PD, Martino R, Craddock C, Caballero D, Chopra R et al. Nonmyeloablative transplantation with or without alemtuzumab: comparison between 2 prospective studies in patients with lymphoproliferative disorders. *Blood* 2002; 100:3121–3127.

18

Alemtuzumab in T-cell malignancies

F. Ravandi, M. Keating

INTRODUCTION

Over the past decade, better understanding of the biology and pathogenesis of various neoplastic disorders, as well as improved supportive care measures and better understanding of the mechanisms of action of therapeutic agents, have led to significant advances in the treatment of a number of malignancies. This has been particularly true for lymphoproliferative disorders where better diagnostic techniques have allowed improved classification and definition of distinct biological subtypes. This has led to identification of tumour-specific targets and as a result, agents with the ability to discriminate between normal and neoplastic cells have been developed.

Monoclonal antibodies targeting specific tumour-related surface antigens have been under investigation in the treatment of both haematological malignancies and solid tumours. However, antibody-based immune therapy has been particularly successful in treating lymphoid neoplasms and a number of these agents have been effective in achieving responses in a variety of B- and T-cell disorders. One of these new antibodies, alemtuzumab, is a humanised monoclonal antibody against CD52, a small glycosylphosphatidylinositol (GPI)-anchored glycoprotein that is highly expressed on normal T and B lymphocytes and on a large proportion of malignant lymphoid cells, but not on haematopoietic progenitor cells. Alemtuzumab has demonstrated significant activity against a number of T-cell malignancies that have traditionally been difficult to treat.

Mature T-cell leukaemias are relatively uncommon neoplasms that are derived from mature or post-thymic T cells [1]. Their tissue counterparts are T-cell lymphomas. These and other T-cell disorders such as peripheral and cutaneous T-cell lymphomas account for a relatively small percentage of lymphoid malignancies (Table 18.1) [1]. Significant geographical and racial differences in the incidence of these disorders have been reported with a higher incidence in East Asia and in individuals of native American descent in Mexico, central and south America [1]. With the availability of modern immunophenotypic and molecular tools, a better distinction of these disorders from their B-cell counterparts has been possible. Similarly, identification of recurrent cytogenetic and molecular abnormalities has shed further light on the pathogenesis of these neoplasms.

In general, T-cell lymphomas and leukaemias are an aggressive group of neoplasms and respond poorly to traditional therapeutic modalities. However, recent development of new therapeutic agents such as alemtuzumab and the reasonable efficacy of nucleoside analogues

Farhad Ravandi, MD, Assistant Professor of Medicine, Department of Leukemia, University of Texas M.D. Anderson Cancer Center, Houston, Texas, USA.

Michael Keating, MD, Professor of Medicine, Department of Leukemia, University of Texas M.D. Anderson Cancer Center, Houston, Texas, USA.

Table 18.1 WHO classification of mature T and natural killer (NK) neoplasms

Disseminated
  T-cell prolymphocytic leukaemia
  T-cell large granular cell leukaemia
  Aggressive NK cell leukaemia
  Adult T-cell leukaemia/lymphoma
Cutaneous
  Mycosis fungoides
  Sezary syndrome
  Primary cutaneous anaplastic
  Large cell lymphoma
  Lymphomatous papulosis
Other extranodal
  Extranodal NK/T-cell lymphoma, nasal type
  Enteropathy-type T-cell lymphoma
  Hepatosplenic T-cell lymphoma
  Subcutaneous panniculitis-like T-cell lymphoma
Nodal
  Angioimmunoblastic T-cell lymphoma
  Peripheral T-cell lymphoma, unspecified
  Anaplastic large cell lymphoma
Neoplasms of uncertain lineage
  Blastic NK cell lymphoma

such as cladribine, 2'deoxycoformycin (DCF) and possibly nelarabine has generated significant interest in devising specific therapeutic strategies for these malignancies. Other potentially useful agents such as denileukin diftitox and forodesine hydrochloride are also under investigation. However, the high response rate of patients with T-prolymphocytic leukaemia (T-PLL) to alemtuzumab has been the cornerstone of development of new therapeutic strategies in this and other T-cell neoplasms. In this chapter we will review the data pertaining to the application of alemtuzumab in treating T-PLL and other malignant T-cell lymphoproliferative disorders.

ALEMTUZUMAB

Alemtuzumab is a humanised monoclonal antibody against the CD52 antigen, which is expressed at high density on the surface of B and T lymphocytes and monocytes but not the haematopoietic stem cells (Figures 18.1 and 18.2) [2]. Initial studies conducted in the laboratory of Hale and colleagues [3] at the University of Cambridge aimed at the identification of strategies to purge T cells from donor cells in order to prevent graft-versus-host disease (GVHD) led to the discovery of murine antibodies capable of lysing human T cells while sparing the haematopoietic stem cells. Campath-1M, a rat IgM antibody capable of binding both T and B lymphocytes as well as fixing human complement was described [3]. Using these antibodies, over 99% of lymphocytes were killed and viable T cells could no longer be detected [3]. Further studies demonstrated the feasibility of *in vivo* administration of Campath-1M antibodies in primates and in patients with advanced lymphoid malignancies [4]. Later research led to the identification of Campath-1G, an antibody of isotype IgG2b, with the same specificity as Campath-1M for CD52 on human lymphocytes and monocytes [5]. In a comparative study of IgM, IgG2a, and IgG2b isotypes, Campath-1M produced transient depletion of blood lymphocytes with consumption of complement but had no effect on solid masses or bone marrow [2]. However, the IgG2b (Campath-1G) produced long-lasting depletion of lymphocytes from blood and marrow and improvement in splenomegaly demonstrating higher

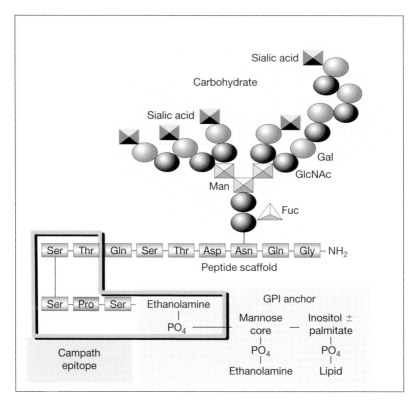

Figure 18.1 The molecular structure of CD52 antigen. The antigen is attached to membrane through a glycosylphosphatidylinositol (GPI) anchor.

efficacy and increased durability of the lympholytic effects of Campath-1G, *in vivo* [2]. In order to avoid the immunogenicity associated with the use of rodent antibodies, Campath-1G was humanised [6]. The recombinant molecule, otherwise known as Campath-1H or alemtuzumab, contains the hypervariable regions of the parent murine antibody inserted into the framework regions of normal human immunoglobulin IgG1 [7].

Alemtuzumab exerts its therapeutic effects through binding to the CD52 antigen on the surface of target cells, which then results in complement-mediated lysis and antibody-dependent cellular cytotoxicity (ADCC) by the activation of natural killer (NK) cells and macrophages through their immunoglobulin G fragment C receptors (FcγR). Other lines of evidence suggest that alemtuzumab can trigger apoptosis in T- and B-lymphoma cell lines and chronic lymphocytic leukaemia (CLL) cells without complement activation [8, 9]. Overall, direct induction of apoptosis, induction of ADCC, and complement-mediated cell death are the mechanisms which contribute to the therapeutic effects of alemtuzumab, particularly the clearance of malignant lymphocytes from the peripheral blood and bone marrow of patients. The effectiveness of ADCC is governed by the susceptibility of tumour cells and the activation of effector cells *via* their FcγR. Several FcγR polymorphisms have been identified that may affect the killing function of NK cells and macrophages. This may be analogous to other monoclonal antibodies, such as rituximab, where recent studies in patients with follicular lymphoma and CLL have implicated a variable role for ADCC and have attempted to correlate high-affinity FcγR polymorphisms with clinical response [10, 11]. However, a report examining the correlation of FcγR3A and FcγR2A polymorphisms with response to alemtuzumab in a series of patients with CLL did not show any such association [12].

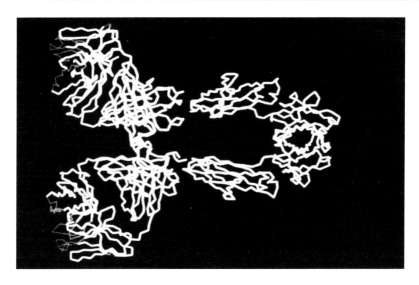

Figure 18.2 Alemtuzumab is a human monoclonal antibody of the IgG1 isotype that has been created by cloning the hypervariable regions of the murine parent Campath-1G into a framework provided by human myeloma proteins.

The U.S. Food and Drug Administration (FDA) has approved alemtuzumab for patients with refractory CLL. Keating and colleagues [13] reported the result of an international study of alemtuzumab in 93 patients with CLL who had failed prior therapy with fludarabine. Alemtuzumab was administered intravenously with a target dose of 30 mg, 3 times weekly for a maximum of 12 weeks. Infection prophylaxis with trimethoprim/sulfamethoxazole and famciclovir or equivalent was administered and continued for at least 2 months after completion of therapy [13]. Objective responses were reported in 33% of patients including 31% partial response (PR) and 2% complete response (CR). The median time to progression was 4.7 months for all patients and 9.5 months for the responders. The median overall survival was 16 months (95% confidence interval (CI) 11.8–21.9 months) for the entire group and 32 months for the responders [13]. Grade 3 or 4 infections were reported in 25 patients (26.9%) including only 3 (9.7%) responders [13]. Other studies have confirmed the efficacy of alemtuzumab in treating patients with relapsed CLL [14–16]. Overall, it appears that alemtuzumab is less efficacious in treating patients with bulky adenopathy and more effective in achieving a bone marrow or peripheral blood response [13].

The principal concern about the use of alemtuzumab is the concomitant reduction of both B and T lymphocytes associated with significant immunosuppression and increased risk of opportunistic infection, particularly in heavily pre-treated patients [13–15, 17]. Of particular concern is the re-activation of cytomegalovirus (CMV). Recently, management guidelines for use of alemtuzumab in CLL have been published and with adherence to these guidelines and adequate prophylaxis, the infectious complications of the drug can be minimised [18].

CLINICAL STUDIES OF ALEMTUZUMAB IN T-CELL NEOPLASMS

The antigen CD52 is expressed on the surface of almost all normal and malignant lymphocytes and alemtuzumab has shown significant activity in patients with lymphoid malignancies of both B- and T cell phenotype. Traditionally, treatment of T-cell neoplasms has been difficult as these disorders have been relatively uncommon, hindering the design and execution of meaningful clinical trials. Furthermore, T-cell malignancies have been resistant to therapy with regimens designed for their B-cell counterparts. For example, therapeutic options for the relatively rare disease T-PLL have been limited as the disease is often resistant to conventional chemotherapy. Nucleoside analogues such as DCF have been used with limited success [19, 20]. In an early study, 68 patients with post-thymic mature T-cell malignancies including 31 patients with T-PLL were treated with DCF 4 mg/m^2 weekly for the first 4 weeks, then every 2 weeks until maximal response [19]. Toxicity was very low with only one death from prolonged neutropaenia. Forty-eight percent of patients with T-PLL responded including 3 patients who achieved a CR and 12 patients with PR. Responses were more likely in patients who had a CD4+/CD8− phenotype in the population as a whole [19].

ALEMTUZUMAB IN T-PLL

T-PLL and probably other mature T-cell leukaemias generally involve the peripheral blood and bone marrow and as such should be excellent candidates for treatment with this antibody. Indeed, alemtuzumab has been used successfully to treat patients with T-PLL (Table 18.2). In an early study, Pawson and colleagues [21] treated 15 patients with T-PLL with alemtuzumab. Most patients had received prior treatment with the purine analogue DCF. Major responses occurred in 11 patients (73%) with a CR rate of 60%. CRs were durable, and re-treatment with the antibody resulted in second CRs in 3 relapsed patients [21].

Dearden and co-workers [22] treated 39 patients with T-PLL with alemtuzumab 30 mg administered intravenously 3 times weekly until maximal response [22]. The overall response rate was 76% with 60% CR and 16% PR. Responses were durable, with a median disease-free interval of 7 months (range, 4–45 months). Survival was significantly prolonged in patients achieving CR compared to PR or no response [22]. Seven patients underwent an autologous stem cell transplant after therapy with alemtuzumab with 3 remaining alive in CR up to 15 months after the transplant. Four patients had an allogeneic transplant from an HLA-identical sibling (n = 3) or matched unrelated donor (n = 1). Two had non-myeloablative conditioning. Three remained alive in CR up to 20 months after the transplant [22]. The authors concluded that although the majority of patients responded to alemtuzumab and many of the CRs were durable (up to 45 months), all but 2 patients followed up for more than 1 year had relapsed at the time of reporting and as such, alemtuzumab could not be considered as curative [22]. The main side-effect of therapy with alemtuzumab was prolonged lymphopaenia with risk of infectious complications such as reactivation of CMV as well as opportunistic infections. Other toxicities included acute infusion-related effects and development of prolonged bone marrow aplasia of unknown etiology in 2 patients, a complication that appears to be more frequent in patients treated with alemtuzumab for T-cell disorders rather than for B-cell CLL [22]. In a follow-up study, Dearden and colleagues [23] administered a standard regimen of alemtuzumab to 11 previously untreated patients with T-PLL. All patients achieved a CR. Response

Table 18.2 Published clinical studies of alemtuzumab in T-prolymphocytic leukaemia

Reference	Patients (n)	Patients with no prior therapy (n)	CR (%)	PR (%)	OR (%)
Pawson et al. [21]	15	0	60	13	73
Dearden et al. [22]	39	2	60	16	76
Keating et al. [23]	66	4	40	11	51
Dearden et al. [24]	11	11	100		100

CR = Complete response; PR = partial response; OR = overall response.

Table 18.3 Published clinical trials of alemtuzumab in T-cell neoplasms

Reference	Patients (n)	Disease	Route of administration	Prior therapy	CR (%)	PR (%)	OR (%)
Lundin et al. [25]	8	Mycosis fungoides	I.V.	Yes	25	25	50
Lundin et al. [26]	22	Mycosis fungoides	I.V.	Yes	32	23	55
Enblad et al. [27]	14	Peripheral T-cell lymphoma	I.V.	Yes	21	14	36

I.V. = Intravenous; CR = complete response; PR = partial response; OR = overall response.

duration was 2–25 months (median 10+ months). After a median follow-up of 12 months (range 4–27 months), 7 patients remained alive and 4 had undergone an autologous stem cell transplant. One patient died from sepsis in CR, 4 patients relapsed at 4–25 months (median 13 months) and died from progressive disease [23]. One of these patients relapsed with CD52-negative T cells and was resistant to further alemtuzumab therapy [23].

More recently, Keating and co-workers [24] reported on 66 patients with T-PLL (including 4 patients with no prior therapy) who received intravenous alemtuzumab 30 mg 3 times weekly for 4–12 weeks. The objective response rate was 51%, with a 39.5% CR rate. The median duration of response was 8.7 months (range, 0.13+ to 44.4 months) and median time to progression was 4.5 months (range, 0.1–45.4 months) compared with 2.3 months after first-line chemotherapy (range, 0.3–28.1 months) [24]. The median overall survival was 7.5 months (14.8 months for patients achieving CR). Treatment-related side-effects were similar as previously reported; 15 infections occurred during therapy in 10 patients including 3 with CMV infections [24].

ALEMTUZUMAB IN PERIPHERAL T-CELL LYMPHOMA (PTCL)

Alemtuzumab has also been evaluated in patients with non-Hodgkin's lymphomas (NHL) including T-cell malignancies (Table 18.3). In the study by Lundin and colleagues [25], 50 patients with relapsed or resistant NHL were treated with alemtuzumab 30 mg administered as a 2-hour intravenous infusion 3 times weekly for a maximum period of 12 weeks. Six patients (14%) with B-cell lymphomas achieved a PR. Patients with mycosis fungoides appeared to respond more frequently (50%; 4/8 patients, including 2 CRs) [25]. Lymphoma cells were rapidly eliminated from blood in 16 of 17 patients (94%). CR in the bone marrow was obtained in 32% of the patients. Lymphoma skin lesions disappeared completely in 4 of 10 patients and partial regression was obtained in 3 patients. Lymphadenopathy and splenomegaly were cleared in only 5% and 15% of patients, respectively [25]. Grade IV neutropaenia occurred in 14 patients (28%) and opportunistic infections were diagnosed in 7 patients. Death related to infectious complications occurred in 3 patients [25].

ALEMTUZUMAB IN CUTANEOUS T-CELL LYMPHOMA (CTCL)

More recently, Lundin and colleagues [26] reported the result of a phase II study of alemtuzumab in 22 patients with advanced mycosis fungoides or Sézary syndrome. The overall response rate was 55% with 32% achieving CR and 23% PR. Sézary cells were cleared from the blood in 6 of 7 (86%) patients, and CR in lymph nodes was observed in 6 of 11 (55%) patients. Median time-to-treatment failure was 12 months (range, 5–32+ months). CMV reactivation occurred in 4 (18%) patients. Enblad and co-workers [27] have also reported their experience in treating 14 patients with relapsed or refractory peripheral T-cell lymphoma. The overall response rate was 36% with 3 patients achieving a CR and 2 PR. The durations of the CRs were 2, 6, and 12 months, respectively. Toxicity included CMV reactivation in 6 patients, which was successfully treated with ganciclovir or foscarnet, pulmonary aspergillosis in 2 patients, and pancytopaenia in 4 patients [27].

SUMMARY

Although Campath antibodies were among the first of a number of novel therapeutic antibodies developed, alemtuzumab has only fairly recently become available for clinical use. Alemtuzumab has demonstrated profound effects on circulating and bone marrow lymphoid cells. As such, it has been found to be an effective therapy for both B- and T-cell leukaemias and for the eradication of residual disease after 'tumour-debulking' using more conventional regimens. The potential toxic effects of alemtuzumab, primarily infections, have become further highlighted with increased clinical use. However, it is likely that with adherence to the published guidelines for management of patients receiving alemtuzumab and with adequate prophylaxis, the infectious complications of the drug can be minimised. New generations of clinical trials investigating the feasibility and safety of combining alemtuzumab with other effective agents, such as nucleoside analogues and other monoclonal antibodies, are emerging. Ongoing clinical trials will demonstrate whether these combinations can overcome the limitations of single-agent alemtuzumab, particularly its relatively low activity against bulky adenopathy. In addition, further understanding of the mechanisms of action of and resistance to alemtuzumab promises to improve our ability to incorporate the drug more logically into our therapeutic armamentarium. The significant response rates observed in patients with T-cell lymphoproliferative disease are likely to provide a basis for the design of more effective regimens that will hopefully improve upon the response rate and duration.

REFERENCES

1. Jaffe ES, Ralfkiaer E. Mature T-cell and NK-cell neoplasms. In: Jaffe ES, Harris NL, Stein H, Vardiman JW (eds). *Tumors of Hematopoietic and Lymphoid Tissues*. IARC Press; Lyon; 2001; pp 189–235.
2. Dyer MJ, Hale G, Hayhoe FG, Waldmann H. Effects of CAMPATH-1 antibodies in vivo in patients with lymphoid malignancies: influence of antibody isotype. *Blood* 1989; 73:1431–1439.
3. Hale G, Bright S, Chumbley G, Hoang T, Metcalf D, Munro AJ *et al*. Removal of T cells from bone marrow for transplantation: a monoclonal antilymphocyte antibody that fixes human complement. *Blood* 1983; 62:873–882.
4. Hale G, Swirsky DM, Hayhoe FG, Waldmann H. Effects of monoclonal anti-lymphocyte antibodies in vivo in monkeys and humans. *Mol Biol Med* 1983; 1:321–334.
5. Hale G, Cobbold SP, Waldmann H, Easter G, Matejtschuk P, Coombs RR. Isolation of low-frequency class-switch variants from rat hybrid myelomas. *J Immunol Methods* 1987; 103:59–67.
6. Riechmann L, Clark M, Waldmann H, Winter G. Reshaping human antibodies for therapy. *Nature* 1988; 332:323–327.
7. James LC, Hale G, Waldmann H, Bloomer AC. 1.9 A structure of the therapeutic antibody CAMPATH-1H fab in complex with a synthetic peptide antigen. *J Mol Biol* 1999; 289:293–301.
8. Rowan W, Tite J, Topley P, Brett SJ. Cross-linking of the CAMPATH-1 antigen (CD52) mediates growth inhibition in human B- and T-lymphoma cell lines, and subsequent emergence of CD52-deficient cells. *Immunology* 1998; 95:427–436.
9. Stanglmaier M, Reis S, Hallek M. Rituximab and alemtuzumab induce a nonclassic, caspase-independent apoptotic pathway in B-lymphoid cell lines and in chronic lymphocytic leukemia cells. *Ann Hematol* 2004; 83:634–645.
10. Cartron G, Dacheux L, Salles G, Solal-Celigny P, Bardos P, Colombat P *et al*. Therapeutic activity of humanized anti-CD20 monoclonal antibody and polymorphism in IgG Fc receptor FcgammaRIIIa gene. *Blood* 2002; 99:754–758.

11. Weng WK, Levy R. Two immunoglobulin G fragment C receptor polymorphisms independently predict response to rituximab in patients with follicular lymphoma. *J Clin Oncol* 2003; 21:3940–3947.

12. Lin TS, Flinn IW, Modali R, Lehman TA, Webb J, Waymer S *et al*. FCGR3A and FCGR2A polymorphisms may not correlate with response to alemtuzumab in chronic lymphocytic leukemia. *Blood* 2005; 105:289–291.

13. Keating MJ, Flinn I, Jain V, Binet JL, Hillmen P, Byrd J *et al*. Therapeutic role of alemtuzumab (Campath-1H) in patients who have failed fludarabine: results of a large international study. *Blood* 2002; 99:3554–3561.

14. Osterborg A, Dyer MJ, Bunjes D, Pangalis GA, Bastion Y, Catovsky D *et al*. Phase II multicenter study of human CD52 antibody in previously treated chronic lymphocytic leukemia. European Study Group of CAMPATH-1H Treatment in Chronic Lymphocytic Leukemia. *J Clin Oncol* 1997; 15:1567–1574.

15. Rai KR, Freter CE, Mercier RJ, Cooper MR, Mitchell BS, Stadtmauer EA *et al*. Brettman L. Alemtuzumab in previously treated chronic lymphocytic leukemia patients who also had received fludarabine. *J Clin Oncol* 2002; 20:3891–3897.

16. Ferrajoli A, O'Brien SM, Cortes JE, Giles FJ, Thomas DA, Faderl S *et al*. Phase II study of alemtuzumab in chronic lymphoproliferative disorders. *Cancer* 2003; 98:773–778.

17. Lundin J, Kimby E, Bjorkholm M, Broliden PA, Celsing F et al. Phase II trial of subcutaneous anti-CD52 monoclonal antibody alemtuzumab (Campath-1H) as first-line treatment for patients with B-cell chronic lymphocytic leukemia (B-CLL). *Blood* 2002; 100:768–773.

18. Keating M, Coutre S, Rai K, Osterborg A, Faderl S, Kennedy B *et al*. Management guidelines for use of alemtuzumab in B-cell chronic lymphocytic leukemia. *Clin Lymphoma* 2004; 4:220–227.

19. Dearden C, Matutes E, Catovsky D. Deoxycoformycin in the treatment of mature T-cell leukaemias. *Br J Cancer* 1991; 64:903–906.

20. Mercieca J, Matutes E, Dearden C, MacLennan K, Catovsky D. The role of pentostatin in the treatment of T-cell malignancies: analysis of response rate in 145 patients according to disease subtype. *J Clin Oncol* 1994; 12:2588–2593.

21. Pawson R, Dyer MJ, Barge R, Matutes E, Thornton PD, Emmett E *et al*. Treatment of T-cell prolymphocytic leukemia with human CD52 antibody. *J Clin Oncol* 1997; 15:2667–2672.

22. Dearden CE, Matutes E, Cazin B, Tjonnfjord GE, Parreira A, Nomdedeu B *et al*. High remission rate in T-cell prolymphocytic leukemia with CAMPATH-1H. *Blood* 2001; 98:1721–1726.

23. Dearden CE, Matutes E, Cazin B, Ireland R, Parreira A, Lakhani A *et al*. Very high response rates in previously untreated T-cell prolymphocytic leukaemia patients receiving alemtuzumab (Campath-1H) therapy. *Blood* 2003; 102:644a.

24. Keating MJ, Cazin B, Coutre S, Birhiray R, Kovacsovics T, Langer W *et al*. Campath-1H treatment of T-cell prolymphocytic leukemia in patients for whom at least one prior chemotherapy regimen has failed. *J Clin Oncol* 2002; 20:205–213.

25. Lundin J, Osterborg A, Brittinger G, Crowther D, Dombret H, Engert A *et al*. CAMPATH-1H monoclonal antibody in therapy for previously treated low-grade non-Hodgkin's lymphomas: a phase II multicenter study. European Study Group of CAMPATH-1H Treatment in Low-Grade Non-Hodgkin's Lymphoma. *J Clin Oncol* 1998; 16:3257–3263.

26. Lundin J, Hagberg H, Repp R, Cavallin-Stahl E, Freden S, Juliusson G *et al*. Phase 2 study of alemtuzumab (anti-CD52 monoclonal antibody) in patients with advanced mycosis fungoides/Sezary syndrome. *Blood* 2003; 101:4267–4272.

27. Enblad G, Hagberg H, Erlanson M, Lundin J, MacDonald AP, Repp R *et al*. A pilot study of alemtuzumab (anti-CD52 monoclonal antibody) therapy for patients with relapsed or chemotherapy-refractory peripheral T-cell lymphomas. *Blood* 2004; 103:2920–2924.

19

Epratuzumab: A new humanised monoclonal antibody to CD22

M. Coleman, R. R. Furman, J. Decter, W. A. Wegener, I. D. Horak, D. M. Goldenberg, J. P. Leonard

CD22 ANTIGEN

The CD22 antigen is a 135-kDa B-lymphocyte-restricted trans-membrane glycoprotein of the immunoglobulin superfamily [1, 2]. It is a member of the sialoglycoprotein group of adhesion molecules that are involved in signal transduction and regulation of B-cell activation (mostly negative), mature B-cell homing, and the interactions of B cells, T cells and antigen-presenting cells [3–6]. The predominant CD22 isoform contains seven extra-cellular domains. CD22 is present in the cytoplasm of developing B cells, but is later expressed on the surface during B cell maturation at the time IgD expression occurs. Most circulating IgM+IgD+ cells express CD22. CD22 is strongly expressed in follicular, mantle and marginal zone B cells but is weakly present in germinal (activated or differentiating) B cells [1, 6, 7]. CD22 is not detected on other normal tissues nor is it expressed by non-lymphatic neoplastic cells. Because the expression of CD22 is lineage restricted, and, in most cases, is not lost during neoplastic transformation, it represents an attractive target for anti-lymphoma immunotherapeutic antibodies [1, 2]. Indeed, in B-cell malignancies, CD22 has been observed in over 80% of evaluated samples [8]. Limited data, however, are available with regard to the expression of different CD22 isoforms in various lymphoma subtypes.

Morton Coleman, MD, Center for Lymphoma and Myeloma and Division of Hematology and Oncology, Department of Medicine, Weill Medical College of Cornell University and New York Presbyterian Hospital, New York, USA.

Richard R. Furman, MD, Weill Medical College of Cornell University and New York Presbyterian Hospital, New York, USA.

Julian Decter, MD, Center for Lymphoma and Myeloma and Division of Hematology and Oncology, Department of Medicine, Weill Medical College of Cornell University and New York Presbyterian Hospital, New York, USA.

William A. Wegener, Immunomedics, Inc., New Jersey, USA.

Ivan D. Horak, MD, Executive Vice President, Research and Development, Immunomedics, Inc., New Jersey, USA.

David M. Goldenberg, Center for Molecular Medicine and Immunology, Garden State Cancer Center, Belleville, New Jersey, Immunomedics, Inc., New Jersey, USA.

John P. Leonard, MD, Medical Director, Oncology Unit, New York Presbyterian Hospital, Assistant Professor of Medcine, Weill Medical College of Cornell University, New York, USA.

A key role of CD22 in B-cell function is suggested by studies showing that CD22-deficient mice have mature B cells which are more susceptible to apoptotic signals, have a shorter cellular lifespan, display a reduced number of B cells in the bone marrow, have a chronic exaggerated antibody response to antigen, and develop autoantibodies [1, 3, 9, 10]. Many of these functions could potentially be modulated by the binding of a specific anti-CD22 antibody (such as epratuzumab) and resultant internalisation and phosphorylation of CD22.

LL2, A MURINE ANTI-CD22 MONOCLONAL ANTIBODY

The humanised anti-CD22 antibody epratuzumab was developed from studies with a mouse monoclonal antibody (mLL2, originally named EPB-2) that specifically binds to the cluster C region of human CD22 [11]. LL2 is a kappa IgG_2 antibody that demonstrates high reactivity to human lymphoma tumour cells with a lack of cross-reactivity to non-lymphatic normal human tissues or tumours. *In vitro* immunohistochemical evaluation demonstrated reactivity of the LL2 antibody with 50 of 51 B-cell lymphoma specimens tested. The hybridoma cell line for LL2 was originally developed by Goldenberg and colleagues [1, 11], through the immunisation of BALB/c mice with Raji cell membranes (Burkitt's lymphoma cell line) and fusion of the spleen cells of these mice with SP210 myeloma cells [2].

EPRATUZUMAB, HUMANISED ANTI-CD22

Epratuzumab (hLL2) is the humanised (complementarity determining region (CDR)-grafted) IgG_1 kappa monoclonal antibody version of LL2 [12]. By replacing a large proportion of the immunoglobulin sequence of murine LL2 monoclonal antibody with constituents of the human immunoglobulin sequences through genetic engineering, epratuzumab was developed potentially to be less immunogenic, to prolong the antibody half-life, and to increase effector function. Competitive binding studies show epratuzumab to have similar binding properties to those of mLL2. Epratuzumab binds to the CD22 antigen present on the surface of most relatively mature B cells and B-cell lymphomas. It reacts across all B-lymphoma subsets, including both indolent and aggressive lymphomas. Preliminary clinical evaluation of epratuzumab labelled with ^{131}I or with ^{111}In/^{90}Y has shown evidence of tumour localisation and accumulation *in vivo* [1, 2, 7, 12]. On the basis of infusion studies, epratuzumab has a mean half-life of 23 days (± 9 days), which is comparable to the half-life of IgG_1 (21 days). Epratuzumab treatment did not affect T-cell levels as measured by CD3+ cell counts, but did decrease B-cell levels (approximately 75% decrease from baseline) for up to 9 months as measured by CD19+ cell counts [13, 14].

Unlike CD20, which remains anchored on the cell surface, binding of epratuzumab with CD22 causes rapid internalisation and phosphorylation of the CD22 cytoplasmic tail. Internalisation is dose-dependent and long-lasting, without reaching irreversibility at clinically meaningful concentrations. Re-expression of CD22 after prolonged epratuzumab treatment, though, appears to follow slow kinetics and requires days (in some cases, over a week) for partial recovery [2].

Preclinical work with anti-CD22 'blocking' monoclonal antibodies (i.e., monoclonal antibodies that prevent CD22 binding to its natural ligand) suggest that modulation of receptor activation has a selective cytotoxic effect on receptor-positive tumour cells. The same ligand-blocking anti-CD22 monoclonal antibody can also trigger primary B-cell proliferation, suggesting that the consequences of CD22 engagement may differ depending on the B-cell stage of differentiation. Epratuzumab binding to CD22 does not block the ligand-binding site on CD22. In contradistinction to the ligand-blocking anti-CD22 monoclonal antibodies, epratuzumab does not show evidence of the ability to directly induce apoptosis nor have studies revealed a significant impact on lymphoma growth *in vitro* [1, 15–17].

It may, nevertheless, have a more significant role *in vivo* that may not be demonstrated in an isolated *in vitro* context. What role epratuzumab plays specifically *in vivo* on the important CD22 functions of adhesion, homing and B-cell receptor activation is still to be elucidated. Another possibility is that CD22 engagement by the antibody and downstream signalling may render a cell more sensitive to pro-apoptotic stimuli and result in anti-proliferative effects.

CLINICAL TRIALS OF EPRATUZUMAB

INDOLENT NON-HODGKIN'S LYMPHOMA (NHL)

Epratuzumab was evaluated at Cornell in a single centre, dose escalation trial using single agent intravenous doses of 120–1,000 mg/m² [13]. Treatment was given weekly for 4 weeks, but, in contrast to rituximab, was given rapidly over 30–60 min. Over 50 heavily pre-treated patients were studied, with half having received at least four prior regimens and with bulky (>5 cm) disease. Epratuzumab produced 18% (95% confidence interval 8–31%) objective responses with 6% complete responses (CRs) over this wide range of doses. In patients with follicular lymphoma, 24% responded including 43% in the 360-mg/m² dose group and 27% in the 480-mg/m² dose group. Median duration of objective response was 79.3 weeks (range, 11.1–143.3 weeks), with a median time-to-progression for responders of 86.6 weeks by Kaplan-Meier estimate. The most frequent toxicity was nausea (22%). Almost all toxicities evaluated were National Cancer Institute (NCI) common toxicity grade 1 or 2. Events occurred less frequently with subsequent infusions. Other common toxicities included fatigue, back pain, anaemia and limb pain. No correlation between the frequency of adverse events and administered dose was observed, and no dose-limiting toxicity occurred. Clinically significant changes in laboratory measures (including haematology values and immunoglobulin levels) or vital signs did not occur and no serious treatment adverse events occurred. No patient developed a human anti-human antibody (HAHA) to the epratuzumab molecule.

AGGRESSIVE NON-HODGKIN'S LYMPHOMA

In a single institution study (again at Cornell), epratuzumab was also administered once weekly for 4 weeks at 120–1,000 mg/m² doses to 56 patients with aggressive lymphoma, 35 of whom had diffuse large B-cell lymphoma [14]. Patients were heavily pre-treated (median, 4 prior therapies), approximately 25% had received prior high-dose chemotherapy with stem cell transplant, and 84% had bulky disease (>5 cm). Across all dose levels, 10% (95% confidence interval 3–21%) responded with 5% CRs. In patients with diffuse large cell lymphoma, 15% demonstrated objective response. Overall 20% of subjects experienced some tumour mass reduction. Median duration of overall responses was 26.3 weeks, and median time-to-progression for responders was 35 weeks. Two responses remained ongoing at ≥34 months, including one rituximab-refractory patient.

Toxicity similar to that encountered with low-grade lymphoma was confined to NCI common toxicity grade 1 and 2. The most frequent toxicities were gastrointestinal and fatigue, and all were minor.

COMBINATION ANTIBODY THERAPY WITH EPRATUZUMAB

PRECLINICAL STUDIES

Given the success of combinations of chemotherapeutic agents with different mechanisms of action and toxicity in order to attack tumour cells 'on multiple fronts', the combined use of multiple monoclonal antibodies against antigens with different signalling pathways and functions would appear to be a logical extension of immunotherapy. Rituximab's notable success in the clinic has prompted laboratory and clinical studies combining it and other anti-CD20 antibodies with epratuzumab [18–21].

In studies using a murine lymphoma model, survival of mice treated with a humanised anti-CD20 monoclonal antibody (IMMU-106) plus epratuzumab was compared with IMMU-106 treatment alone. Although the combined treatment did not improve median survival, an increased proportion of long-term survivors was observed. An enhanced anti-proliferative effect was also observed *in vitro* in SU-DHL-6 cells when the IMMU-106 anti-CD20 antibody was combined with epratuzumab. These findings were consistent with the *in vitro* demonstration of up-regulation of CD22 expression observed after pre-treatment of lymphoma cells with IMMU-106 [18].

In vitro immunohistochemical studies, however, demonstrate an overlapping expression of CD20 and CD22 in B-cell lymphoma specimens. Mechanistically, epratuzumab has not been found to cause B-cell killing by apoptosis or complement-mediated cytotoxicity, but has shown modest antibody-dependent cellular cytotoxicity when tested on lymphoma cell lines. In contrast, all three mechanisms have been shown with anti-CD20 antibodies [18]. Internalisation, though, is not a feature of anti-CD20 antibodies, a putative mechanism in the anti-neoplastic activity of epratuzumab.

CLINICAL TRIALS OF COMBINATION ANTIBODY THERAPY WITH EPRATUZUMAB

In a single institutional trial, 23 patients with recurrent, antibody-naïve B-cell lymphoma received epratuzumab 360 mg/m^2, followed by rituximab 375 mg/m^2 infused over 4–6 h on the same day [19, 20]. Infusions were administered for 4 consecutive weeks. Sixteen patients had indolent histologies (15 with follicular lymphoma) and 7 had diffuse large cell lymphoma. The subjects with indolent lymphoma had received a median of 1 (range 1–6) prior treatment, with 31% refractory to their last therapy and 81% with high-risk follicular lymphoma international prognostic index (FLIPI) scores. Patients with diffuse B large cell lymphoma had a median of 3 (range 1–8) prior regimens (14% resistant to their last treatment) and 71% had high-intermediate or high-risk international prognostic index (IPI) scores. All patients were rituximab-naïve.

Treatment was well tolerated, with toxicities principally infusion-related and predominantly NCI grade 1 or 2. Ten (67%) patients with follicular NHL achieved an objective response, including 9 of 15 (60%) with CRs. Four of six evaluable subjects (67%) with diffuse B-cell lymphoma achieved an objective response, including 3 (50%) CRs. Median time-to-progression for all indolent lymphoma patients was 17.8 months. In a subsequent multi-centre trial of rituximab-sensitive *or* naïve patients with indolent lymphoma, overall response rate was 58% with 28% CRs. Time-to-progression was not reached in the rituximab-naïve group (though they had a lower response rate), while the overall response rate was 75% in the rituximab-relapsed group (despite a shorter time-to-progression). The differences in results may relate to the disparate patient subgroups enrolled in the study (with small patient numbers in each), as well as the variations in patient selection. These studies differed in prior treatment exposure (rituximab), and additionally, the multi-centre trial may have included a group with some unfavourable prognostic features, such as elevated LDH (in half of the subjects), which is relatively less common in indolent lymphoma. In order to clearly establish any potential benefit of combination antibody therapy (epratuzumab + rituximab) over single-agent therapy, a randomised trial (with a comparison group of rituximab alone) is necessary. Modifications in dose and schedule of treatment may impact results. For instance, preclinical laboratory data suggest that rituximab may up-regulate the expression of the CD22 molecule in some systems [18]. Further evaluation of a combination antibody approach is being conducted by Micallef and colleagues, who have a combination trial of epratuzumab plus rituximab plus CHOP (cyclophosphamide, adriamycin, vincristine, prednisone) chemotherapy currently underway in diffuse large B-cell lymphoma. Initial results suggest that this regimen is associated with acceptable toxicity, while efficacy analysis is ongoing (22).

RADIOIMMUNOTHERAPY WITH EPRATUZUMAB

Both ^{90}Y and ^{131}I radioisotopes have been used successfully in combination with anti- CD20 murine antibodies as part of a radioimmunotherapeutic approach. Radiolabelled ^{90}Y ibritumomab and ^{131}I tositumomab, both murine agents, have been approved for clinical use in the USA for the treatment of recurrent indolent or low-grade NHL [22–24]. Recent studies, though, have suggested that radioimmunoconjugates are also highly effective in untreated patients [25, 26]. Radioimmunotherapy has been especially convenient to use since therapy is completed in 1–2 weeks, and both short- and long-term toxicities have been manageable. Goldenberg and colleagues [27], using the ^{131}I-anti-CD22 (LL2), reported in 1991 that a patient receiving a trace amount of antibody could respond (with tumour shrinkage), suggesting that lymphoma could be exquisitely sensitive to radiation delivered in this fashion. Since only a few milligrams of antibody were administered, the effect was believed to relate primarily to the radiation and less to the antibody component.

Rhenium-186 (^{186}Re) has favourable physical characteristics for radioimmunotherapy. It has medium energy beta emissions and low-abundance gamma photons with ideal energy (137 kV) for scintigraphic imaging [28]. The radioisotope was combined with epratuzumab in a dose-escalation study. In contrast to the usual practice with radioimmunotherapy (generally pre-dosing with unlabelled monoclonal antibody), the humanised ^{186}Re-epratuzumab was directly infused over 45 min in a dose escalation study of 0.5, 1.0, 1.5 and 2.0 GBq/m^2. No cold (unlabelled) 'pre-dosing' was required. Only one grade 4 haematological toxicity was observed. Of the 15 patients, one-third had an objective response including 1 CR and 4 partial responses (PRs). Responses ranged from 3 to 14 months.

A fractionated radioimmunotherapy dose schedule with ^{90}Y-labelled epratuzumab has been employed in a few selected patients. Fractionated dosing was utilised based on the hypothesis that a decrease in tumour mass (which may occur rapidly during therapy) will significantly increase the calculated absorbed dose, and that fractionating the dose may potentially provide a more tailored approach [29]. Chatal and co-workers [30] recently summarised an ongoing multi-centre phase I/II study which examined a fractionated approach. This study employed small weekly doses of ^{90}Y-epratuzumab. Although the maximum tolerated dose has not yet been reached, the investigators reported an overall response rate of 50% (13 of 26 patients with various forms of B-cell NHL, except CLL) with 10 of the 13 responses being CR or unconfirmed CR (CRu). Studies of both labelled and unlabelled epratuzumab are continuing, and these and other planned studies should establish the potential role of this anti-CD22 antibody in lymphoma therapy.

SUMMARY

Epratuzumab, anti-CD22 monoclonal antibody, is currently in development for the treatment of B-lymphoproliferative disorders. It has several features which differentiate it from other antigen targets used for therapeutic antibodies, such as CD20 and CD52. For example, CD22 is expressed on a relatively small proportion of normal cells, which limits the potential toxicity; antibody bound to CD22 is rapidly internalised, which might facilitate its use as a vehicle for radioimmunotherapy; and epratuzumab has a different mode of action to rituximab, facilitating combination approaches.

REFERENCES

1. Coleman M, Goldenberg DM, Siegel AB *et al*. Epratuzumab: targeting B-cell malignancies through CD22. *Clin Cancer Res* 2003; 9:3991S–3994S.
2. Carnahan J, Wang P, Kendall R *et al*. Epratuzumab, a humanized monoclonal antibody targeting CD22: characterization of *in vitro* properties. *Clin Cancer Res* 2003; 9:3982S–2990S.
3. Nitschke L, Carsetti R, Ocker B *et al*. CD22 is a negative regulator of B-cell receptor signalling. *Curr Biol* 1997; 7:133–143.
4. Sato S, Tuscano JM, Inaoki M *et al*. CD22 negatively and positively regulates signal transduction through the B lymphocyte antigen receptor. *Semin Immunol* 1998; 10:287–297.
5. Engel P, Nojima Y, Rothstein D *et al*. The same epitope of CD22 of B lymphocytes mediates the adhesion of erythrocytes, T and B lymphocytes, neutrophils, and monocytes. *J Immunol* 1993; 150:4719–4732.
6. Tedder TF, Tuscano J, Sato S *et al*. CD22, a B lymphocyte specific adhesion molecule that regulates antigen receptor signaling. *Annu Rev Immunol* 1997; 15:481–504.
7. Dorken B, Moldenhauer G, Pezzoto A *et al*. HD39(B3), a B lineage-restricted antigen whose cell surface expression is limited to resting and activated human lymphocytes. *J Immunol* 1986; 136:4470–4479.
8. Cesano A, Gayko U, Brannan C *et al*. Differential expression of CD22 by indolent and aggressive NHLs: implications for targeted immunotherapy. *Blood* 2002; 100:3500.
9. Otipoby KL, Andersson KB, Braves KE *et al*. CD22 regulates thymus-independent responses and the lifespan of B cells. *Nature* 1996; 34:634–637.
10. O'Keefe TL, Williams GT, Davies SL *et al*. Hyperresponsive B cells in CD22-deficient mice. *Science* 1996; 274:798–801.
11. Pawlak-Byczkowska EJ, Hansen HJ, Dion AS *et al*. Two new monoclonal antibodies, EPB-1 and EPB-2, reactive with human lymphoma. *Cancer Res* 1989; 79:4568–4577.
12. Leung SO, Goldenberg DM, Dion AS *et al*. Construction and characterization of a humanized, internalizing, B cell (CD22)-specific, leukemia/lymphoma antibody, LL2. *Mol Immunol* 1995; 32:1413–1427.
13. Leonard JP, Coleman M, Ketas JC *et al*. Phase I/II trial of epratuzumab (humanized anti-CD22 antibody) in indolent non-Hodgkin's lymphoma. *J Clin Oncol* 2003; 16:3051–3059.
14. Leonard JP, Coleman M, Ketas JC *et al*. Epratuzumab, a humanized anti-CD22 antibody, in aggressive non-Hodgkin's lymphoma: phase I/II clinical trial results. *Clin Cancer Res* 2004; 10:5327–5334.
15. Tuscano JM, Riva A, Tuscano SN *et al*. CD22 cross-linking generates B cell antigen receptor-independent signals that activate the JNK/SAPK signaling cascade. *Blood* 1999; 94:1382–1392.
16. Shan D, Press OW. Constitutive endocytosis and degradation of CD22 by human B cells. *J Immunol* 1995; 154:4466–4475.
17. Shin LB, Lu HH, Xuan H *et al*. Internalization and intracellular processing of an anti-B cell lymphoma monoclonal antibody, LL2. *Int J Cancer* 1994; 56:538–545.
18. Stein R, Qu Z, Chen S *et al*. Characterization of a new humanized anti-CD20 monoclonal antibody, Immu-106, and its use in combination with the humanized anti-CD22 antibody, epratuzumab, for the therapy of non-Hodgkin's lymphoma. *Clin Cancer Res* 2004; 10:2868–2878.
19. Leonard J, Coleman M, Matthews J *et al*. High complete response rate following epratuzumab (anti-CD22) and rituximab (anti-CD20) combination antibody therapy in follicular non-Hodgkin's lymphoma. *Ann Oncol* 2002; 13:38.
20. Leonard JP, Coleman M, Ketas J *et al*. Combination antibody therapy with epratuzumab (humanized anti-CD22 antibody) and rituximab (chimeric anti-CD20 antibody) in relapsed/refractory non-Hodgkin's lymphoma (NHL), submitted.
21. Emmanouilides C, Leonard JP, Schuster SJ *et al*. Multicenter phase II study of combination antibody therapy with epratuzumab plus rituximab in recurrent low grade NHL. *Blood* 2003; 102:69a.
22. Kaminski MS, Zelenetz AD, Press OW *et al*. Pivotal study of iodine I 131 tositumomab for chemotherapy-refractory low-grade or transformed low-grade B-cell non-Hodgkin's lymphomas. *J Clin Oncol* 2001; 19:3918–3928.
23. Coleman M, Kaminski MS, Knox SJ *et al*. The Bexxar therapeutic regimen (tositumomab and iodine-I-131 tositumomab) produced durable complete remissions in non-Hodgkin's lymphoma patients with relapsed/refractory disease and rituximab-naïve. *Blood* 2003; 111:29a.
24. Witzig T, Gordon L, Cabanillas F *et al*. Randomized controlled trial of yttrium-90-labeled ibritumomab tiuxetan radioimmunotherapy versus rituximab immunotherapy for patients with relapsed or

refractory low-grade, follicular, or transformed B-cell non-Hodgkin's lymphoma. *J Clin Oncol* 2002; 20:2453–2463

25. Kaminski MS, Tuck M, Estes J *et al*. 131-I-tositumomab therapy as initial treatment for follicular lymphoma. *N Engl J Med* 2005; 252:441–449.

26. Leonard JP, Coleman M, Kostakoglu L *et al*. Abbreviated chemotherapy followed by tositumomab and iodine I-131 tositumomab for untreated follicular lymphoma. *J Clin Oncol*, in press.

27. Goldenberg DM, Horowitz JA, Sharkey RM *et al*. Targeting, dosimetry, and radioimmunotherapy of B-cell lymphoma with iodine-131-labeled Ll2 monoclonal antibody. *J Clin Oncol* 1991; 9:548–561.

28. Postema EJ, Raemaekers JMM, Oyen WJG *et al*. Final results of a phase I radioimmunotherapy trial using [186]Re-Epratuzumab for the treatment of patients with non-Hodgkin's lymphoma. *Clin Cancer Res* 2003; 9:33995S–4002S.

29. Hindorf C, Linden O, Stenberg L *et al*. Change in tumor-absorbed dose due to decrease in mass during fractionated radioimmunotherapy in lymphoma patients. *Clin Cancer Res* 2003; 9:4003S–4006S.

30. Chatal JF, Harousseau JL, Trumper LH *et al*. Radioimmunotherapy in non-Hodgkin's lymphoma (NHL) using a fractionated schedule of DOTA-conjugated, 90-Y-radiolabeled, humanized anti-CD22 monoclonal antibody, epratuzumab. *Cancer Biother Radiopharm* 2004; 19:525a.

20

Education and management of patients undergoing immunotherapy and radioimmunotherapy

N. L. Tuinstra

INTRODUCTION

Immunotherapy is used in haematological cancers to induce an immune response against the tumour cells, to produce active or passive immunity to tumour cells with vaccines, or to target the tumour cell with a monoclonal antibody. This chapter will focus on nursing care and education of patients being treated with monoclonal antibodies. Monoclonal antibodies are custom-made immunoglobulins produced in the laboratory to a specific cell surface antigen. These antibodies, when injected into patients, will attach to a specific target and kill the cell by inducing apoptosis or direct the patient's immune system to attack the tumour cell by a process called antibody-dependent cellular cytotoxicity.

Immunotherapy with monoclonal antibodies can be divided into two categories – unlabelled or 'cold' antibodies and radiolabelled or 'hot' antibodies. To form a radioimmunoconjugate, a radioisotope is attached to the antibody so that the target cells also receive radiation. This process is called radioimmunotherapy (RIT) [1–3]. The advantage of immunotherapy and RIT over chemotherapy is that they are more targeted than chemotherapy. In general, chemotherapy is less selective and is often toxic to normal organs as well as the cancer itself. Antibodies can have toxicity too because the antigen they target is often found on some normal cells. In the case of RIT, the highest amount of radiation is delivered to the tumour cell with the only toxicity being myelosuppression (Figure 20.1).

PATIENT EDUCATION

When a patient is anticipating immunotherapeutic treatment for lymphoid cancers, it is important that they understand all aspects of these treatments to reduce anxiety and ensure the safest and most effective treatment possible. This teaching is typically performed by the treatment nurse. Most patients have had experience with chemotherapy and it is important for the patient to understand the similarities and differences between immunotherapy and chemotherapy. Common side-effects of chemotherapy include alopecia, nausea, vomiting, diarrhoea, constipation, stomatitis, cardiomyopathy, and neuropathy – all of which are uncommon with immunotherapy. Chemotherapy often produces myelosuppression, which produces anaemia, neutropaenia, and thrombocytopaenia with the consequent risk

Nancy Lou Tuinstra, RN, Mayo Clinic College of Medicine, Nuclear Medicine, Rochester, Minnesota, USA.

Chemotherapy   Antibody therapy

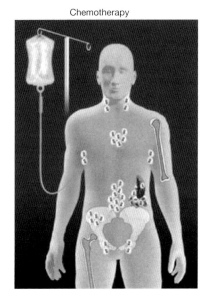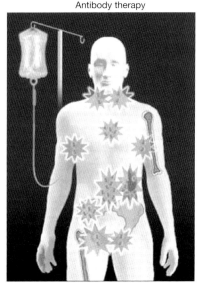

Figure 20.1   Antibody therapy by nature is more selective than chemotherapy in targeting tumour cells. Used by permission from Biogen IDEC (San Diego, CA and Cambridge, MA).

of fatigue, infection, and bleeding. However, a common side-effect of immunotherapy not often seen with chemotherapy is infusion-related toxicity including fever, chills, rigors, bronchospasm, urticaria, and hypo- or hypertension. These symptoms can occur suddenly and be severe, and if the patient and staff are not knowledgeable about these reactions, they can be very frightening for the patient and the nursing staff alike. Cold antibodies such as rituximab and alemtuzumab target lymphoid cells such that infection is a risk – more so with alemtuzumab than rituximab. Radiolabelled antibodies definitely produce myelosuppression that predictably occurs at about 4–8 weeks. In summary, before the patient receives monoclonal antibody treatment, the issue of infusion-related issues and risk of myelosuppression and immunosuppression should be reviewed with the patient and their family.

Cold antibodies that have been approved by the U.S. Food and Drug Administration (FDA) for use in lymphoid malignancies include rituximab, tositumomab, ibritumomab, and alemtuzumab; tositumomab and ibritumomab are only approved for use in RIT. There are other antibodies undergoing clinical investigation (Table 20.1).

RITUXIMAB

Rituximab is a monoclonal antibody directed against the CD20 antigen. The typical schedule is $375\,mg/m^2$ weekly for 4 weeks [4]. Rituximab is diluted to achieve a concentration of $1\,mg/ml$. The initial infusion is initiated at $50\,ml/h$ and increased by $50\,ml/h$ every 30 min if there are no adverse reactions. Rituximab should never be given as intravenous push or bolus. Subsequent infusions are given at a rate of $100\,ml/h$ and increased by $100\,ml/h$ every 30 min to a maximum of $400\,ml/h$. Vital signs should be recorded every 15 min for the first hour and then hourly for the remainder of the infusion.

The pre-medication for rituximab and the treatment for rituximab reactions can be considered the paradigm for monoclonal antibody administration. Alemtuzumab is an exception

Table 20.1 Monoclonal antibodies in clinical use or clinical trials and their respective target antigen

Monoclonal antibody	Target
Approved by the FDA	
Rituximab	CD20
Tositumomab	CD20
Ibritumomab	CD20
Alemtuzumab	CD52
Investigational	
Epratuzumab	CD22
IDEC-114	CD80
TRM-1	Death-receptor 4
MDX-060	CD30
MDX-010	CD4

and will be discussed separately. Patients are pre-medicated with acetaminophen 650–1,000 mg PO and diphenhydramine 25–50 mg PO or IV. Despite these pre-medications, infusion reactions to rituximab are common and consist of fever, rigors, nausea, pruritus, angioedema, asthenia, hypotension, headache, bronchospasm, throat irritation, rhinitis, urticaria, rash, vomiting, myalgia, dizziness, and hypertension. The most common reactions for patients are fever, rigors, sensation of fullness in the throat, hypotension, and nausea [5]. It is important for the nursing staff to be prepared for these reactions and to educate the patient to inform the nurse if these symptoms begin to develop. The sudden rigors are especially frightening for patients and the nurse should reassure the patient that this side-effect is transient and treatable. The most severe reactions typically occur on the first treatment of each cycle and the reactions are usually minor on subsequent doses of each cycle. The nursing staff must be prepared to treat these reactions quickly as they happen, typically 60–90 min into the infusion. Rigors should be treated by stopping the infusion and administering meperidine 25 mg IV and, if necessary, an additional dose of diphenhydramine. Rigors are usually accompanied by chills, and warm blankets will help make the patient more comfortable. In the pivotal studies of rituximab, corticosteroids were not permitted because it was important to learn if the rituximab was producing the anti-tumour activity [4]. If the patient has a severe reaction that is not adequately treated by stopping the infusion, IV fluids, diphenhydramine and meperidine, then methylprednisolone 100 mg IV (or equivalent) should be given. After the reaction subsides, the rituximab can usually be re-started and completed. In our experience it is very unusual for these patients to be unable to complete the entire prescribed dose of rituximab. In some cases, the reactions markedly prolong the infusion time and the patient does not complete the entire dose of rituximab before the out-patient unit is scheduled to close. In these situations, the patient can be transferred to an in-patient bed to complete the infusion. If a patient has a reaction to the extent that they require IV corticosteroids, then consideration should be given for pre-medicating with corticosteroids at the time of the next rituximab infusion. This can be with methylprednisolone IV or the patient can be instructed to take prednisone PO at home on the day of their treatment [6].

Throat irritation is also a common reaction. This reaction can be usually be treated by slowing the infusion rate until the symptoms resolve. If the problem continues, the infusion should be stopped until the symptoms completely resolve and then re-started at the highest previously-tolerated rate.

Hypotension can also result from rituximab infusions. If the patient is on anti-hypertensive drugs, it is recommended that patients do not take their daily anti-hypertensive medication medicine prior to the rituximab infusion. If hypotension is anticipated or begins to develop during rituximab administration, infusing 0.9% normal saline at 100 ml/h will improve blood pressure readings and the rituximab can be continued. If systolic pressure drops below 90 mmHg the nurse should consider interrupting the rituximab and increasing (or starting) IV saline infusion at a rate of 500 ml/h. If this is not effective at increasing the blood pressure then the patient should be given IV methylprednisolone as described above. This works the majority of the time and the rituximab can be restarted at 50 mg/h. Because of this potential for anaphylactic and other hypersensitivity reactions related to the administration of proteins to patients, medications for the treatment of such reactions, such as epinephrine, antihistamines, and corticosteroids, should be readily available during the administration of the rituximab [7]. Epinephrine is reserved for life-threatening situations and in our experience of over 8 years we have never needed to use it.

The other monoclonal antibodies (Table 20.1) are infused at a constant rate. The following investigational antibodies have variable infusion times. For example, epratuzumab is infused over 60 min; TRM-1 over 120 min; and MDX-060 and MDX-010 over 90 min. All investigational antibodies should be infused with caution and constant vigilance for unforeseen infusion-related reactions. These rates and infusion recommendations may change if they are eventually FDA-approved.

ALEMTUZUMAB

Alemtuzumab is directed against CD52 and is approved for relapsed B-cell chronic lymphocytic leukemia (CLL) [8]. CD52 is also expressed on T cells; therefore, alemtuzumab induces T-cell depletion making the patient susceptible to infections and re-activation of cytomegalovirus (CMV) [9, 10]. Prior to starting the alemtuzumab regimen, the patient should begin prophylaxis with trimethoprim/sulfamethoxazole (one double-strength tablet twice daily 3 times a week) and an anti-viral such as acyclovir or valaciclovir to reduce the risk of serious opportunistic infections. Patients who have serological evidence of having been exposed to CMV (as evidenced by a IgG antibody to CMV) should be monitored every 2 weeks during therapy with a blood test for CMV viral load. If the patient develops evidence of re-activation of CMV infection, then specific anti-viral therapy for CMV (such as ganciclovir or foscarnet) should be initiated. These patients are also at risk of developing fungal infections but anti-fungal prophylaxis is not currently recommended [11]. This regimen should continue for 2 months after completion of alemtuzumab therapy or until the CD4 count is >200 cells/μl – whichever occurs later.

Alemtuzumab is approved for IV administration. The patient should be pre-medicated with acetaminophen 650 mg and diphenhydramine 50 mg PO or IV 30 min prior to infusion. Infusion-related events associated with alemtuzumab include hypotension, rigors, fever, shortness of breath, bronchospasm, chills, and rash. The most common reactions are rigors and rash. This rash can occur hours after the infusion. In addition to pre-medication, alemtuzumab should be initiated at a low dose with a gradual increase of doses, as tolerated, up to the effective dose. The initial dose is 3 mg, administered as a 2-hour infusion (IV) daily, increased to 10 mg daily, and finally the maintenance dose of 30 mg every other day or 3 times weekly. A typical course is 12–18 weeks. Alemtuzumab should never be given by bolus or push intravenous infusion.

Alemtuzumab can also be given as subcutaneous injection and patients should be pretreated in the same way as for intravenous infusion [12]. In the first 1–2 weeks the patients are dose-escalated to the 30 mg dose by starting at 3 mg, then 10 mg and finally 30 mg; no more than 90 mg should be given over a one-week period. The 30 mg 3-times-weekly maintenance dose is given for up to 18 weeks. With the subcutaneous dosing, skin rash is common for the first few weeks and then usually resolves. Patients normally require the acetaminophen and diphenhydramine for several weeks and then may discontinue it. Patients should have complete blood counts monitored throughout therapy and alemtuzumab therapy should be

Table 20.2 Dose modification recommendations for alemtuzumab

Haematological toxicity	Dose modification and re-initiation of therapy
For first occurrence of ANC <250/μl and/or platelet count ≤25,000/μl	Withhold alemtuzumab therapy. When ANC ≥ 500/μl and platelet count ≥50,000/μl, resume alemtuzumab therapy at same dose. If delay between dosing is ≥7 days, initiate alemtuzumab therapy at 3 mg and escalate to 10 mg and then to 30 mg as tolerated
For second occurrence of ANC <250/μl and/or platelet count ≤25,000/μl	Withhold alemtuzumab therapy. When ANC ≥ 500/μl and platelet count ≥ 50,000/μl, resume alemtuzumab therapy at 10 mg. If delay between dosing is ≥7 days, initiate alemtuzumab therapy at 3 mg and escalate to 10 mg only
For third occurrence of ANC <250/μl and/or platelet count ≤25,000/μl	Discontinue alemtuzumab therapy permanently
For a decrease of ANC and/or platelet count to ≤50% of the baseline value in patients initiating therapy with a baseline ANC ≤ 500/μl and/or a baseline platelet count ≤ 25,000/μl	Withhold alemtuzumab therapy. When ANC ≥ 500/μl and platelet count ≥50,000/μl return to baseline value(s), resume alemtuzumab therapy. If delay between dosing is ≥7 days, initiate alemtuzumab therapy at 3 mg and escalate to 10 mg and then to 30 mg as tolerated

Reproduced from the package insert. ANC = Absolute neutrophil count.

discontinued during serious infections or if grade 3 or 4 haematological toxicity develops. If therapy is interrupted for 7 or more days, alemtuzumab should be re-instituted with gradual dose escalation. Alemtuzumab therapy should be permanently discontinued if evidence of autoimmune anaemia or thrombocytopaenia appears (Table 20.2).

RADIOIMMUNOTHERAPY

RIT is another treatment for lymphoid malignancies. The goal of RIT is to use the monoclonal antibody to target radiation to the tumour cells while sparing the normal organs. There are several requirements for RIT to be successful – a good monoclonal antibody, an antigen that is expressed on tumour cells, a commercially available radionuclide, and a radiosensitive tumour. Lymphomas are good tumours for RIT because most express CD20, the CD20 is only on B cells, and non-Hodgkin's lymphoma (NHL) is known to be radiosensitive. There are currently two FDA-approved radioimmunoconjugates for cancer and both are for NHL. Ibritumomab tiuxetan (Zevalin™, BiogenIdec) chelates [111]Indium (^{111}In) for imaging and dosimetry and [90]Yttrium (^{90}Y) for therapy. Tositumomab (Bexxar™, GlaxoSmithKline) uses [131]Iodine (^{131}I) for imaging, dosimetry, and therapy. Both treatment programs give a single dose of the radioimmunoconjugate and the entire treatment program is complete in 1–2 weeks as an out-patient making this treatment very convenient for the patient.

To successfully perform RIT, several team members are involved. These include the Haematologist/Oncologist, the Nuclear Medicine Physician or Radiation Oncologist, Nuclear Medicine Technologist, Nurse, Radiopharmacist, Pharmacist, and the Hospital Radiation Safety Officer (Figure 20.2). The haematologist/oncologist identifies the patient as a candidate for RIT and performs the blood tests, bone marrow, and CT scans required for RIT. Radioisotope therapies in the USA are regulated by the U.S. Nuclear Regulatory

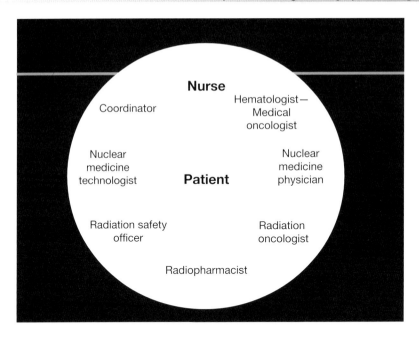

Figure 20.2   Team needed to perform successful radioimmunotherapy. Reproduced with permission from BiogenIDEC.

Commission and all states must be in agreement with the regulations given by this commission. Some states also have more stringent regulations than those given by the commission [7, 13]. The administration of Zevalin or Bexxar must be performed by a physician licensed by the Nuclear Regulatory Commission to handle and administer radioactive compounds; therefore, RIT is usually administered in either the Nuclear Medicine or Radiation Oncology department. This physician will order the RIT and essentially handle the patient for one week. Once the RIT is delivered, the patient returns to the care of the haematologist/oncologist. The rituximab (in the case of Zevalin) can be administered by the haematologist/oncologist or by the Nuclear Medicine nursing staff. In the case of Bexxar, the cold tositumomab is typically given in the same area as the ^{131}I-Bexxar.

All team members involved prior to, during, and following the use of RIT treatments, must be familiar with the safety measures required for RIT. There are some differences in patient education depending on whether the patient is receiving Zevalin or Bexxar. Zevalin uses ^{90}Y, a pure beta emitter, which has a 5-mm path length and penetrates only through to the dermis; there is no gamma radiation with Zevalin. Bexxar uses ^{131}I, which emits beta and gamma radiation; the latter penetrates through the subcutaneous tissue (Figure 20.3). Prior to giving RIT, the patient should be given oral and written instructions regarding the exposure of family, friends and the general public (Table 20.3).

ZEVALIN

Zevalin dosing is based on the patient's body weight and pre-treatment platelet count. A dose of 0.4 mCi/kg is given for a pre-treatment platelet count of 150,000 or greater and a dose of 0.3 mCi/kg is given for a pre-treatment platelet count between 100,000–150,000. The Zevalin treatment regimen (Figure 20.4) consists of rituximab 250 mg/m^2 on day 1 followed by an injection of ^{111}In labelled to a small amount of Zevalin for the purpose of imaging and tracking the uptake of Zevalin. Images are performed at 2–24 h, 48–72 h, and if the results are

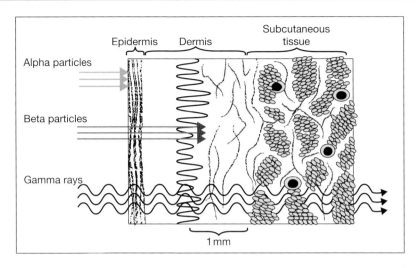

Figure 20.3 Differences in depth of penetration of radiation by type of radiation emitted. The ^{90}Yttrium emitted from Zevalin is pure beta and thus once in the bloodstream does not penetrate past the dermis. The ^{131}I attached to Bexxar has gamma radiation and can thus penetrate through the skin. Adapted from Wootton R, Radiation Protection of Patients 1993. Reproduced with permission from Biogen IDEC.

Table 20.3 Differences in patient education between beta-emitting radioimmunoconjugates, such as Zevalin, and gamma-emitting radioimmunoconjugates, such as Bexxar

Safety restrictions for beta and gamma emitters	
Beta emission	**Gamma emission**
Perform pregnancy tests before treatment, and do not breastfeed during treatment period and for approximately 12 months following treatment	Perform a pregnancy test before treatment, and do not breastfeed during treatment period and for approximately 12 months following treatment
Wash hands well after using the toilet, and flush the toilet twice with the lid down for 3 days following treatment.	Wash hands well after using the toilet, and flush the toilet twice with the lid down, per instructions from the treatment team (usually for 1–2 weeks following treatment).
Interact with family members without any restrictions (radiation exposure is similar to normal background radiation)	Limit the time spent in close contact with others and maintain a distance of 6 feet from other individuals. Limit exposure to others to 20 min per 8-hour period. Avoid contact with pregnant woman and small children
May sleep in same bed as partner. Use condoms for sexual relations for one week following treatment	Must sleep in separate bed
Inform family members or caregivers to wear gloves when a risk exists of contact with stool, urine, emesis, or other bodily fluids.	Use a separate bathroom. Use your own towels, washcloths, and toiletries. Inform family members or caregivers to wear gloves when a risk exists of contact with stool, urine, emesis, or other bodily fluids.
	Undergo reproductive counseling before treatment if you are of childbearing age

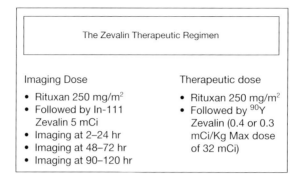

The Zevalin Therapeutic Regimen

Imaging Dose
- Rituxan 250 mg/m^2
- Followed by In-111 Zevalin 5 mCi
- Imaging at 2–24 hr
- Imaging at 48–72 hr
- Imaging at 90–120 hr

Therapeutic dose
- Rituxan 250 mg/m^2
- Followed by ^{90}Y Zevalin (0.4 or 0.3 mCi/Kg Max dose of 32 mCi)

Figure 20.4   Zevalin therapeutic regimen.

inconclusive a third image can be taken at 90–120 h. The amount of ^{111}In given for imaging is low enough that no side-effects occur and no radiation restrictions apply. On day 8 the patient receives a second dose of rituximab 250 mg/m^2 followed by ^{90}Y-Zevalin over 10 min by slow IV push and at least 10 ml of normal saline. Zevalin should not be given as an intravenous bolus. Only plastic shielding is required for the ^{90}Y infusion. If lead shielding is used it could cause bremsstrahlung radiation so the lead must be covered with plastic. Because beta radiation from ^{90}Y only travels 5 mm, Zevalin can be safely administered as an outpatient [7]. The patient can leave the treatment centre and return to their home without risk to family members [14]. Patients should be reminded to follow good hygienic practices, such as not sharing eating utensils, good hand washing, and cleaning up any spilled body fluids. These restrictions should be in effect for one week. Men should use condoms for sexual relations for one year. However, radiation restrictions will vary in different treatment facilities and it is important to follow the restrictions as given in each facility (Table 20.3).

Since rituximab is given before Zevalin, the patient should be pre-medicated as indicated above for any rituximab-related infusion side-effects. Since Zevalin (both ^{111}In and ^{90}Y) is given at the end of the rituximab, it is almost unheard of to see any additional infusion-related side-effects to the 10-min infusion of Zevalin; therefore, the patient can be dismissed as soon as the infusion is complete. The most important late effects of Zevalin are related to the myelosuppression that occurs at the beginning of 4 weeks with the nadir occurring between 6 and 8 weeks post-^{90}Y-Zevalin. Neutropaenia increases the risk of infection but in previous studies the actual incidence of serious infections was low [15]. Prophylactic white blood cell (WBC) growth factors were never used in the pivotal studies of Zevalin; however, some patients have received growth factors at the time of neutropaenia with a prompt increase in the WBC count. If severe thrombocytopaenia occurs, the patient is at increased risk of bleeding. While the blood counts are low it is important to instruct patients to watch for signs of infection, such as fever, and easy bruising. Patients should be instructed to refrain from taking aspirin, non-steroidal inflammatory agents, heparin, or coumadin. In general, if the patient is on long-term coumadin, it should be temporarily discontinued when the platelet count drops below 75,000.

TOSITUMOMAB (BEXXAR)

Bexxar is a murine monoclonal antibody to CD20 that is linked to ^{131}I and used for RIT of NHL. There are several differences in patient treatment and education with Bexxar compared with Zevalin (Table 20.3). Because of the presence of ^{131}I and since iodine is absorbed by the thyroid gland, an oral iodine thyroprotective medication must be given 24 h prior to starting the treatment and continued daily for 2 weeks after the therapeutic dose is given.

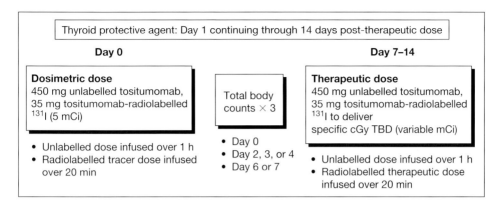

Figure 20.5   Bexxar treatment schema. TBD = Total body dose.

The therapeutic regimen is as follows: 450 mg of cold tositumomab is diluted in 100 ml of normal saline and infused over one hour at a constant rate followed by 5.0 mCi of ^{131}I administered IV over 20 min. Tositumomab requires similar pre-medication and treatment of reactions as rituximab; however, although infusion reactions to tositumomab are common, they are usually mild and rarely require changes in, or interruption of, the infusion rate [16]. Since ^{131}I emits gamma radiation, lead shielding is required. Following this infusion, gamma camera images are acquired every 3 days for 3 images to determine the body-clearance of the radioisotope. These measurements are then used for calculation of the therapeutic dose that is given 7–14 days following the first imaging dose. On the day of treatment, cold tositumomab 450 mg is administered followed immediately by therapeutic dose IV over 20 min (Figure 20.5). In most states, Bexxar can be administered as an out-patient; however, this may vary by state or country depending on the dose given and the ability and willingness of the patient to comply with these restrictions. These restrictions include sleeping in a separate room, not travelling more than 4 h with others, and limiting time spent with small children and pregnant women. According to the U.S. Nuclear Regulatory Commission, if the radiation dose to the family and others is less than 5 mrem, treatment can be performed as an out-patient; if the patient is treated in the hospital, the same criteria are applied for discharge. Because radioactivity is excreted through the kidneys, it is important to drink extra fluids to allow for excretion of the radioactivity in approximately one week. RIT should not be given to patients that are pregnant or nursing. Patients who receive Bexxar can develop a flu-like illness that occurs about 2 weeks after the therapeutic dose of Bexxar. This is characterised by fevers, arthralgias, and myalgias and usually resolves in 3–4 days. In a recent Bexxar study, this illness occurred in 26% of patients [16].

SUMMARY

It is imperative that patients are thoroughly educated regarding the treatments they are given for their lymphoma. This is necessary to provide a safe and effective treatment. This also provides the patient with a complete understanding of their treatment, what to expect, and what to be prepared for. A well-educated patient is also a more compliant patient.

REFERENCES

1.   Cheson BD. Radioimmunotherapy of non-Hodgkin lymphomas. *Blood* 2003; 101:391–398.
2.   Friedberg JW. Radioimmunotherapy for non-Hodgkin's lymphoma. *Clin Cancer Res* 2004; 10:7789–7791.

3. Dillman RO. Radiolabeled anti-CD20 monoclonal antibodies for the treatment of B-cell lymphoma. *J Clin Oncol* 2002; 20:3545–3557.

4. McLaughlin P, Grillo-Lopez AJ, Link BK, Levy R, Czuczman MS, Williams ME *et al.* Rituximab chimeric anti-CD20 monoclonal antibody therapy for relapsed indolent lymphoma: half of patients respond to a four-dose treatment program. *J Clin Oncol* 1998; 16:2825–2833.

5. Kanelli S, Ansell SM, Habermann TM, Inwards DJ, Tuinstra N, Witzig TE. Rituximab toxicity in patients with peripheral blood malignant B-cell lymphocytosis. *Leuk Lymphoma* 2001; 42:1329–1337.

6. Sehn L, Donaldson J, Filewich A, Fitzgerald CA, Gill KK, Runzer N *et al.* Rapid infusion rituximab in combination with steroid containing chemotherapy can be given safely and substantially reduces resource utilization. *Blood* 2004; 104:Abstract 1407.

7. Wagner HN, Jr, Wiseman GA, Marcus CS, Nabi HA, Nagle CE, Fink-Bennett DM *et al.* Administration guidelines for radioimmunotherapy of non-Hodgkin's lymphoma with (90)Y-labeled anti-CD20 monoclonal antibody. *J Nucl Med* 2002; 43:267–272.

8. Keating MJ, Flinn I, Jain V, Binet JL, Hillmen P, Byrd J *et al.* Therapeutic role of alemtuzumab (Campath-1H) in patients who have failed fludarabine: results of a large international study. *Blood* 2002; 99:3554–3561.

9. Faderl S, Thomas DA, O'Brien S, Garcia-Manero G, Kantarjian HM, Giles FJ *et al.* Experience with alemtuzumab plus rituximab in patients with relapsed and refractory lymphoid malignancies. *Blood* 2003; 101:3413–3415.

10. Rai KR, Freter CE, Mercier RJ, Cooper MR, Mitchell BS, Stadtmauer EA *et al.* Brettman L. Alemtuzumab in previously treated chronic lymphocytic leukemia patients who also had received fludarabine. *J Clin Oncol* 2002; 20:3891–3897.

11. Enblad G, Hagberg H, Erlanson M, Lundin J, MacDonald AP, Repp R *et al.* A pilot study of alemtuzumab (anti-CD52 monoclonal antibody) therapy for patients with relapsed or chemotherapy-refractory peripheral T-cell lymphomas. *Blood* 2004; 103:2920–2924.

12. Lundin J, Kimby E, Bjorkholm M, Broliden P-A, Celsing F, Hjalmar V *et al.* Phase II trial of subcutaneous anti-CD52 monoclonal antibody alemtuzumab (Campath-1H) as first-line treatment for patients with B-cell chronic lymphocytic leukemia (B-CLL). *Blood* 2002; 100:768–773.

13. Carrico JB, White AC, Collins DJ, Piskura DA, Prendergast KM, Nellis DO. Consolidated guidance about materials licenses program: specific guidance about industrial radiography licenses. Washington D.C. U.S. Nuclear Regulatory Commission, 1998.

14. Wiseman G, Leigh B, Witzig T, Gansen DN, White C. Radiation exposure is very low to the family members of patients treated with yttrium-90 Zevalin™ anti-CD20 monoclonal antibody therapy for lymphoma. *European Journal of Nuclear Medicine* 2001; 28:1198.

15. Witzig TE, White CA, Gordon LI, Wiseman GA, Emmanouilides C, Murray JL *et al.* Safety of Yttrium-90 ibritumomab tiuxetan radioimmunotherapy for relapsed low-grade, follicular, or transformed non-Hodgkin's lymphoma. *J Clin Oncol* 2003; 21:1263–1270.

16. Kaminski MS, Tuck M, Estes J, Kolstad A, Ross CW, Zasadny K *et al.* ^{131}I-Tositumomab therapy as initial treatment for follicular lymphoma. *N Engl J Med* 2005; 352:441–449.

21

Antibody therapy for chronic lymphocytic leukaemia

J. C. Byrd, K. A. Blum, T. S. Lin

INTRODUCTION

Chronic lymphocytic leukaemia (CLL) is one of the most common types of adult leukaemia. The majority of CLL patients are not symptomatic at diagnosis, but the majority will develop symptoms from the disease at some time point. Therapy for CLL has evolved significantly. Alkylator therapy has been shown to be inferior to fludarabine in randomised phase III studies [1–3]. Following this, promising phase II data [4, 5] with fludarabine and cyclophosphamide led to initiation and recently reported complete phase III studies demonstrating that this combination is superior to fludarabine monotherapy with respect to response rate, complete response rate (CR) and progression-free survival (PFS) [6, 7]. Thus, phase III studies have taken the field of CLL forward, but it is uncertain that further addition of chemotherapy to these regimens will either be possible relative to toxicity or beneficial with respect to improvement in response duration and overall survival (OS). Indeed, if progress is to be appreciated we will likely need to utilise therapeutic agents that work differently in CLL.

Monoclonal antibodies represent such a therapy. Like most effective anti-cancer therapies, monoclonal antibodies have the potential to recruit several different cytotoxic pathways through antibody-dependent cellular cytotoxicity (ADCC), complement-mediated cytotoxicity (CDC) and direct induction of apoptosis through initiation or disruption of signal transduction. This review will focus both on monoclonal antibodies that have already demonstrated benefit in CLL and those for whom significant promise exists in preclinical or early phase I testing.

RITUXIMAB

Rituximab is a chimeric monoclonal antibody that targets an external epitope of the CD20 antigen. CD20 is broadly and selectively expressed on B cells, not modulated, and therefore

John C. Byrd, MD, Associate Professor of Medicine and Medicinal Chemistry, D. Warren Brown Professor in Leukemia Research, Director of Hematologic Malignancies, Division of Hematology and Oncology, The Ohio State University, Columbus, Ohio, USA.

Kristie A. Blum, MD, Assistant Professor of Internal Medicine, Division of Hematology and Oncology, The Ohio State University, Columbus, Ohio, USA.

Thomas S. Lin, MD, PhD, Assistant Professor of Internal Medicine, Division of Hematology and Oncology, The Ohio State University, Columbus, Ohio, USA.

represents a good therapeutic target for a therapeutic monoclonal antibody. The function of CD20 is uncertain, but it appears to act as a calcium channel that interacts with the B-cell immunoglobulin receptor complex [8, 9]. Data on the shedding of CD20 in CLL and related non-Hodgkin's lymphoma (NHL) is controversial, with one group having noted significant levels of soluble CD20 in the sera of patients with both of these diseases. In each case, increased levels of soluble CD20 correlated with poorer survival [10–12]. Utilising an alternative, more direct anti-CD20 assay, another group failed to confirm the presence of significant soluble CD20 in CLL or related B-cell malignancies [13]. Therefore, both the presence and clinical impact of soluble CD20 must be further explored to resolve these conflicting results.

Understanding how rituximab mediates cell death in CLL will improve our ability to develop it. Like most other therapeutic antibodies, rituximab has been proposed to utilise several mechanisms including ADCC, CDC, and a direct pro-apoptotic effect. In lymphoma, where the CD20 target is generally expressed at a more abundant copy number, both *in vitro* and *in vivo* experiments support the importance of ADCC as a major mechanism of action [14]. In contrast, CLL has more dim expression of CD20 and represents a genetically different disease than NHL. Data derived from *in vitro* and *in vivo* studies with primary CLL cells suggest that apoptosis may contribute more to the mechanism of cell clearance in this disease [15, 16]. *In vitro*, Pedersen and colleagues [16] demonstrated that CLL cells in the presence of rituximab and a cross-linking F(ab)(2) fragment resulted in dose- and time-dependent induction of apoptosis [16]. Cross-linking of rituximab induced strong and sustained phosphorylation of the three mitogen-activated protein (MAP) kinases c-Jun NH_2-terminal protein kinase, extracellular signal-regulated kinase and p38 [16]. In this study, inhibition of p38 with SB203580 significantly decreased anti-CD20-induced apoptosis [16]. In conjunction with a clinical trial of rituximab administration in CLL, our group demonstrated *in vivo* induction of apoptosis through the intrinsic (caspase 9) pathway of CLL in patients who showed a significant decline in their peripheral blood lymphocyte counts [15]. This observation does not diminish the potential importance of complement or ADCC as a potential contributor to the mechanism by which rituximab mediates its cytotoxic effect, but suggests that several mechanisms of cell killing are actively involved in CLL cell elimination [17, 18].

CLINICAL STUDIES: SINGLE-AGENT WEEKLY RITUXIMAB

Initial phase I clinical studies of rituximab in NHL utilised the empiric dose of $375\,mg/m^2$ given by intravenous (IV) infusion weekly for 4 doses that produced an overall response rate (ORR) of 48% in the pivotal licensing study with a median response duration of 12 months [19]. Subsequent analysis of this study showed that patients with indolent follicular centre B-cell NHL had an ORR of 60%, while only 4 of 30 patients with small lymphocytic lymphoma (SLL) (13%) responded. Collective studies in relapsed CLL following this (reviewed in [20]) have demonstrated that weekly rituximab administered using the NHL schedule has limited activity in previously treated CLL. This contrasts with a study in previously untreated patients [21] where a 51% (CR 4%) response was noted, which improved with maintenance therapy to 58% (CR 9%). However, the median PFS for all patients was 19 months, significantly shorter than the >3-year PFS seen with follicle centre NHL [21]. These studies collectively point to a difference in rituximab response when administered weekly for 4 weeks early vs. late in the course of the natural treatment history of CLL.

CLINICAL STUDIES: ALTERNATIVE DOSING SCHEDULES OF RITUXIMAB

Given the modest activity of rituximab in previously treated CLL, we and others hypothesised that the large intravascular burden of circulating CLL cells may alter the pharmacokinetics of rituximab and result in accelerated clearance of antibody from plasma. This was in part supported by data from the initial pivotal study of rituximab where lower trough concentrations were observed in SLL patients [22]. Utilising this rationale, two studies were initiated to overcome these pharamacokinetic limitations.

O'Brien and colleagues [23, 24] reported a study of 50 patients with previously treated CLL (n = 40) or other B-cell leukaemias (n = 10) who received weekly rituximab dose-escalated to a maximum of 2,250 mg/m^2 per week. Although no CR was noted, the partial response rate (PR) was 40%, and a statistically significant dose-response relationship was observed with 22% of patients treated with 500–850 mg/m^2 as compared to 75% of patients treated with 2,250 mg/m^2. The higher dose was complicated by a higher frequency of non-dose limiting fatigue.

In an alternative approach, our group studied 33 patients with relapsed or refractory SLL/CLL where we administered rituximab three times per week at 250 mg/m^2 (n = 3) or 375 mg/m^2 (n = 30) for 4 weeks [25]. Patients received 100 mg over 4 h on the first day of therapy as a 'stepped up' dose in an attempt to minimise infusion-related toxicity, shorten overall infusion time on day 1, and prevent wasting non-administered rituximab if toxicity was noted early in treatment. While non-stepped up dosing is also acceptable practice, our group continues to do this for the reasons mentioned above. Outside of infusion toxicity, few other adverse events were noted. In terms of efficacy, this study demonstrated a 45% response rate with one CR (3%) and a median response duration of 10 months. These two studies using higher overall doses of rituximab with different schedules in SLL/CLL established a role for this agent in the treatment of relapsed CLL. Subsequent studies by our group have demonstrated that the subset of CLL patients with del(17p13.1) in relapse do not respond to even dose-intensive rituximab [26]. It is therefore our practice to screen for del(17p13.1) in relapsed CLL patients before administering monotherapy with rituximab.

RITUXIMAB COMBINATION THERAPY

Several published studies have combined rituximab with fludarabine- or pentostatin-based therapies in previously untreated CLL [27–29]. To date, these studies have all been phase II studies that limit comparison to previously reported studies with chemotherapy. A multi-centre European phase II study of concurrent fludarabine and rituximab in 31 evaluable patients with CLL achieved an ORR of 87% (CR 32%) with a median duration of response of 75 weeks [29]. The responses in this study were similar in previously treated (ORR 91%, CR 45%) and untreated patients (ORR 85%, CR 25%). Overall, toxicity was manageable in this study with only one potential treatment-related death due to prolonged cytopaenia and subsequent bleeding [29].

Another large randomised multi-institutional phase II study [27] was undertaken by the Cancer and Leukemia Group B (CALGB). This study included only symptomatic, previously untreated patients who received 6-monthly courses of standard-dose fludarabine with or without concurrent rituximab. Two months later, all patients received four weekly doses of rituximab for consolidation therapy. One hundred and four patients were randomised to the concurrent (n = 51) or sequential (n = 53) regimens. The ORR with the concurrent regimen was 90% (47% CR, 43% PR; 95% CI 0.82–0.98) compared with 77% (28% CR, 49% PR; 95% CI 0.66–0.99) with the sequential regimen. Early evaluation of response duration demonstrated no difference between the two arms. Toxicity was similar between the two arms of treatment with the exception that patients receiving the concurrent regimen experienced more grade 3 or 4 neutropaenia (74 vs. 41%) and grade 3 or 4 infusion-related toxicity (20 vs. 0%), compared with the sequential arm. A subsequent update of this study was performed which also examined the outcome of the 9,712 CLL patients treated with fludarabine and rituximab with that of patients enrolled on CALGB 9011 [2] who were treated with fludarabine monotherapy as initial therapy [30]. The eligibility requirements for these studies were similar and pre-treatment features of the 104 patients enrolled on CALGB 9712 and 179 patients enrolled on CALGB 9011 treated with fludarabine monotherapy were not different. Analysis of PFS and OS in this study demonstrated a highly significant difference between the outcomes of fludarabine monotherapy and fludarabine combined with rituximab [30]. Adjustment for pre-treatment clinical variables associated with altered treatment outcome was performed and did not alter these results. This follow-up analysis provides preliminary evidence that the addition of rituximab to fludarabine therapy for symptomatic, previously untreated CLL may improve both PFS and OS when compared with fludarabine therapy alone.

Another study undertaken by the MD Anderson group [31] in previously untreated CLL patients added rituximab (R) ($375\,mg/m^2$ with the first cycle and $500\,mg/m^2$ for subsequent cycles) to a slightly attenuated dose of fludarabine (F) ($25\,mg/m^2$ IV, days 1–3) and cyclophosphamide (C) ($250\,mg/m^2$ IV, days 1–3) for six cycles. This study included 224 patients who completed treatment; 70% CR and 95% OR rates were noted [31]. Toxicity was acceptable other than a higher frequency of neutropaenia, compared with previous studies by the same group with fludarabine and cyclophosphamide at identical doses. Two thirds of the patients assessed for minimal residual disease by two-colour flow cytometry had <1% CD5/CD19+ cells and had a prolonged remission duration as compared to those with evidence of minimal residual disease. Overall, 70% of patients remained disease free at 4 years [31]. This group has also reported on 177 patients who received this same regimen (FCR) in relapse with an ORR of 73% including a CR rate of 25% [32]. Toxicity associated with this regimen included myelosuppression and infections. In addition, 4 patients developed therapy-related acute myelogenous leukaemia (AML) or myelodysplatic syndrome (MDS).

The promising data outlined above from phase II studies [30–32] have provided valuable leads to be pursued in subsequent phase III multi-institutional studies with rituximab. Overall, these data with rituximab combinations provide a strong rationale for such studies and suggest that it has significant promise for improving outcome for patients with CLL.

ALEMTUZUMAB

Alemtuzumab (Campath-1H) is a humanised anti-CD52 monoclonal antibody that effectively fixes complement and depletes normal lymphocytes and lymphoma cells [33–35]. CD52 is a 21 to 28-kD glycopeptide expressed on the surface of nearly all human lymphocytes, monocytes and macrophages [36–38]. CD52 is expressed on a small subset of granulocytes, but CD52 is not expressed on erythrocytes, platelets or bone marrow stem cells. CD52 is expressed on all CLL cells, indolent B-cell NHL cells and the majority of adult ALL cases [39, 40]. The physiological function of alemtuzumab is uncertain, but cross-linking of CD52 on B-cell and T-cell lymphoma cell lines resulted in growth inhibition [38] and similar ligation in CLL cells results in apoptosis. The ubiquitous expression of CD52 on normal lymphocytes and monocytes also results in profound immunosuppression with alemtuzumab as compared to rituximab. Indeed, prior to alemtuzumab's known therapeutic efficacy in CLL, it was initially developed as an immunosuppressive therapy for rheumatoid arthritis and allogeneic stem cell transplant.

ALEMTUZUMAB FOR PREVIOUSLY TREATED CLL

The initial schedule optimisation of alemtuzumab occurred in CLL and NHL patients. These studies have never been published, but empirically established a dose of 30 mg IV three times per week for 4–12 weeks as the most effective schedule of administration of alemtuzumab. Several clinical studies established the efficacy of alemtuzumab in relapsed and refractory CLL that ultimately lead to its approval for marketing to treat fludarabine-refractory CLL [41–44]. A multi-centre, European phase II study administered alemtuzumab

30 mg three times per week for up to 12 weeks to 29 recurrent and refractory CLL patients where a 42% response rate was observed with only one patient (4%) attaining a CR [44]. The pivotal licensing trial administered the same alemtuzumab regimen to 93 heavily pre-treated, fludarabine-refractory CLL patients where a 33% response rate was observed, although only 2 (2%) patients achieved a CR [42]. Median time to progression for responders was 9.5 months, with a median OS of 16 months for all patients and 32 months for responders. In general, alemtuzumab worked better against blood, spleen and bone marrow disease. While 74% of all patients with nodal disease responded, patients with lymph nodes greater than 5 cm did significantly poorer with only 12% attaining a PR. All patients on this trial received prophylactic anti-bacterial and anti-viral agents, and infectious toxicity was manageable. However, patients with an Eastern Cooperative Group performance status of 2 did markedly worse, with no patients responding. A subsequent multi-institutional study in 136 patients with fludarabine-refractory B-CLL [45] noted similar response rates of 40% (CR 7%) with a median PFS and OS of responders being 7.3 and 13.4 months, respectively. As a result of this pivotal CAM211 study, alemtuzumab was approved for the treatment of flu-darabine-refractory CLL in the United States.

Alemtuzumab administration IV is associated with significant infusion toxicity, whereas preliminary reports have suggested subcutaneous dosing may decrease these in patients with previously untreated CLL. Until recently, there have been no data demonstrating either the feasibility of this approach in relapsed CLL or that 12 weeks as opposed to 18 weeks, as reported in previously untreated CLL patients, is efficacious. The German CLL study Group recently reported a phase II study, where subcutaneous (SC) alemtuzumab at a dose of 30 mg was administered three times per week for a maximum of 12 weeks in fludarabine-refractory CLL after IV dose escalation (3, 10, 30 mg) [46]. The response rate in the first 50 patients with enrollment characteristics similar to the initial pivotal study included an ORR of 36% with one patient (2%) attaining a CR. The median PFS time was 9.7 months and median OS time for all patients was 13.1 months. Responses were similar among patients with high-risk genetic features such as del(17p13.1) compared with those patients without these aberrations. These results, combined with those observed by others [47], provide justification for utilising alemtuzumab earlier in the treatment course of CLL patients with del(17p).

INITIAL ALEMTUZUMAB THERAPY IN PREVIOUSLY UNTREATED PATIENTS

A phase II clinical trial administered SC alemtuzumab to 41 previously untreated patients with CLL. In this study, patients received a prolonged course of alemtuzumab 30 mg SC three times per week for up to 18 weeks. The ORR was 87% in the 38 patients who received at least 2 weeks of treatment, and the intent-to-treat ORR was 81% [48]. This study established the safety of alemtuzumab in previously untreated CLL and the potential benefit in terms of infusion toxicity of administering this agent subcutaneously.

ALEMTUZUMAB FOLLOWING CYTOREDUCTIVE THERAPY

An alternative method of administering alemtuzumab is by giving lower doses following cytoreductive therapy to target residual bone marrow disease; this has been piloted by two groups in small studies [49, 50] and three other groups in more definitive studies (reviewed in [20]) [51–53]. These studies collectively have demonstrated that alemtuzumab is effective at eliminating minimal residual disease that is not eradicated after fludarabine-based therapy. Toxicity with this approach is acceptable, but the total dose of alemtuzumab administered and the proximity to chemotherapy must be considered. This approach is particularly attractive following cytoreduction for patients with del(17p13.1) or p53 mutations, where alemtuzumab has demonstrable clinical activity [46, 54].

ALEMTUZUMAB IN COMBINATION WITH OTHER EFFECTIVE THERAPIES

A small study of combined fludarabine and alemtuzumab in 6 CLL patients, refractory to fludarabine alone and alemtuzumab alone, yielded an 83% ORR (CR 17%) [55]. This important study prompted several investigators to add alemtuzumab to other effective chemotherapies for CLL as had previously been done with rituximab. In one of these studies, small amounts of alemtuzumab were given in combination with fludarabine [56]. Specifically, this study administered a short dose escalation of alemtuzumab in week 1 followed by fludarabine 30 mg/m^2/day IV and alemtuzumab 30 mg IV, both on days 1–3 monthly for up to six cycles. Of the 34 patients evaluable at the time of an updated report [57], the response rate was 85%, with 10 (29%) patients achieving a CR and 19 (56%) patients a PR. Overall toxicity including infections was manageable. A second study integrated low-dose alemtuzumab into the FCR regimen described previously [58]. This study was performed in previously treated patients where alemtuzumab was administered at 30 mg on day 1, 3 and 5 with standard FCR as previously reported administered on day 3–5. A total of 31 patients were reported, of whom 21 were evaluable for response with a 52% ORR and 14% CR. Twelve of these twenty-one patients were alive at the time of this report with a median follow-up time of 21 months. Toxicities consisted predominately of cytopaenias and infections, but were on the whole manageable. While additional follow-up on these combination strategies [57, 58] will be required, these results in relapsed and refractory patients are quite promising.

Two studies indicate that the combination of alemtuzumab and rituximab can be given safely and may have clinical activity in patients with relapsed CLL [59, 60] The largest of these administered rituximab, 375 mg/m^2 weekly for four doses, with alemtuzumab 30 mg on days 3 and 5 of each week, to 48 patients with relapsed or refractory lymphoproliferative disorders, including 32 patients with CLL and 9 patients with CLL/PLL [60]. The ORR was 52% (CR 8%), with a median time to progression of 6 months. Toxicity on the whole was acceptable. Thus, the administration of weekly rituximab to alemtuzumab allowed for dramatic reduction in the dose of both antibodies with effective short-term palliation in refractory CLL patients.

HU1D10 AND OTHER HLA-DR ANTIBODIES

Hu1D10 (Apolizumab, Remitogen) is a humanised murine IgG monoclonal antibody whose antigenic epitope is a polymorphic determinant on the MHC class II HLA-DR beta chain [61]. Preclinical studies against primary CLL cells demonstrate that Hu1D10 mediates apoptosis through a novel caspase-independent manner. These preliminary data and those by others with second-generation HLA-DR-directed antibodies promoted initiation of clinical trials in CLL with Hu1D10. A phase I dose escalation study of apolizumab three times per week was recently reported using 'stepped-up' dosing, in 18 patients with relapsed CLL (17) and ALL (1). Fifteen heavily pre-treated CLL patients were evaluable for response with one patient with del(17)(p13.1) having a PR, 9 with stable disease, and 5 progressing within 2 months of completing therapy. Studies with apolizumab are ongoing and the development of other improved second generation HLA-DR–directed antibodies is warranted.

LUMILIXIMAB

CD23 is expressed at high density on the cell surface of certain B-cell malignancies, including CLL. Lumiliximab is a macaque-human chimeric anti-CD23 monoclonal antibody for which preclinical studies demonstrated induction of apoptosis, CDC and ADCC against CD23-bearing lymphoid cells including primary CLL cells. More importantly, l lumiliximab mediates synergy with both fludarabine and rituximab against primary CLL cells. A phase I multicentre study of single-agent lumiliximab in 46 patients with relapsed or refractory

CLL was reported [62]. This dose escalation study of weekly and then three times per week dosing for 4 weeks (maximum dose 500 mg/m^2) noted minimal infusion toxicity, with only 15% patients experiencing grade 3 or 4 adverse events. Decreases in absolute lymphocyte count (ALC) $\geq 50\%$ were observed in 11 of 40 (28%) patients enrolled at 375 mg/m^2/week or higher. Similarly, of the 37 patients evaluated for change in lymphadenopathy, reductions were observed in 22 (59%). Ongoing clinical studies are assessing the potential of lumiliximab in combination with fludarabine-cyclophosphamide-rituximab (FCR) in previously treated CLL patients based upon preclinical synergy with these agents.

OTHER ANTIBODIES FOR CLL

A variety of antibodies are in early phase I clinical trials or are reaching late preclinical development and have promising data that complement current agents being employed in CLL.

CHIR-12.12 is a fully humanised antibody directed at human CD40 that blocks interaction with CD40 ligand, a known anti-apoptotic stimuli to CLL cells [63]. In one preliminary study, primary CLL cells incubated with CD40L were resistant to spontaneous apoptosis that was reversed by co-incubation with CHIR-12.12 antibody [64]. CHIR-12.12 was also demonstrated to mediate ADCC against primary CLL cells *in vitro*. Based upon these promising studies, successful xenograft lymphoma studies, and acceptable toxicity *in vivo*, a phase I study of CHIR-12.12, has recently been initiated in relapsed and refractory CLL. Another CD40-directed antibody, SGN40, is also being used in clinical trials at this time in low-grade NHL and multiple myeloma.

TGN1412 is a humanised super-agonistic anti-CD28 antibody [65]. Ligation of CD28 can activate human T cells *in vitro* without concurrent engagement of the T-cell antigen receptor. Soluble TGN1412 that was cultured with CLL cells demonstrated polyclonal T-cell activation including proliferation, cytokine production and induction of activation markers concurrent with modulation of CLL cell antigens including HLA-DR, CD95, CD80 and CD86. Additionally, TGN1412-activated T cells exhibited enhanced cytotoxic T-lymphocyte (CTL) activity against primary B-CLL cells. Based upon these studies, early clinical trials TGN1412 are being considered for CLL.

Tru 16.4 is a single-chain protein with a modified CD37-binding Fv domain linked to a modified human IgG1 hinge, CH2 and CH3 domains and is a member of a novel composition class called small modular immunopharmaceuticals (SMIP) [66]. Preclinical studies with Tru 16.4 have demonstrated that it binds to CD37 on primary CLL cells surface and induces caspase-independent apoptosis. Further modifications of Tru16.4 are underway to enhance ADCC mechanisms against primary CLL cells for future clinical trials targeting CD37.

ACKNOWLEDGEMENTS

This work was supported by the National Cancer Institute (P01 CA95426–01A1, TL and JCB), the Sidney Kimmel Cancer Research Foundation (JCB), The Leukemia and Lymphoma Society of America (JCB) and The D. Warren Brown Foundation (JCB, KB and TL).

REFERENCES

1. Johnson S, Smith AG, Loffler H *et al.* Multicentre prospective randomised trial of fludarabine versus cyclophosphamide, doxorubicin, and prednisone (CAP) for treatment of advanced-stage chronic lymphocytic leukaemia. The French Cooperative Group on CLL. *Lancet* 1996; 347:1432–1438.
2. Rai KR, Peterson BL, Appelbaum FR *et al.* Fludarabine compared with chlorambucil as primary therapy for chronic lymphocytic leukemia. *N Engl J Med* 2000; 343:1750–1757.
3. Leporrier M, Chevret S, Cazin B *et al.* Randomized comparison of fludarabine, CAP, and ChOP in 938 previously untreated stage B and C chronic lymphocytic leukemia patients. *Blood* 2001; 98:2319–2325.

4. O'Brien SM, Kantarjian HM, Cortes J *et al.* Results of the fludarabine and cyclophosphamide combination regimen in chronic lymphocytic leukemia. *J Clin Oncol* 2001; 19:1414–1420.
5. Flinn IW, Jemiai Y, Bennett JM *et al.* Fludarabine and cyclophosphamide achieves high complete response rate in patients with previously untreated chronic lymphocytic leukemia: ECOG 1997. *Blood* 2001; 98:633a.
6. Eichhorst BF, Busch R, Hopfinger G *et al.* Fludarabine plus cyclophosphamide (FC) induces higher remission rates and longer progression free survival (PFS) than fludarabine (F) alone in first line therapy of advanced chronic lymphocytic leukemia (CLL): results of a phase III study (CLL4 Protocol) of the German CLL Study Group (GCLLSG). *Blood* 2004; 102:72a.
7. Flinn IW, Kumm E, Grever MR *et al.* Fludarabine and cyclophosphamide produces a higher complete response rate and more durable remissions than fludarabine in patients with previously untreated CLL: Intergroup Trial E2997. *Blood* 2004: 104:475a.
8. Bubien JK, Zhou LJ, Bell PD *et al.* Transfection of the CD20 cell surface molecule into ectopic cell types generates a Ca^{2+} conductance found constitutively in B lymphocytes. *J Cell Biol* 1993; 121:1121–1132.
9. Leveille C, Al-Daccak R, Mourad W: CD20 is physically and functionally coupled to MHC class II and CD40 on human B cell lines. *Eur J Immunol* 1999; 29:65–74.
10. Vose JM, Giles FJ, Manshouri T *et al.* High levels of soluble CD20 (sCD20) in patients with non-Hodgkin's lymphoma (NHL): correlation with clinical behavior and contrast with patients with Hodgkin's disease (HD). *Blood* 2001; 98(abstract #3196):767a.
11. Keating MJ, O'Brien S, Albitar M: Emerging information on the use of rituximab in chronic lymphocytic leukemia. *Semin Oncol* 2002; 29:70–74.
12. Manshouri T, Do KA, Wang X *et al.* Circulating CD20 is detectable in the plasma of patients with chronic lymphocytic leukemia and is of prognostic significance. *Blood* 2003; 101:2507–2513.
13. Beum PV, Kennedy AD, Taylor RP: Three new assays for rituximab based on its immunological activity or antigenic properties: analyses of sera and plasmas of RTX-treated patients with chronic lymphocytic leukemia and other B cell lymphomas. *J Immunol Methods* 2004; 289:97–109.
14. Eisenbeis CF, Caligiuri MA, Byrd JC. Rituximab: converging mechanisms of action in non-Hodgkin's lymphoma? *Clin Cancer Res* 2003; 9:5810–5812.
15. Byrd JC, Kitada S, Flinn IW *et al.* The mechanism of tumor cell clearance by rituximab *in vivo* in patients with B-cell chronic lymphocytic leukemia: evidence of caspase activation and apoptosis induction. *Blood* 2002; 99:1038–1043.
16. Pedersen IM, Buhl AM, Klausen P *et al.* The chimeric anti-CD20 antibody rituximab induces apoptosis in B-cell chronic lymphocytic leukemia cells through a p38 mitogen activated protein-kinase-dependent mechanism. *Blood* 2002; 99:1314–1319.
17. Farag SS, Flinn IW, Modali R *et al.* Fc gamma RIIIa and Fc gamma RIIa polymorphisms do not predict response to rituximab in B-cell chronic lymphocytic leukemia. *Blood* 2004; 103:1472–1474.
18. Bannerji R, Kitada S, Flinn IW *et al.* Apoptotic-regulatory and complement-protecting protein expression in chronic lymphocytic leukemia: relationship to *in vivo* rituximab resistance. *J Clin Oncol* 2003; 21:1466–1471.
19. McLaughlin P, Grillo-Lopez AJ, Link BK *et al.* Rituximab chimeric anti-CD20 monoclonal antibody therapy for relapsed indolent lymphoma: half of patients respond to a four-dose treatment program. *J Clin Oncol* 1998; 16:2825–2833.
20. Lin TS, Byrd JC: Monoclonal antibody therapy in lymphoid leukemias. *Adv Pharmacol* 2004; 51: 127–167.
21. Hainsworth JD, Litchy S, Barton JH *et al.* Single-agent rituximab as first-line and maintenance treatment for patients with chronic lymphocytic leukemia or small lymphocytic lymphoma: a phase II trial of the Minnie Pearl Cancer Research Network. *J Clin Oncol* 2003; 21:1746–1751.
22. Berinstein NL, Grillo-Lopez AJ, White CA *et al.* Association of serum Rituximab (IDEC-C2B8) concentration and anti-tumor response in the treatment of recurrent low-grade or follicular non-Hodgkin's lymphoma. *Ann Oncol* 1998; 9:995–1001.
23. Keating MJ, O'Brien S: High-dose rituximab therapy in chronic lymphocytic leukemia. *Semin Oncol* 2000; 27:86–90.
24. O'Brien SM, Kantarjian H, Thomas DA *et al.* Rituximab dose-escalation trial in chronic lymphocytic leukemia. *J Clin Oncol* 2001; 19:2165–2170.
25. Byrd JC, Murphy T, Howard RS *et al.* Rituximab using a thrice weekly dosing schedule in B-cell chronic lymphocytic leukemia and small lymphocytic lymphoma demonstrates clinical activity and acceptable toxicity. *J Clin Oncol* 2001; 19:2153–2164.

26. Byrd JC, Smith L, Hackbarth ML *et al*. Interphase cytogenetic abnormalities in chronic lymphocytic leukemia may predict response to rituximab. *Cancer Res* 2003; 63:36–38.

27. Byrd JC, Peterson BL, Morrison VA *et al*. Randomized phase 2 study of fludarabine with concurrent versus sequential treatment with rituximab in symptomatic, untreated patients with B-cell chronic lymphocytic leukemia: results from Cancer and Leukemia Group B 9712 (CALGB 9712). *Blood* 2003; 101:6–14.

28. Keating MJ, O'Brien S, Lerner S *et al*. Combination chemo-antibody therapy with fludarabine (F), cyclophosphamide (C) and rituximab (R) achieves a high CR rate in previously untreated chronic lymphocytic leukemia (CLL). *Blood* 2000; 96:514a.

29. Schulz H, Klein SK, Rehwald U *et al*. Phase 2 study of a combined immunochemotherapy using rituximab and fludarabine in patients with chronic lymphocytic leukemia. *Blood* 2002; 100:3115–3120.

30. Byrd JC, Rai K, Peterson BL *et al*. Addition of rituximab to fludarabine may prolong progression-free survival and overall survival in patients with previously untreated chronic lymphocytic leukemia: an updated retrospective comparative analysis of CALGB 9712 and CALGB 9011. *Blood* 2005; 105:49–53.

31. Keating MJ, O'Brien S, Albitar M *et al*. Early results of a chemoimmunotherapy regimen of fludarabine, cyclophosphamide, and rituximab as initial therapy for chronic lymphocytic leukemia. *J Clin Oncol* 2005; Mar 14 [Epub ahead of print].

32. Wierda W, O'Brien S, Wen S *et al*. Chemoimmunotherapy with fludarabine, cyclophosphamide, and rituximab for relapsed and refractory chronic lymphocytic leukemia. *J Clin Oncol* 2005; Mar 14 [Epub ahead of print].

33. Flynn JM, Byrd JC: Campath-1H monoclonal antibody therapy. *Curr Opin Oncol* 2000; 12:574–581.

34. Hale G, Bright S, Chumbley G *et al*. Removal of T cells from bone marrow for transplantation: a monoclonal antilymphocyte antibody that fixes human complement. *Blood* 1983; 62:873–882.

35. Hale G, Dyer MJ, Clark MR *et al*. Remission induction in non-Hodgkin lymphoma with reshaped human monoclonal antibody CAMPATH-1H. *Lancet* 1988; 2:1394–1399.

36. Treumann A, Lifely MR, Schneider P *et al*. Primary structure of CD52. *J Biol Chem*. 1995; 270:6088–6099.

37. Domagala A, Kurpisz M. CD52 antigen: a review. *Med Sci Monit* 2001; 7:325–331.

38. Rowan W, Tite J, Topley P *et al*. Cross-linking of the CAMPATH-1 antigen (CD52) mediates growth inhibition in human B- and T-lymphoma cell lines, and subsequent emergence of CD52-deficient cells. *Immunology* 1998; 95:427–436.

39. Hale G, Swirsky D, Waldmann H *et al*. Reactivity of rat monoclonal antibody CAMPATH-1 with human leukaemia cells and its possible application for autologous bone marrow transplantation. *Br J Haematol* 1985; 60:41–48.

40. Salisbury JR, Rapson NT, Codd JD *et al*. Immunohistochemical analysis of CDw52 antigen expression in non-Hodgkin's lymphomas. *J Clin Pathol* 1994; 47:313–317.

41. Bowen AL, Zomas A, Emmett E *et al*. Subcutaneous CAMPATH-1H in fludarabine-resistant/relapsed chronic lymphocytic and B-prolymphocytic leukaemia. *Br J Haematol* 1997; 96:617–619.

42. Keating MJ, Flinn I, Jain V *et al*. Therapeutic role of alemtuzumab (Campath-1H) in patients who have failed fludarabine: results of a large international study. *Blood* 2002; 99:3554–3561.

43. Osterborg A, Fassas AS, Anagnostopoulos A *et al*. Humanized CD52 monoclonal antibody Campath-1H as first-line treatment in chronic lymphocytic leukaemia. *Br J Haematol* 1996; 93:151–153.

44. Osterborg A, Dyer MJ, Bunjes D *et al*. Phase II multicenter study of human CD52 antibody in previously treated chronic lymphocytic leukemia: European Study Group of CAMPATH-1H Treatment in Chronic Lymphocytic Leukemia. *J Clin Oncol* 1997; 15:1567–1574.

45. Rai KR, Coutre S, Rizzieri D *et al*. Efficacy and safety of alemtuzumab (Campath-1H) in refractory B-CLL patients treated on a compassionate basis. *Blood* 2001; 98:365a.

46. Stilgenbauer S, Winkler D, Kröber A *et al*. Subcutaneous Campath-1H (alemtuzumab) in fludarabine-refractory CLL: interim analysis of the CLL2h Study of the German Cll Study Group (GCLLSG). *Blood* 2004; 104:140a.

47. Lozanski G, Heerema NA, Flinn IW *et al*. Alemtuzumab is an effective therapy for chronic lymphocytic leukemia with p53 mutations and deletions. *Blood* 2004; 103:3278–3281.

48. Lundin J, Kimby E, Bjorkholm M *et al*. Phase II trial of subcutaneous anti-CD52 monoclonal antibody alemtuzumab (Campath-1H) as first-line treatment for patients with B-cell chronic lymphocytic leukemia (B-CLL). *Blood* 2002; 100:768–773.

49. Dyer MJ, Kelsey SM, Mackay HJ *et al*. *In vivo* 'purging' of residual disease in CLL with Campath-1H. *Br J Haematol* 1997; 97:669–72.

50. Montillo M, Cafrq AM, Tedeschi A *et al*. Safety and efficacy of subcutaneous Campath-1H for treating residual disease in patients with chronic lymphocytic leukemia responding to fludarabine. *Haematologica* 2002; 87:695–700.
51. Rai KR, Byrd JC, Peterson B A phase II trial of fludarabine followed by alemtuzumab (Campath-1H) in previously untreated chronic lymphocytic leukemia (CLL) patients with active disease: Cancer and Leukemia Group B (CALGB) Study 19901. *Blood* 2002; 101:205a.
52. Ferrajoli A, Thomas DA, Albitar M *et al*. Alemtuzumab for minimal residual disease in CLL. *Proc Am Soc Clin Oncol* 2003; 2290a.
53. Wendtner CM, Ritgen M, Fingerle-Rowson G *et al*. High efficacy but considerable toxicity of campath-1H consolidation therapy in CLL patients responding to fludarabine – results of a randomized phase III trial. *Proc Am Soc Clin Oncol* 2003; 2330a.
54. Lozanski G, Heerema NA, Flinn IW *et al*. Alemtuzumab is an effective therapy for chronic lymphocytic leukemia with p53 mutations and deletions. *Blood* 2004; 103:3278–3281.
55. Kennedy B, Rawstron A, Carter C *et al*. Campath-1H and fludarabine in combination are highly active in refractory chronic lymphocytic leukemia. *Blood* 2002; 99:2245–2247.
56. Elter T, Borchmann P, Reiser M *et al*. Development of a new, four-weekly schedule (FluCam) with concomitant application of Campath-1H and Fludarabine in patients with relapsed/refractory CLL. *Proc Am Soc Clin Oncol* 2003; 22:580.
57. Elter T, Borchmann P, Schulz H FluCam—a new, 4-weekly combination of fludarabine and alemtuzumab for patients with relapsed chronic lymphocytic leukemia. *Blood* 2004; 104:690a.
58. Wierda W, Faderl S, O'Brien S *et al*. Combined cyclophosphamide, fludarabine, alemtuzumab, and rituximab (CFAR) is active for relapsed and refractory patients with CLL. *Blood* 2004; 104:101a.
59. Nabhan C, Tallman MS, Riley MB *et al*. Phase I study of rituximab and Campath-1H in patients with relapsed or refractory chronic lymphocytic leukemia. *Blood* 2001; 98:365a.
60. Faderl S, Thomas DA, O'Brien S, *et al*. Experience with alemtuzumab plus rituximab in patients with relapsed and refractory lymphoid malignancies. *Blood* 2003; 101:3413–3415.
61. Kostelny SA, Link BK, Tso JY *et al*. Humanization and characterization of the anti-HLA-DR antibody 1D10. *Int J Cancer* 2001; 93:556–565.
62. Byrd JC, O'Brien S, Flinn I *et al*. Safety and efficacy results from a phase I trial of single-agent lumiliximab (anti-CD23 antibody) for chronic lymphocytic leukemia. *Blood* 2004; 104.
63. Kitada S, Zapata JM, Andreeff M *et al*. Bryostatin and CD40-ligand enhance apoptosis resistance and induce expression of cell survival genes in B-cell chronic lymphocytic leukaemia. *Br J Haematol* 1999; 106:995–1004.
64. Tong X, Georgakis GV, Li L *et al*. *In Vitro* activity of a novel fully human anti-CD40 antibody CHIR-12.12 in chronic lymphocytic leukemia: blockade of CD40 activation and induction of ADCC. *Blood* 2004; 104:abstrac #2504, page 687a.
65. Lin CH, Kerkau T, Gutermann C *et al*. Superagonistic anti-CD28 antibody TGN1412 as a potential immunotherapeutic for the treatment of B cell chronic lymphocytic leukemia. *Blood* 2004; 104:abstract #2519, page 690a.
66. Zhao XB, Biswas S, Mone A *et al*. Novel anti-CD37 small modular immunopharmaceutical (SMIP) Induces B-cell-specific, caspase-independent apoptosis in human CLL cells. *Blood* 2004; 104:abstract #2515, page 689a.

Index